HEALTH CARE
MARKET STRATEGY

From Planning to Action

FOURTH EDITION

STEVEN G. HILLESTAD, BA, MA
Advisor, Business Owner
Adjunct Professor, School of Public Health
University of Minnesota
Minneapolis, Minnesota

ERIC N. BERKOWITZ, PhD
Professor of Marketing
Isenberg School of Management
University of Massachusetts
Amherst, Massachusetts

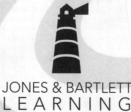

JONES & BARTLETT
LEARNING

World Headquarters
Jones and Bartlett Learning
5 Wall Street
Burlington, MA 01803
978-443-5000
info@jblearning.com
www.jblearning.com

Jones & Bartlett Learning books and products are available through most bookstores and online book-sellers. To contact Jones & Bartlett Learning directly, call 800-832-0034, fax 978-443-8000, or visit our website, www.jblearning.com.

Substantial discounts on bulk quantities of Jones & Bartlett Learning publications are available to corporations, professional associations, and other qualified organizations. For details and specific discount information, contact the special sales department at Jones & Bartlett Learning via the above contact information or send an email to specialsales@jblearning.com.

Production Credits
Publisher: Michael Brown
Editorial Assistant: Chloe Falivene
Production Assistant: Leia Poritz
Senior Marketing Manager: Sophie Fleck Teague
Manufacturing and Inventory Control
  Supervisor: Amy Bacus

Composition: Laserwords Private Limited
Cover Design: Kristin E. Parker
Cover Image: © Ximagination/Dreamstime.com
Printing and Binding: Edwards Brothers Malloy
Cover Printing: Edwards Brothers Malloy

Library of Congress Cataloging-in-Publication Data
Hillestad, Steven G.
Health care market strategy: from planning to action / Steven Hillestad, Eric Berkowitz—4th ed.
  p. ; cm.
Includes bibliographical references and index.
ISBN 978-0-7637-8928-2 (pbk.)—ISBN 0-7637-8928-3 (pbk.)
I. Berkowitz, Eric N. II. Title.
[DNLM: 1. Marketing of Health Services. W 74.1]

362.1068'8—dc23

2012005236

6048

Printed in the United States of America
16 15 14 13 12   10 9 8 7 6 5 4 3 2 1

CONTENTS

PREFACE

Too often, we value the process of creating strategy while paying little attention to our results.

The healthcare industry is increasingly a focal point of public interest regarding access to care, quality, and affordability. Employers are becoming overwhelmed by health insurance costs, Medicare is a major stress on federal budgets, and there is an increasing concern about the total percentage of the GDP spent on health services. In spite of these national concerns, at the local level, healthcare organizations have continued to develop strategies around the assumption of increasing the number of programs, services, and facilities without regard to the possibility of reaching the limits of the public tolerance in terms of paying for these ever-expanding healthcare services.

Healthcare delivery changes are taking root in the 21st century that often challenge the conventional way health care is delivered. With so many financial resources going into health care, strong perceived profit margins, and demand for services likely to increase as the population ages, many entrepreneurs see opportunities to challenge conventional delivery of care. At the same time, policymakers are demanding that the medical community begin to seriously examine efficiency and efficacy of care, and business leaders are working hard to create incentives for employees to make more prudent financial decisions regarding their personal health care in an effort to control cost and reduce utilization. All of these forces have significant impact on strategic decisions for healthcare organizations.

In short, entrepreneurs who have historically operated outside of the healthcare arena now see this environment as having enormous potential financial opportunity, while others see health care in need of dramatic cuts in terms of economic costs. In either case, hospitals, clinics, physicians, and other providers are going to see more pressure to provide better, more efficient care, often using new methods of delivery that could shrink the need for existing and expensive facilities.

Many traditional providers such as hospitals and clinics will survive, but others will likely fail if they do not embrace changes such as concentrated specialty centers, web-based doctor visits, or voucher-style payment systems. Every business school student is taught about the theory and practice of S-curve thinking. S-curve theory is based on the idea that services have a natural pattern of initial, often slow, introduction followed by a growth pattern where the new idea begins to eclipse the more mature and recognizable service. Sometimes the mature service or product offering is ultimately replaced or fails by what at one time was considered a new or breakthrough concept. Some call this concept *creative disruption*, and we see the concept in practice all around us every day. For example, the passenger train was eclipsed by the airplane, Main Street has been eclipsed by the big box retailer, and brick-and-mortar bookstores are disappearing as a result of the e-reader and tablet technology. Health care is not immune to the same kinds of upheaval, as primary care physician visits are being disrupted by care being delivered in grocery and drugstores, credible orthopedic care is being delivered to Americans willing to travel to Thailand, and web-based physician visits are, in turn, replacing urgent care and traditional doctor visits. All of these changes are examples of creative disruption that brings about new services, which modify or replace old clinical programs with new and different clinical service offerings. The key for a healthcare executive is to learn how to recognize that change and new ideas are unstoppable, and to figure out how to work with both existing and new concepts to manage successfully into the future.

We see individuals within healthcare organizations spending countless hours in discussions, committee meetings, retreats, and analyses to create a strategy. Often, however, such strategies are only partially successful because of a lack of crisp focus and a gap between strategic decisions and tactical implementation at the marketing level. In our view, such plans often fail because: (1) the leadership does not recognize the changing environment where there is a new demand for different services that are delivered in a different way, (2) the organization has made intuitive judgments about the marketplace that are not accurate, (3) the strategies lack clear focus and direction, (4) they are strategically or tactically weak, (5) the organization is unable or unwilling to identify a clear value add or unique organizational advantage, or (6) the action portion of the plan is not precise and powerful enough to be successful.

Healthcare strategy development has become very complex. In the past, a hospital would estimate admissions and units of care delivered, calculate costs, prepare a budget, and then pass the cost increase on to insurers and other payers. But that model is gone. New, nontraditional competitors are figuring out how to take volume from hospitals and doctors' offices by offering a different service at a lower cost. Others are creating models such as accountable care organizations (ACOs) that require hospitals to essentially offer a service at a fixed cost and guarantee the outcome of the service. As health care continues to be a large and still growing economic power, existing players will see even more "outsiders" looking at new ways of providing good patient care, while, at the same time, taking a share of the economic opportunity. As we move forward, anyone involved in healthcare management will need to be much more focused, strategic, analytical, and tactical than we have ever seen in the past.

This text provides a market-focused method to fill the gap between strategy design and tactical implementation. It offers a useful, step-by-step method for implementing and connecting the strategic plan along with the tactical implementation at the marketplace level. Furthermore, individuals who have read an introductory textbook on marketing or strategic management and want to know what to do next will find this book useful as an immediate follow up as they begin to implement strategic and marketing concepts.

The major contribution this text makes to health care is in linking strategic thinking to appropriate market tactics. We call this tactical model the *strategy/action match*. Using this model, the reader will have confidence when choosing the tactics to employ in many different situations. In addition, we emphasize the mindset that successful strategy requires. We call it the *strategic mindset*.

Since the publication of the third edition of this text, we have had the opportunity to work with hundreds of organizations, both large and small. As a result, we believe more than ever that great emphasis needs to be placed on creating an atmosphere or culture that is open to honestly examining where an organization fits within the competitive marketplace. Sometimes these conversations and decisions are very difficult. This text provides tools to help health-related entities have robust and honest conversations, so that failure can be minimized.

Finally, this text attempts to clarify relationships—relationships among managers within a healthcare company, and relationships between each of those managers and strategic planners and marketing staff—so conflict can be avoided and teamwork can be established. In this edition, we have significantly expanded the discussions of strategy and strategic planning in order to clarify how strategy, business plans, and marketing relate. We have also added tools to help health organizations have balanced discussion around strategic issues that allows for participation by all relevant decision makers.

Chapter 1 provides an overview of strategy and the importance of strategy in the organization. In this chapter, the reader will become grounded in strategic thinking at the highest level and develop a mindset that is conducive to strategy development at the leadership level. Chapter 2 details the more precise task of understanding how the process of strategic planning, business planning, and marketing work connect.

Both strategic planning and market planning start with an understanding of the environment. Chapter 3 looks at the environment and discusses how it is changing and its impact on strategy. Chapter 4 offers ideas around the next logical step: analyzing in detail internal capability and external factors. Here the reader will learn about market research and other tools that can be used to get a fair-and-balanced view of the situation facing the organization.

Chapter 5 explores the importance of a vision to the organization and it examines the other elements of a strategic plan. This chapter also provides models and tools to help executives manage a strategic conversation, understand the framework of what a strategic plan should accomplish, and compare and contrast good strategic visions with less desirable ones.

Chapter 6 is the cornerstone of this text. It provides a model from which the reader can use data and theory to develop the framework of a reasonable connection between strategy and specific tactics. We call this the strategy/action match. In this chapter, we examine the product lifecycle and look at tactics that can be used depending on where an organization's product is in its lifecycle or S-curve.

From this point on in the book, we take a tactical look at tools used to accomplish the organization's vision. In Chapter 7, we look at traditional marketing concepts including pricing, advertising, distribution, and product development from a healthcare point of view. Chapters 8 and 9 are about making the marketing plan an integral part of the organization and using tools to monitor items such as financial progress and sales performance.

The appendix material is designed to show the reader what questions might be important throughout this process. We have also updated and clarified a model market plan so that the reader will have a clear understanding of what such a plan should look like.

This text is a bridge. It bridges theory with practical applications. It connects strategic thinking from the corporate office to tactical application at the clinical business unit. It connects modern business strategic and tactical thinking with application to healthcare organizations such as hospitals, doctors' offices, blood banks, organ donor programs, rural healthcare co-ops, and weight-loss services.

Steven G. Hillestad
Eric N. Berkowitz

ABOUT THE AUTHORS

Steven G. Hillestad, BA, MA trained at the University of Wisconsin–Madison in business and public administration. He led marketing efforts at the Fairview System in Minneapolis in the late 1970s, when the first edition of this book was published. Until 1998, he led marketing, strategy, acquisitions, and business-development efforts at Abbott Northwestern Hospital, LifeSpan, and Allina Health System, all located in Minneapolis. He provides consulting support to healthcare organizations in strategic planning and market research. He has been active in professional organizations and has published frequently. He was awarded the Frank Weaver Leadership Award and the Corning Award from the American Hospital Association, where he served as President of the Society for Healthcare Strategy and Market Development. Hillestad teaches part-time at the University of Minnesota, co-owns an upscale lodge on the shores of Lake Superior, and provides consultation to organizations involved in healthcare delivery. Currently, he is working with not-for-profit boards to help them improve performance so they can achieve their vision. He resides in the Twin Cities area.

Eric N. Berkowitz, PhD is Professor of Marketing, Isenberg School of Management, University of Massachusetts Amherst. He served as Associate Dean of Professional Programs for the Isenberg School of Management. He also acted for 11 years as chair of the Marketing Department. Previously, Dr. Berkowitz served on the faculty of the University of Minnesota, holding an appointment in the School of Management and the Center for Health Services Research. Dr. Berkowitz received his PhD from the Ohio State University.

Dr. Berkowitz has consulted frequently on marketing and market research for a wide range of healthcare organizations. A frequent speaker for medical staff meetings and retreats, Dr. Berkowitz also serves as a core faculty member for the American College of Physician Executives. Dr. Berkowitz has also been a frequent speaker at meetings of the Medical Group Management Association, the American Hospital Association, the Association of Community Cancer Centers, and the American Academy of Orthopaedic Surgeons, among others. Dr. Berkowitz has taught in the Executive Management Programs of the University of Minnesota, Health Systems Management Center at Case Western Reserve University, Carnegie Mellon University, ITAM in Mexico City, and for the University of Connecticut.

Professor Berkowitz has published extensively in both marketing and health care. He is an author of six books: *Essentials of Health Care Marketing* (3rd ed., Jones & Bartlett, 2011); *Marketing* (7th ed., McGraw-Hill, 2002); *Marketing* (6th ed., Canadian Edition, McGraw-Hill, 2006); *Health Care Market Strategy* (4th ed., Jones & Bartlett, 2013); *Strategic Planning in Health Care Management: Marketing and Finance Perspectives* (Aspen, 1981); *Healthcare Market Research* (McGraw-Hill, 1997).

Dr. Berkowitz is a past editor of the *Journal of Health Care Marketing*. He also served as Chairperson of the Alliance for Healthcare Strategy and Marketing, and as the editor of *TrendWatch* for the Alliance for Healthcare Strategy and Marketing. Professor Berkowitz is listed in *Who's Who in American Industry and Finance, Who's Who in Education* (6th ed., 2004–2005), and *Who's Who Among Emerging Leaders*. While on the faculty of the University of Minnesota, Professor Berkowitz was twice named the outstanding teacher in the School of Management. In 1998, he received the outstanding teacher award in the School of Management at the University of Massachusetts. In 1985, Dr. Berkowitz was named an honorary member of the American College of Physician Executives, and in 1988, he received the Frank J. Weaver Leadership Award from the Alliance for Healthcare Strategy and Marketing for his contributions to the advancement of healthcare marketing.

CHAPTER 1

STRATEGY DEVELOPMENT AND THE STRATEGIC MINDSET

WHAT YOU WILL LEARN

- Devising a strategy is not a lock-step process that belongs to a committee or staff department.
- An important characteristic of a good strategy is that it is focused and clear.
- Before an organization can do effective market-based business planning, it needs to have a market-based mindset.
- Strategy devised in the boardroom should connect with tactics employed in the marketplace.
- There is no single correct strategy; multiple alternatives abound.

WHAT IS STRATEGY?

The ultimate purpose of any strategy is to help an organization realize its objectives. Since the publication of Kenneth Andrews's book, *The Concept of Corporate Strategy*, in 1971, strategy exploration in the classroom and boardroom has exploded.[1] General strategy models and specific strategies around benchmarking, Five Forces theory, total quality management, Blue Ocean Strategy, and value chain theory are just a few of the concepts found in modern strategy discussions. But in spite of all the attention paid to this area, success is not assured. Porter studied 33 large companies and found that they had entered more than 80 new industry areas, and by 1986 they had abandoned more than half of these diversification strategies.[2] In 2002, an important article in the *Journal of Business Strategy* suggested that execution, not the strategy itself, was the key to business success.[3] But in the *Harvard Business Review*, Porter argued that both operational effectiveness and strategy are essential to superior performance.[4]

Although strategy is critical to the business planning effort, it is neither a concrete methodology nor a guarantee of success. What then is strategy? Developing a strategy to attain a goal is useful in business, athletics, personal financial planning, and a variety of other activities. In the 1960s strategy was viewed as the "silver bullet" for management. But over the years we have discovered that strategy is not a silver bullet or even a precise recipe from which to get from point A to point B. As Mintzberg points out in an article entitled "The Fall and Rise of Strategic Planning," strategy development cannot be fit into an event or activity that one attends once a month for 5 or 6 months.[5] Rather, successful organizations allow for an environment where strategy is constantly discussed, shaped, and supported by experts who help gather data, study options, and provide overall general direction. Strategy does not belong to the planners or to the planning committee, and it does not fit into an artificial timeline that magically ends on December 31. Healthcare executives often treat strategy as a theatrical performance culminating in the fall of the year with a retreat at a beautiful resort with the board and senior management team. At the retreat, outside speakers are brought in to inform and entertain, and the strategy of the organization is discussed using beautiful PowerPoint presentations filled with broad general initiatives. All of this might be acceptable if, at the end of the day, the strategy is based on data and each executive and board member can specifically articulate what the organization is intending to accomplish, but too often this is not the case. However, strategy is a constant journey, winding back and forth and involving the organization as a whole, with ideas and theories brought forward by many sources. It does not come from a planner operating in a dark room; strategy is not an event, nor is it a performance. Strategy is the core underlying job of the executives and board to work on day after day.

Upsetting and Reestablishing the Competitive Equilibrium

The use of strategy in a business environment takes on a special interpretation, as outlined by Bruce Henderson of the Boston Consulting Group: "Any useful strategy must include a means of upsetting the competitive equilibrium and reestablishing it again on a more favorable basis."[6] The foundation for Henderson's statement is the assumption that the organization wishes to grow. Because the other organizations that compete in the same territory or service area also wish to grow, many organizations are attempting to reach the same potential endpoint (growth) at the same time. Thus, to succeed, an organization must often change the competitive situation and attempt to dominate it by using strategies that are favorable to its own goals. As shown in **Figure 1.1**, sometimes changes in the environment upset the equilibrium for virtually everyone. For example, by 2008, as the Internet grew, the equilibrium of the way news was delivered changed and newspapers across the country declined or went bankrupt; similarly, by 2011, bookstore giant Borders' failure to move to e-readers and online distribution models, among other factors, caused it to go out of business.

In developing a useful growth strategy, it is necessary, first, as Henderson points out, to upset the competitive equilibrium. Within most communities, a competitive equilibrium exists among hospitals, clinics, insurance carriers, and other health-related businesses. The hospital with a strong reputation 10 years ago usually has a strong reputation today, and the health plan that was the leader then is often the leader now. Many physicians consider these organizations members of a medical fraternity. As a result, physicians or hospitals may compete with one another, but they would rather avoid the use of an overt and aggressive competitive strategy. In recent years, the use of aggressive advertising has made overt competitive tactics more common than they once were; however, because of the recognition of the medical fraternity, groups are often reluctant to try new ideas that are outside the bounds of traditional practice. Creating an online patient appointment system and opening a separate for-profit heart center are examples of concepts that have often met with resistance from the medical community. For the same reason, hospitals are often unwilling to make dramatic competitive moves against other institutions. If a strategy is to be useful, however, physicians and executives of healthcare organizations must understand the need to upset the competitive equilibrium.

Upsetting the equilibrium has happened in the world of routine pediatric care. Typically pediatric care is offered in a standard clinical office,

FIGURE 1.1

Upsetting the Equilibrium

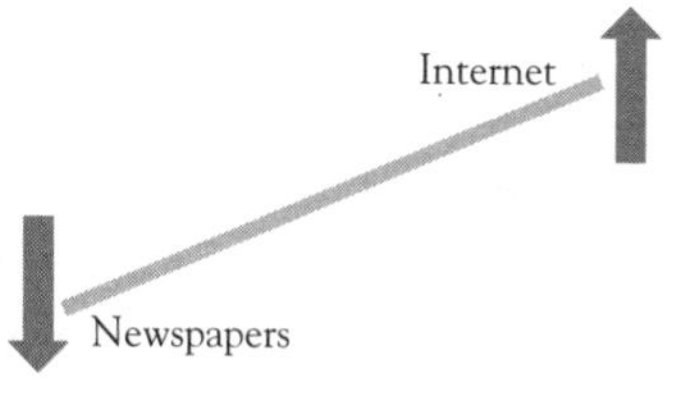

likely located in a multi-practice medical building. The office has physicians, nurses, billing, scheduling, and medical records staff. A routine school physical exam might cost $150–200. This is the way pediatrics has been practiced; equilibrium among pediatricians has been firmly in place. But along came stores like Target, CVS, and Walmart with a new model where routine school physical exams are provided by a nurse inside the store, in a space no larger than 200 square feet—with no receptionist, no appointment desk, no billing office, no medical records room. The fee is as low as $29. This is a new model of care, with new assumptions—a classic example of equilibrium upset.

After upsetting the equilibrium, according to Henderson, it is then necessary to "reestablish the equilibrium on a more favorable basis."[7] Strategies may be developed to promote new concepts, ideas, and product offerings, or to serve markets that have not been considered before or that have not been thought to be worthwhile. Within this area, innovation can be expected. For example, an organization might reestablish the equilibrium on a basis more favorable to itself by offering a new service. Such an organization could establish an urgent-care center that would compete with the traditional hospital emergency room, or it could station a nurse practitioner in a supermarket next to the pharmacy in order to steal market from the hospital by providing even more convenient and low-cost care. It would be difficult for a hospital to make a retaliatory response.

Creating a Difference

Thornhill and White provide additional insight into what strategy is all about. In essence, the strategy must include a unique advantage that is difficult, if not impossible, for others to compete against. Looking at more than 2,300 companies, they concluded that the greater a firm's strategic purity (competitive advantage) the greater the profitability—with cost leadership at one end of the spectrum of strategic purity and product differentiation at the other.[8] These two options represent strategic purity. Many organizations, however, choose to operate somewhere in the middle, providing no clear distinction for their service with no clear cost distinction. Failure to have a point of difference typically relegates an organization to competing on price alone; it thereby creates a commodity market subject to the ups and downs of supply and demand, much like the coffee, sugar, and wheat futures.

If strategy is about being different, it stands to reason that no two strategies for a given market need to be or should be alike and that no single strategy is the correct one for achieving success in that market. Often, when students are given a case study about a business problem, they are eager to give the "right" answer and are often quick to change their strategy when they learn that another group has a different strategy that sounds better. However, even though Walmart, Target, Kmart, and Costco are all in the discount retail market, each has adopted different strategies, and all have experienced successes (and setbacks) over the years. Today, as health care is trying to integrate services (including doctors, hospitals, home care, and health plans), many businesses are moving away from integration toward virtual organizations. For example, rivals Motorola and IBM use parts from each other, and Chrysler and Mitsubishi develop cars together even though they are competitors. Abbott Northwestern and North Memorial Medical Center of Minneapolis have in the past invested together in technology and buildings even though they competed aggressively as separate organizations. Healthcare organizations tend to be lemmings; if one goes to integrated care, everyone tends to go to integrated care—or to physician health organizations (PHOs), managed care, or accountable care organizations (ACOs). Even though competitive advantage as a strategy does not necessarily involve following everyone else, being different is not easy, especially for large or established organizations.

Hamel and Prahalad explain that organizations fail because they are unable to escape the past and to invent the future.[9] Hospitals get trapped being traditional hospitals and often cannot change from being bureaucratic organizations with high overhead and salary structures in order to compete with more nimble retail-style competitors in the areas of day surgery, eye care, cardiac disease, or other opportunities. Likewise, health maintenance organizations (HMOs) are committed to "the movement" and have trouble jumping to a future where the HMO might no longer work. **Figure 1.2** explores the reasons why it is so difficult for established firms to change, and therefore why it is so likely that new organizations will enter the market and upset the equilibrium.

Because strategy is about creating a difference in an environment of constant inquiry, it cannot be an artificial, calendar-based process in which June is the month for ideas and July is the month for tactics. The strategy process is the framework around which an organization allows strategy to percolate. The role of the strategist is to assist in maintaining an environment that allows for the exploration of ideas and options as a daily part of organizational life.

Once an organization begins to develop a strategy and related marketing plans, it becomes clear that the strategy and the plans are not passive entities; they are appropriate for a changing competitive environment. They are also action oriented. Competitive actions are necessary for achieving organizational goals. Here, numerous decisions have to be made, such as

FIGURE 1.2

Why Do Great Companies Fail?

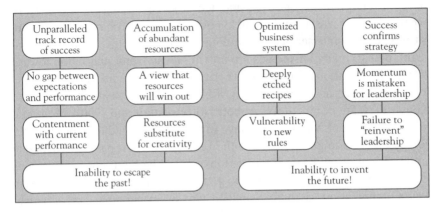

Source: Hamel, G., & Prahalad, C. K. (1994). *Competing for the future.* Boston, MA: Harvard Business School Press; p. 17.

which services to offer; which markets to serve; which methods to use in providing the services (e.g., centralized or decentralized); which pricing strategies to use for different markets, services, and marketplace conditions; and which promotional strategies to adopt.

Building Strategy into the Organization

Starting with the corporate office at Walmart, the company has a strategy to be a low-cost discount retailer. The strategy that is articulated at the corporate level is to save people money. This is a strategy that is embedded within the board, officers, and employees of the organization, but it does not end there. It is driven into the depths of the organization and is implemented daily via multiple tactics, not the least of which is a dose of advertising that constantly focuses on Walmart price cuts on a variety of products. This is a perfect example of a strategic focus at the top of the organization with a matching tactical focus at every level, including the day-to-day advertising on television, and in print. A constant theme of this text is to focus on making sure that strategy at the corporate level and tactics at the detailed level connect. Unfortunately, this is often not the case.

In health care it is not unusual to observe intense and well-meaning conversations about mission, vision, strategy, and tactics, but often the results of these efforts are generic with no specific outcome, and the general statements made in the corporate office do not connect with the tactics employed at the clinic level. Organizations must be more precise at the boardroom strategy level and more specific and connected at the tactical level. For example, if in the boardroom it is determined that your medical group will have the highest quality surgeons, one would expect that only top-quality doctors with medical board certification would be accepted on the staff. However, if a high-revenue surgeon who is not board certified is accepted on the staff, then the strategic statements become only window dressing, creating a disconnect between the strategy at the corporate level and the reality in the everyday operation of the clinic. This leads to confusion and a discrediting of the strategic process.

Search for the Driving Force[10]

Healthcare professionals are trained to serve and help. They have difficulty saying no. Therefore, it is not unusual that hospitals tend to want to "do it all," and their strategies often include a broad spectrum of clinical, community health, and social initiatives. But Robert argues that successful companies have a strategic area that is the heartbeat of the company, and that is what gives the organization a strategic edge in the marketplace.[11] Robert is echoing the idea of clear focus, and he suggests that the identification of this focus will ultimately shape the look and profile of the clinic. An organization's heartbeat could be cardiac services or obstetrics or easily accessible clinics in every community or first-generation technology or a host of other options. The point is that greater success will be had by focusing attention on a narrow range of clinical skill versus attempting to be the leader in public health, education, clinical care, and outreach clinics. The task, therefore, is to figure out at the strategic level what the heartbeat of the organization is—that is, what it is that a clinic brings to the market that is that particular clinic's core distinctive capability.

Treacy and Wiersema are even more direct.[12] They suggest that entities must choose one of three options: customer intimacy, product leadership, or operational excellence. Again, the idea is that at the strategic level every effort should be made to focus on the piece of the competitive landscape where the entity has the greatest expertise and capability. The Ritz-Carlton Hotel chain focuses on customer intimacy and service, Apple has a focus on innovative product leadership, and FedEx focuses on operational excellence involving the delivery of packages as quickly as possible.

University-controlled hospitals tend to be known for a product focus that translates into technology and extraordinary levels of clinical advancement, but they are not usually well known for operational excellence involving scheduling, referral systems, or efficient staffing. Likewise, while health-care entities in general do a good job of providing clinical care, they are not at the forefront of providing top-notch personal service. Treacy and Weirsema would suggest that more successful organizations will know what they are good at, and will concentrate on that feature of their enterprise in order to gain business success.

The Possibility of Failure

Organizations that move through the process of developing strategic plans, business plans, and marketing plans frequently fail. Sometimes this failure is the result of (1) failure to gather appropriate data, (2) errors in analyzing the data, (3) lack of specific objectives, or (4) failure to adopt the appropriate tactics to marketplace conditions. Stated another way, failure may be caused by the inability to match strategy with action tactics or market conditions. Healthcare organizations, particularly hospitals, often lack information on consumers, referring physicians, and competitive pricing strategies; and this type of analysis with incomplete data often leads to failure. Another source of failure is the lack of specific objectives and the logistical tactics necessary to meet those objectives. This text explains the correct progression from gathering information and establishing firm objectives to developing the appropriate tactics.

Marketing planning often fails in industry.[13] A study based on a profile of 40 United Kingdom companies categorized by products, sales, and employees, found that 29% of the companies did not have specific objectives for product sales, and 32% did not have objectives for their marketing plans. Many companies, both in and out of the healthcare industry, fail to set targeted, measurable objectives that would facilitate the control and evaluation of ultimate success or failure. It is essential to identify market segments and to outline the appropriate strategy for each group. An objective of this text is to provide the necessary detail for healthcare organizations to be able to address relevant market questions, establish workable objectives, and develop tactics that meet those objectives. These approaches create the greatest chance of healthcare organizational success.

DEVELOPMENT OF THE STRATEGIC MINDSET

Before the organization begins the process of strategy development and ultimately the production of a marketing plan, there must be an atmosphere within the organization that we call the "strategic mindset." A number of factors must be in place and understood by all parties if strategy development and implementation are to be effective. These factors include the attitudes of the key participants, as well as their understanding of the basic concepts of marketing and strategy development. Each element of the strategic mindset is reviewed in this section.

CLEAR VISION, FOCUSED STRATEGY, AND UNDERSTANDING BY THE LEADERSHIP

Indicating that the hospital is world class, low cost, easily accessible, and focused on community health is great for general conversation, but this is usually not good strategy. Additionally, it is likely not an honest statement of what anyone really believes. Yet, this kind of statement can be found in the boardrooms of countless clinics, hospitals, and medical organizations across the country. At the foundation of good strategy design is an honest view of where the enterprise really wants to go that includes a specific handful of strategies on how to get there. Fortune 500 companies demand precision at the highest level, and health care needs the same rigor. Is the local hospital's focus public health, primary care, or something else? Is it really "world class" or should its focus be on providing basic inpatient care with board-certified doctors? Successful organizations know what they do best and everyone in the group understands what the organization is really all about. In the end, strong organizations have a clear vision and will create a clear competitive advantage, which results in a corresponding brand that has meaning in the community.

But a vision and strategy are only good if those who need to execute the plan understand them. It is not unusual for the chief executive officer (CEO) to have a vision, but the board and management team are not sure what it is, or the team has different interpretations of what the strategy is. At a minimum, every board member and every person on the management team should be able to articulate the vision and the strategy of the organization.

FOCUS ON THE CUSTOMER

An important element in resolving any marketing problem is thinking about and trying to understand the customer. Customers would obviously include patients, but they could also be physicians who send referrals to a particular hospital, health plan executives who decide which physicians are on the provider list, social workers who help decide where to send patients for treatment, and many other customer categories. In any case, the most important and seemingly simple step is to think about the people who need the organization's services. This concept is often transformed into the somewhat cold notion of markets, although understanding the customers as people is emphasized to every marketing student from the first day of class.

A healthcare institution must understand the needs of its customers, whether they are patients, referral physicians, or social workers. The initial step in reaching this understanding is market research—talking with customers, thinking like the customers, and, above all, keeping an open mind. Researchers should not assume that they know what potential customers will do, how customers think, or how they make purchase or referral decisions. One hospital's senior marketing director overlooked this lesson of customer focus. In a presentation to a Fortune 500 company about the hospital's healthcare program for executives, the marketing director described all the therapies involved and the team that would provide all the wonderful executive services. The people at the Fortune 500 company, including its vice president, were polite as the hospital representative droned on and showed them a succession of slides he thought they would like. Finally, the hospital representative asked if there were any questions. The vice president at the Fortune 500 company had only one: When would the executive in this program be able to go back to work after treatment or other services? The hospital representative had no answer. Having believed that the company was concerned primarily with therapy, surgical outcome, and cost, the hospital representative was prepared to answer questions related only to those concerns. In retrospect, if the representative had talked to corporate decision makers responsible for health benefits before developing the presentation, the issues that were important to the company would have become clear. The presentation would have focused not only on the surgical and therapeutic care, but also on the time required to return a worker to productivity. After all, the program may be efficient, with an average length of stay of only 6 days, but if it takes an executive 6 additional weeks to return to work, the total cost to the company may be far greater than the cost of the 6-day length of stay. Understanding customers and the criteria on which they base their evaluations is ultimately the key to effective marketing.

When interviewing people for marketing jobs, it is important to discuss different types of problems to see to what extent the candidate under-stands the true market-based concept. For example, a candidate's response to a hypothetical situation in which a group of five physicians are think-ing of opening a new clinic in a new community can be revealing. After suggesting that the candidate has been invited out to dinner with the five doctors to discuss how the new clinic "can be marketed," the interviewer should ask the candidate for recommendations about what to do next. If the candidate starts talking about a direct-mail strategy, signage for the clinic, the advantages to be gained if the physicians join the Rotary, or any of the other hundred marketing tactics, the candidate is not the right person for the job. The answer the candidate should provide is a series of questions: Who are the possible customers? How do they make decisions? Where do they get care now? What are their needs?

In the business press, Peters and Austin have popularized the idea of knowing customers by talking to them.[14] Although this method may seem somewhat simple for sophisticated healthcare organizations, talking to customers can have incredible value. Market research with relevant sample sizes is important, but it is also important to take a personal, close-up approach and, most of all, to adopt a customer-focused philosophy.

In the parking lot of many hospitals, a sign posted next to the spot closest to the front door is marked "Administrator." It is odd in the healthcare industry that the administrator parks next to the front door while those who are sick, often elderly, are asked to park farther away. In contrast, at most hotels, people are greeted at the front door; someone takes their bags, escorts them to the front lobby, and parks their car. The hotel staff parks away from the facility, and the guests park next to it. This example does not demonstrate everything about marketing, but it does give an insight into such an organization's attitude toward its patients or toward its markets. Marketing is about listening carefully to customers, understanding their needs, and providing the best possible service to meet those needs before implementing tactics.

An example of the nonmarketing approach in health care can be found in a chemical-dependency program that was known for its quality and for its high cost. During "family week," the patients were reunited with their families at the treatment facility. In one such gathering, approximately 14 different family members were sitting on comfortable couches. Several were drinking coffee purchased from a vending machine located in the basement at a cost of $1.50. The counselor, however, walked in with a china cup filled with coffee obviously poured from a coffeepot somewhere else in the building. This is a minor detail, but in a market-driven organization, family members rather than the counselor should have coffee in a china cup. Family members are part of the customer group; counselors are part of the production line.

Complex articles, seminars, books, and meetings may cloud the meaning of marketing. In the healthcare industry, marketing has created its own culture, succumbing to analysis paralysis by constant emphasis on data and research. Some administrators consider market research so critical that they do not make decisions without voluminous information. Yet, they can often obtain the best data by meeting customers in the lobby and on the units.

In working with customers, it is important to focus on their questions and concerns, their expectations of the institution, and their decision-making processes. Sometimes marketers need to sit in the emergency room for hours, blending in and talking with families. They need to sit at the nurses' station or watch TV in the lounge with families. Sometimes they need to get in the car with a group of subspecialists (who are often key customers at a hospital), driving with them to their monthly clinic at a family-practice facility 2 hours away (their customer), and simply finding out how they perceive the hospital.

This approach may not be scientific, but it brings the data to life in a way that no amount of formal market research can. Former President George H. W. Bush realized the importance of "meeting the people" and used this methodology during the 1988 presidential campaign. During the summer of 1988, Democratic candidates Michael Dukakis and Jesse Jackson were fighting a battle to become the Democratic nominee. Throughout the Democratic primaries, Dukakis was viewed as the conservative; Jackson, as the liberal. The Republican nomination was not nearly so exciting, nor did it capture the attention of the voters the way the Democratic nomination did. After the Republicans had officially nominated Bush and the Democrats had officially nominated Dukakis, the campaign was ready to get under way after the Labor Day break. Bush's advisers were disturbed by national polls that showed Dukakis easily walking over the Republicans. They were finding it difficult to develop a strategy that might be effective against Dukakis—difficult, that is, until candidate Bush watched a couple of focus-group videotapes taken in a middle-class Roman Catholic community in Paramus, New Jersey. These people were Reagan Democrats, the people Bush needed if he had any hope of winning in November. As the tapes rolled, Bush was horrified to see that the group perceived him as more liberal than Dukakis because Dukakis had positioned himself as the broad-based Democrat against the "wild liberalism" of Jackson.

Out of these focus-group sessions came the decision to reposition Bush, but this time by keeping Bush where he was and moving Dukakis back to the left. In the words of *Newsweek* magazine, it was decided to "portray Dukakis as a bona fide, double-dip, frost belt, [George] McGovern style liberal whose most basic values were alien to most of America."[15] Thus a basically negative campaign was born, during which the case of Willie Horton, a murderer allowed out of a Massachusetts prison on furlough during Governor Dukakis's tenure, was drummed into the minds of the electorate from September through November until his name became the one most closely associated with Dukakis. The focus-group information told Bush how to win the election. So it is with a marketing plan.

CHANGE IS RELENTLESS

Services cannot remain static; change is inevitable. Many forgotten products, goods, and services illustrate how today's successes can be in mothballs tomorrow. The marketplace is constantly changing; its needs and desires are dynamic and technology is making products obsolete at an ever-quickening rate. Some not-for-profit groups embrace change, like the church in Houston, Texas that has a McDonald's on the property, or the church in Arizona that has a bookstore and a mortuary. Meanwhile, some resist change, such as small towns across the country that have watched Walmart move into the outskirts of the town because local leaders and business people refused to work with the retail giant, fearing that the downtown area would change. In many cases the downtown area did change—the businesses died because existing community leaders refused to understand and work through the Walmart dilemma.

Organizations that take a narrow view of their products may miss opportunities for growth in tomorrow's market, while those that resist change may find themselves with no market to serve. Tuberculosis hospitals, slide rulers, and landline-based telephones and fax machines are examples of products and services that are no longer needed or wanted by the modern consumer. This same concern pertains to hospitals and clinics. Urgent-care clinics may, in large part, replace emergency rooms. The group practice may replace the solo practice and personal physician, and a nationwide chain of clinics may replace the group practice. The Internet is in the process of transforming the demand for primary care, and as most subspecialists can attest, the Internet provides patients with extensive information about disease that is often new to the physicians themselves. The clinic at the pharmacy may replace the doctor's offices, while the specialty eye hospital of Brazil may replace the eye clinic in small-town America. The laser surgeon may replace the general surgeon, the surgical robot may replace the rural surgeon, and genome science may revolutionize all medical services. In developing strategy, it is dangerous to say, "We've been doing it this way for 30 years, and there's no reason to change." Physicians, hospitals, and businesses must dare to create a vision for tomorrow with change as a fundamental ingredient. Those who are not willing to change to meet customer needs are not ready for effective marketing planning.

SEARCH FOR A BETTER WAY

There is often a better way, and the competition will find it. Product and service innovation is a cornerstone of U.S. business as well as medicine. Today, innovations from business and medicine are coming together in the form of better approaches to organizing practices, better ways of paying for services, better technologies to help patients stay out of the hospital, and, for the consumer, better ways of getting treatment (e.g., clinics in shopping malls, evening hours, and family settings). As a result, when individuals within an organization sit down to develop strategy, they should not assume that they have a lock on the best hospital, the best clinic, the best location, or the best physicians. These are risky assumptions. IBM used to be the undisputed leader in software; now Microsoft has taken the lead position. Hilton hotels used to be first in the deluxe-hotel category; now several chains including Ritz-Carlton and Marriott have supplanted Hilton. Blue Cross was in the lead position for health insurance; now companies such as United Health Care are leading the way. No one in the United States had ever heard of a Kia automobile prior to the 2000s; now it is one of the major automotive nameplates in the country. Pediatricians used to provide most school and camp physical exams, and now it appears that Target Clinic is stealing that business. Never assume that the historical reputation of your organization will stand forever—it will stand only if it provides value relative to other alternatives available in the marketplace.

DECISION-MAKING ROLE OF THE MARKETPLACE

That the marketplace has a decision-making role in helping to direct the future course of a business is often difficult to impress on professionals who take daily responsibility for decisions on behalf of their customers. It is correct and appropriate that physicians assume such responsibility for their patients, but many times patients should have the opportunity to make their own decisions regarding health care. As mentioned earlier, one of the most important elements in designing successful marketing strategies is to ask consumers how they can be better served and what their needs are. Their answers are often helpful in establishing office hours, fee ceilings, clinic locations, and a host of other elements. Basically, the types of decisions that consumers make regarding health care are the same types of decisions that healthcare professionals and other consumers make in the retail and commercial environment.

Consumers, if not asked in advance, make their judgments known by requesting some physicians in a group practice more often than others, by regularly seeking care at certain clinic locations, or by joining particular HMOs because the services provided are more suited to their needs than those offered in other HMOs or fee-for-service alternatives. Therefore, the involvement of potential customers in determining strategy is fundamental to the process of developing marketing plans.

NEED FOR A CHAMPION

To ensure the best possible result, a program or service needs a champion—someone who is totally committed to making the idea work. The importance of this factor has become clear in profiling successful plans. Great program leadership will in all probability equal excellent results. At this stage in the marketing process, if the organization is unable or unwilling to find the necessary champion-style leadership, the program should be put on hold. The chances of failure are too great.

Peters and Austin noted that thousands of ideas are discussed every day in the United States, but that an idea needs leadership—a champion.[16] A champion is determined to succeed, customer oriented, energetic, willing to tout the idea to anyone, focused on success, always looking for new and better ways, and sometimes a gadfly, but always a believer.

Steve Jobs was the champion for Apple computers. He started the company in 1977, and it flourished. When he then left the company in 1987, it languished until his return in 1996 to bring new growth to the company with products such as the iPod, iPhone, and iPad. Debbie Fields worked diligently for Mrs. Fields cookies. Sam Walton was absolutely immersed in making sure that success happened at Walmart. At any given hospital, everyone recognizes three or four department managers as successful. These managers commonly create a high return on investment, new ideas, and requests for more capital; they are service champions. They believe in what they do, they are willing to look at new ideas, and they enjoy working with their customers. Somehow, the business grows.

The same holds true for physicians. In every large clinic or on every medical staff, a couple of physicians are outstanding. They are good, respected, energetic, and service oriented, and they are thinking about the future. Their practices seem to grow faster and better than other practices. Peters and Austin called their attitude a passion.[17] Every major marketing effort or service line needs a champion, a shepherd, someone who has the respect of others, but who also has the passion to be successful. Such an individual has the drive to create the best possible program with the highest possible return and can maneuver through the jungle of bureaucracy to put that program in front of the customer.

Most consultants and executives who work with troubled businesses cite the lack of leadership and failure to anticipate capital needs as the two leading reasons for business failure. Without a champion, the probability of success is limited. Collins and Porras describe high-performance organizations such as Walmart, Nordstrom, Disney, and others as having a "cult-like" feel: Leadership, and therefore the entire organization, exhibits similar characteristics.[18] These important characteristics include extensive indoctrination, tightness of fit, and elitism. As discussed by Collins and Porras, extensive indoctrination includes training, hiring, and close mentoring to create a passion around customers. Tightness of fit involves being an IBMer at IBM or a Nordie at Nordstrom. This sense of family involves working together and also recognizing that one is part of the same organization day in and day out. Elitism refers to a feeling of superiority; the organization is able to convince employees that they, in fact, work for a special company. This is not to imply that the best leadership style is paternalistic. However, the leadership style of top organizations includes a passionate view of the business along with strong attempts to build a sense of family, involvement with the organization, and a strong commitment to customers.

TRADEOFFS IN COURSES OF ACTION

It is impossible to use all available strategies at the same time. By the same token, multiple strategies are often in conflict with one another. As **Figure 1.3** suggests, a strategy of high growth through additional volume generated by an aggressive sales program conflicts with a strategy of high profitability. Simply stated, tremendous growth may not be compatible with maximum profitability in the short run. Dramatic growth costs money.

On a short-term basis, in order to achieve growth, profits may have to be diminished. In a growth phase, profits may decline because capital is required for new clinics and related costs, such as staffing. Such a tradeoff can be an obstacle, because individuals in the partnership who are approaching retirement may not want to sacrifice income for growth.

FIGURE 1.3

Strategies Force Tradeoffs

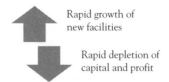

Rapid growth of new facilities

Rapid depletion of capital and profit

BEWARE OF GROWING AND SHRINKING AT THE SAME TIME–MARKET SHARE IS THE KEY

An interesting book published in 2002, *Four's a Crowd*, suggests that in a mature business, on average, only the top three market-share leaders are successful, and that usually these three will account for or control 70–90%

of the market.[19] An organization's market share is an important indicator of performance. Common measures of a healthcare program's success are number of patient days, number of new patients, net revenue, or average daily census. These measures are all appropriate and valuable. As health care becomes increasingly competitive, however, these measures can provide a false sense of security. Each has one major limitation—it is an absolute and does not take into account the competition. The Hampton clinic example provides a good understanding of volume versus market share insight.

Hampton Orthopedic Group

	Year 1	Year 2	Year 3	Year 4
Hampton Volume	50	75	80	90
Other Clinics' Volume	0	25	80	150
Hampton Market Share	100%	75%	50%	38%

The patient volume (or net revenue) of the Hampton Orthopedic Group, for example, steadily increased from year 1 to year 4. In year 1, Hampton had 100% of the market in the new emerging suburban market, in part because it had no competitors. In year 2, with competition in the market, Hampton had 75% of market share, and by year 4, its market share had dipped to less than 38%. In each year it was growing in volume, but at the same time becoming less important in the market from a market-share point of view. In fact, this group's common response to any suggested change in its strategy or tactics was, "No, we've never done better!" In year 1, these absolute measures were sufficient indicators of success. In the past, many hospitals and groups had little or no competition. Few healthcare organizations today, however, could describe their environment as noncompetitive. Even the rural parts of the United States now see competition, as large tertiary facilities offer helicopter service as a way to attract patients.

But an absolute measure may not reveal the truth. Although there was a steady growth in patient volume at Hampton, its market share of referrals from primary care physicians in its service area during those same years decreased. How could this be, and what does it mean? New orthopedists moved in; some of these physicians had more convenient locations than Hampton, which provided better access. Thus, Hampton is becoming a less important player in the market. If a new managed-care organization enters the market and contracts only with the market-share leader for specialty referrals, Hampton will lose. The time may have passed when it should have made strategic changes to remain a market leader.

Once a healthcare organization has competitors for its service or program, it must broaden its measures of performance and success. While absolute measures (e.g., net profit, volume) are valuable, a relative index (relative to the competition) is also essential. Plotting and tracking market share may keep an organization from being left with an unprofitable segment of the business as the demand for the service matures.

FORCE AND FOCUS

Normally, in the for-profit world, force and focus would be part of the formal marketing process. Yet, these two items seem to cause tremendous difficulties for marketing plans in healthcare organizations, as not-for-profits have a difficult time being seen as competitive. A common mistake in the marketing tactics of many healthcare providers is the failure to provide enough *force* (resources) to a marketing program. Usually, they allocate just enough advertising dollars for a 6- to 8-week image campaign, a half-time salesperson, or a part-time product manager. This tactic amounts to a partial commitment with a full expectation of success. It is essential to provide necessary resources or to save the capital altogether. With the typical consumer seeing more than 2,000 advertising messages per day in the United States, the chances of success for a poorly funded, understaffed, and inadequately promoted healthcare program are slim.

Figure 1.4 describes how health systems and hospitals tend to dabble in 5 to 20 different strategies simultaneously, while often not being able to offer sufficient resources to each strategy. Successful organizations tend

FIGURE 1.4

Focus and Force versus Diverse and Dabble

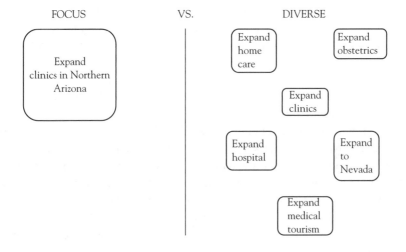

to focus their efforts. One successful national retailing executive, when asked about his strategy, indicated that the single most important notion was market force. The organization concentrated on its core business, offering products and services in high-traffic malls (strategy), and always entered new markets with the goal of becoming the dominant retailer in its product area (the force). Therefore, this company, rather than opening one store in 20 cities in a given year, opened 20 stores in one city and became the dominant player in that city before moving to the next.

It makes little sense for a company to enter a market with a new product unless it intends to be the dominant player in the market. Hospitals often enter many markets (clinical programs), however, and end up as minor players in all of them. They do not become preeminent in any major clinical area or service. This is the central reason why much of the expansion anticipated from marketing in the 1990s failed to materialize. An aggressive position to capture a market was missing. Hospitals and clinics need to think about becoming forceful—forceful in spending capital, forceful in dominating the market, and forceful in advertising. Once they have decided to enter a market, they need an aggressive strategy with supporting tactics.

As healthcare institutions consider their options, they often find it necessary to narrow those options—to *focus*—both from a business-line perspective and from the perspective of marketing strategy. A lack of focus will result in what one marketing expert, Tom Bonoma, calls "bunny marketing"—hopping from one strategy to another while having minimal impact with any of them.[20] Once an institution can focus its marketing and general business strategy, it can place greater force behind that strategy. Such force includes money, people, and strategic thinking—critical elements in a successful marketing program.

An analysis of diversification attempts by the top 200 of the Fortune 500 corporations showed that only a few businesses (18%) achieved profits in their first few years of diversification.[21] New ventures need, on average, 8 years to reach profitability and approximately 12 years to reach cash flows similar to those of a mature business. Clearly, extrapolating these data directly to the healthcare environment would be foolhardy, but the Fortune 500 companies from which these data were drawn are among the most well-managed organizations in the United States; their administrators often have a greater knowledge of diversification than do most administrators of healthcare organizations.

The extent to which an organization chooses to emphasize a target market or key service, or the extent to which it chooses to function in multiple businesses is its focus. Often this focus is described as vertical or horizontal integration. Vertically integrated companies seek to function within related businesses. For example, if Theodore General buys Aaron Supply Company and Wayzata Nursing Home, Inc., this is considered a vertically integrated organization. However, a hospital that purchases another hospital and adds yet a third is horizontally integrated. Usually, it is easier to operate horizontal businesses because of prior knowledge and expertise that can transfer from one like entity to the next in the product category. The problems in this area are complex, however.

Some executives seem to take a Las Vegas approach to developing focus. They note that if 70% of business lines fail, some are sure to work. Similarly, a person who throws 10 balls in the air at the same time will surely be able to catch a couple. Those who take this approach believe that it must be more risky to throw only one ball up in the air or to place only one or two bets. The difference between Las Vegas and business is the management time and attention that must be given to manage risk, direct resources, and provide service. Managers cannot throw money down and watch it passively. Managers have to participate, make decisions, try to manage risk, and try to maximize return. Thus, they must be concerned about force and focus.

The hottest management rage in the healthcare industry in the late 1970s and early 1980s was acquiring and operating multiple lines of business. Each month the management journals published articles about the grandiose plans of this system or that system. They reviewed complex organization structures, along with the myriad businesses that hospitals seemed to be entering. Hospital managers without diversified businesses felt old fashioned; it seemed that the landscape of the hospital industry was forever changed as managers attended seminars on diversification. The following experience is typical.

A hospital trade publication ran an announcement by Libertyville General Hospital's CEO that the hospital had established a holding company and would be entering a multitude of different businesses. The CEO was quoted as saying that because of the difficult times ahead for hospitals, it was necessary to seek revenue sources from alternative new businesses, including a health-food store, a home healthcare agency, and franchised dental centers, as well as from new healthcare programs. The hospital planned to establish 30 chemical-dependency programs around the United States within 3 years. The article noted that a major partner in a national accounting firm had been hired as the hospital's chief financial officer (CFO) to assist in this business-development and acquisition process. Two years later, in the Help Wanted section of the same magazine, an advertisement appeared for a CFO for the Libertyville General holding company. After the company's dismal record in establishing chemical-dependency programs and the collapse of other businesses, the new CEO and CFO of Libertyville General Hospital announced a new strategy at their first board meeting—getting back to basics.

Some organizations, such as St. Joseph's Hospital of Ottumwa, Iowa, have been able to accommodate diversification nicely. This organization has diversified into hospitals, rehabilitation facilities, family recovery programs, skilled-nursing facilities, and wellness programs.[22] Other companies had a dramatic drop in stock value in late 1985, largely because of investor concerns about the organizations' failure to diversify into managed healthcare systems. For example, Hospital Corporation of America became less attractive to the investor community because it was operating only hospitals.

At the other end of the spectrum, well-known management writers such as Tom Peters suggested that it was time to get back to the basics of business.[23] Events at other giants, such as the collapse of Enron and the sale of diversified, not-for-profit, Philadelphia-based Allegheny Health System by a bankruptcy court in 1998, caused management experts to reevaluate the whole concept of horizontal and vertical growth. The histories of many large corporations, including banks, automobile manufacturers, and airlines show numerous failures as these companies tried to expand. Integrated health systems such as the not-for-profit Henry Ford Health System lost more than $90 million in 2001. Further, hospitals across the country have found it difficult to make their medical clinic practice purchases work. Organizations such as these have sold or are thinking about selling businesses that are not core—sometimes the hospital, sometimes the doctors' group, and sometimes the health plan. Finally, a telltale sign of this new stick-to-the-knitting focus appears in conversations among CEOs, who talk about their need to develop the base business. This view is in sharp contrast to the articles about national expansion that these same CEOs wrote just a few years ago.

This is not to say that expansion or diversification is not a viable strategy and cannot be used effectively. For example, the Mayo Clinic's expansion into Arizona, Florida, and the Middle East has been successful because the Mayo Clinic has the reputation, the brand name, the manpower, the force, and the focus. Long-term commitment to a primary business also helps make such a venture successful. Such success would be impossible for most others, however.

The key is to develop strategy thoughtfully within the realistic capability of the firm. Health care is complex. The Las Vegas approach is simply too difficult to manage and sustain for most healthcare providers. Each organization needs to *focus* on a comfortable set of services and apply those key marketing strategies that can help bring them about with *force*.

UNIQUE SELLING PROPOSITION

Every organization needs a unique selling proposition, a combination of what its customers "give it" and those services or enhancements that the organization wants to add. Usually, the unique selling proposition is one or two attributes that, over time, become the institution's claim to fame or point of distinction from the competition. For IBM, it is maintenance availability; for Frito-Lay, it is freshness; for the Cleveland Clinic, it is comprehensive technology; for Nordstrom, it is an absolute commitment to service; and for Google, it is about preeminent information search.

Consumers' Perspective

Customers determine, in part, the unique selling proposition because they have views and perceptions about alternative healthcare providers, even though they may have no personal experience with them. For example, if customers view an emergency room as the most convenient, that is a powerful, unique selling proposition—one that the customers have "given" the organization.

Consumers have a difficult time determining the competence of various physicians and hospitals, but they have little difficulty perceiving such characteristics as high-tech or high-touch approaches, convenience, safe neighborhood, and friendly staff. Most hospitals like to think that their unique selling proposition is high quality, and consumers expect a hospital to provide high-quality care. As consumers consider the purchase of a durable product such as a TV set, for example, they recognize that they can pay less than $100 for a portable, small-screen TV to a few thousand dollars for a wide-screen LED-LCD TV with Internet and the latest apps. Within each category, consumers expect to purchase quality. It is the same with health care. Pahrom said it best: "Quality is the tar baby of health care competition. Nearly everyone vows or claims to compete on this dimension . . . but there are real problems with [this] approach."[24] He goes on to point out that service quality, not clinical quality, will be the competitive dimension of the future.

The consumer assumes that if a hospital has a license, nurses, physicians, and all the other trappings, it must provide quality—to at least a minimal standard. In a competitive strategy, quality is the cost of entry; it is the given. Saying "we are the quality hospital" is a little like saying "our pizza tastes good" or "our accountants know the tax law." The *New England Journal of Medicine* published findings from a study of patients who changed doctors. Only 25% cited incompetence. In several proprietary studies (conducted by Steven Hillestad and Eric Berkowitz) provided to clients in 2011, the results remain basically the same: Most consumers who switch physicians base their decisions on personality, style, cleanliness, and poor communication skills—"It was clear that competence was taken for granted."[25]

Some organizations on a national level and, to a greater extent, on a regional level have achieved superior quality status. Johns Hopkins, the Cleveland Clinic, and the Mayo Clinic fall into this category. The interesting aspect of this status is that the organization, not an individual physician, has gained the recognition based on the perception of quality. A study conducted by the Strategic Planning Institute and the Harvard Business School of the Profit Impact of Market Strategy (PIMS) of more than 450 companies and 3,000 business units found that relative perceived quality and profitability are strongly related.[26] The link between relative perceived quality and return on investment is clear in the PIMS data (**Figure 1.5**).

Whether the measure is return on sales or return on investment, superior perceived quality leads to superior performance. Few people (relative to those who have expressed opinions) have experienced care at these centers, however, and on the surface it is difficult to determine what these centers have done specifically to achieve their quality position. The consumer assumes quality; he or she will not knowingly visit a bad hospital. How then does a consumer differentiate between "quality" hospitals in a given community?

FIGURE 1.5

Relative Quality Perception as Related to Integration of Services

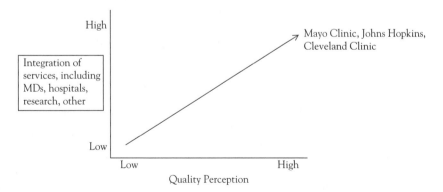

From the consumer's perspective, the primary product to be purchased is the expertise of physicians, nurses, and staff, along with the accompanying technology (**Figure 1.6**). The primary product is the core of healthcare service just as the engine is the core of the car or airplane. The primary product gives a healthcare organization its quality, or technical component—the cost of entry. It must work, just as an engine must start. It is expected. But it is not the differential advantage for business consumers; they differentiate one hospital from another on the basis of the generic product—components such as breadth of services, image, price, and attitude of the staff. Although "healthier" is a complex notion, the evaluation of the consumer often rests on seemingly simple parameters such as wait times and written materials and instructions. Likewise, the automobile is complex, but some consumers make purchase decisions based on the availability of cup holders. They infer quality from such components, and they can make this inference even if they have never experienced the service or used the product. Therefore, instead of emphasizing general quality in a marketing plan, a hospital may find it more valuable to focus on the physicians and the special training that they have—assuming that this is indeed a unique selling proposition.

Determinant Attribute

It is important in building a unique selling proposition to focus on a component of the service that may be a determinant attribute. Such a component is one that consumers feel is important (e.g., breadth of services) and that they perceive as a difference from the competition. If one hospital in a community has taken convenience as its unique selling proposition, another hospital will probably not be able to counteract it with, "we are

FIGURE 1.6

Health Care as a Primary and Generic Product

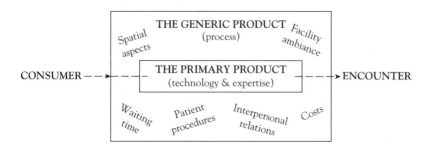

quality." Because most consumers see all hospitals as providing some reasonable level of quality, the convenience factor comes up time and again as one of the most powerful and sustainable unique selling propositions available to a hospital or to a physician. In order to overcome this unique selling proposition, another organization must have a strategy that goes beyond convenience and quality.

If quality cannot be used as a unique selling proposition, it may be possible to use price, particularly a low price. The use of pricing strategies as a unique selling proposition is untested in the healthcare arena, however, and it is probably one of the most dangerous strategies for at least two reasons. First, competitors can often easily match this strategy, at least for a short period of time, unless the price package includes unique benefits to the buyer. If a competitor matches your low price, in effect it takes away the unique selling proposition and sets up the possibility of a price war. Classic price wars have taken place among hundreds of companies and have sometimes changed the entire structure of an industry. Throughout the 1980s, for example, the airline industry was in a price war to such an extent that discount prices came to be expected; this expectation drove profit margins down, drove bankruptcies up, and ultimately led to a massive consolidation that resulted in sharp price increases as competitors were eliminated.

Second, price is one of the ways that consumers judge quality, and organizations try to position the quality of their services through the use of price strategies. As a rule of thumb, setting a higher price and bundling benefits with that price help position a product as a higher quality item. Setting a lower price may cheapen the product and attract a different market. For example, consumers are likely to perceive the skills of tax preparers who advertise their services for $19 as poor, particularly if they know that a national certified public accounting firm would charge $275. For most products and services, there is a perceived price–quality relationship. These discount accountants may have graduated at the top of their classes, but the pricing system they use may raise concerns about the quality of the service delivered. The situation is similar for hospitals and physicians. Most patients do not want their surgery done by the cheapest surgeon in the cheapest hospital. Instead, they want good care, a great outcome, and a responsible price. Being known as the "Kmart of hospitals" may be all right for such products as school physicals, health education, and other low-risk services, but it could be dangerous for others.

Although quality and price may not be appropriate competitive advantages or unique selling propositions, no service needs to be a commodity—as long as points of difference between competitors can be highlighted.

Some of these differentiations or unique selling propositions may seem trivial or small, but they may be just enough to set an organization apart from the competition. A certified public accountant is generally assumed to be competent, for example. Others are also competent, so consumers can shop around every year to get the best deal on their tax preparation. The clients of one particular accountant seldom change, however, because of a small service that he or she provides as a byproduct of preparing tax forms. The accountant may use a computer-generated model to complete the forms because it is fast, it is accurate, and it allows the accountant to check on significant variances from one year to the next that may indicate a client's error in reporting information. As a byproduct of this process, the accountant may provide a nicely packaged 3-year comparative history of income, deductions, and significant financial transactions, complete with a folder that can be easily filed with other personal financial information. The customer does not receive an extra charge for this added service and perceives it as unique and convenient. Providing such a service also keeps the customer, because switching to another accountant (who has the same services, if not more) would interrupt this series of comparative financial reports. Therefore, the accountant not only has a unique selling proposition (comparative reports), but also provides it in such a way as to lock in a satisfied customer.

Add-Ons

Often, add-ons become unique selling propositions. A surgeon's generic service is his or her ability to skillfully examine, operate, and manage the patient's postoperative care. A routine add-on service is talking to the family immediately and calling the referral physician. Although the routine service is not part of the generic product, it is important to the extent that it helps differentiate one surgeon from another. The surgeon can go even further—to an extraordinary add-on product that is above and beyond the routine. Services in this category might be a telephone call from the surgeon to the referral physician or the patient 10 days later to make sure everything is all right, or a fax from the surgeon to the referral source immediately with information about the case.

Other services or add-ons are designed to keep the institution in the forefront. A surgeon may have an invitation-only Saturday morning seminar for referral sources, after which the group attends a university football game. Another surgeon may invite referral physicians to scrub for two or three cases to see a new laser technique in use so that they can better explain the procedure to their patients. Service thus includes the generic, routine, and extraordinary dimensions, which will change. Today's extraordinary services can become tomorrow's routine services.

Differential Advantage

A differential advantage is a core feature that makes you different from the competition. It is your unique advantage to your customers. Some call this concept your strategic heartbeat or your core driver. Most differential advantages are derived from one of three broad categories: a cost, a product, or a market driver. A differential advantage achieved through cost is self-explanatory. For example, many freestanding surgi-centers, which have low overhead, have been able to achieve a differential advantage on price over hospital-based surgery programs, which must pay a significant portion of the plant's overhead operating expenses. In order to obtain a cost-based differential advantage, organizations turn to a few basic approaches. First, an organization may create a no-frills product. Some managed healthcare plans have entered the market at a significant cost advantage by offering coverage with high deductibles or by providing care through lower-cost providers, such as physician extenders rather than physicians, at the first point of patient intervention. Second, the experience may lead to a cost advantage. As an individual or organization performs a task more and more frequently, the result should be increased efficiency. Some organizations charge more than $1,000 for Lasik vision correction, while others with large volumes of business charge under $500. Third, organizations may obtain a cost-based differential advantage through expense control.[27] Ideally, an organization may have an actual cost advantage over competitors, but not find it necessary to use this advantage in the marketplace. Creating a differential advantage on cost often requires extremely good expense control, and it is achieved at the sacrifice of the profit margin. Unfortunately, to some extent, buyers of healthcare services are choosing among competing providers based on this differential advantage.

Organizations can achieve product-based advantages from several factors, such as name or image, a demonstrably higher-quality service, innovations involving getting clinic information appointments online, or by being willing to constantly review and update their business model to stay competitive with changing clinical and economic conditions.[28] An organization gains a market-based differential advantage by offering a relatively narrow product line, focusing on a targeted market segment, or having a strong geographical focus. For example, the Joslin Clinic has historically been strongly positioned in the area of diabetes research and treatment, giving it a strong market-based differential advantage. In recent years, several hospitals, such as Abbott Northwestern Hospital, have attempted to achieve a differential advantage among women by promoting specialized women's healthcare services (**Figure 1.7**).

FIGURE 1.7

Advertisement for Women's Healthcare Services

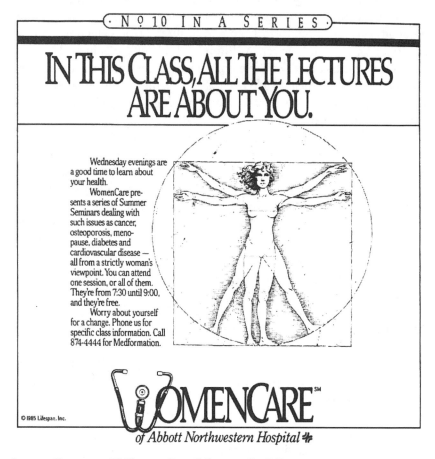

Source: Courtesy of Lifespan, Inc., Minneapolis, Minnesota.

Finally, many large, multispecialty group practices have aggressively expanded by means of primary care satellite networks in an attempt to establish a strong geographical differential advantage. In the 1970s, the Scott and White Clinic in Temple, Texas had no primary care satellites; by 1989, it had established multiple satellites in a wide geographical radius. Similarly, the Geisinger Clinic in Pennsylvania rapidly increased the number of its satellite clinics over a 10-year period in order to have wide geographical dispersion. Soon after, most hospitals and large medical centers were trying this model. But by 2000, after failing to achieve economic return from the expansion of clinic sites, many hospitals began to unload clinics as fast as possible.

CREATING BARRIERS FOR COMPETITORS' ENTRY AND MINIMIZING BARRIERS FOR SELF EXIT

In developing a competitive strategy, an organization's ultimate goals should be to create barriers that discourage competitors from entering the market and to minimize barriers that hinder its own exit.

There are several sources of *barriers to entry*. Size can create economies of scale and make competition difficult. The consolidation within a prepaid business may discourage new competitive entries, for example. A prepaid plan with a membership of 2–3 million obviously has a risk base that may allow for more aggressive pricing than is possible for an independent physician association plan with 35,000–40,000 members. In essence, market share can be a formidable barrier to entry. Another valuable barrier to the entry of competitors is the consumers' switching cost. The goal is to link the consumer to the hospital or other healthcare providers in such a way that switching to a new provider may cost too much in information lost, hardware made obsolete, or, ultimately, financial resources. A large advertising budget provides a competitive advantage beyond the impression of the organization that it gives potential buyers. Any new competitor must at least match the advertising budget to compete for awareness among potential buyers. Capital requirements can also create a useful barrier to entry. A financial consultant may wince at the thought, but expensive projects have a market advantage in their very expensiveness. They prevent many competitors from entering the market because they lack the financial resources to do so. The ideal barrier to a competitor's market entry is product differentiation. The service provided must, however, be superior in some characteristic that is both perceived and valued by the potential buyer. In health care today, as technology pervades the system and the skill levels of physicians increase, product differentiation is difficult to achieve.

As important as it is to consider creating barriers to market entry, it is also useful to *minimize barriers to market exit*. In considering competitive plans for services or programs, an organization should attempt to maximize its ability to leave the market. The first barrier to exit that must be minimized is high fixed costs; once a lot of money has been approved for a project, it is difficult to drop. The second barrier to exit that must be minimized is psychological commitments. Senior management may believe that too much has been invested in a project to consider dropping it.

DIVERSION AND DISSUASION

Some organizations use diversion strategies; they try to make it appear as though they will not invest in a given opportunity or that the opportunity in which they have invested is so unimportant that it does not warrant attention.[29] Dissuasion strategies lead competitors to believe that, in direct competition, the organization will be able to crush them because of the resources the organization will pour in. These tactics are common in business and are used to diminish the probability that a competitor will open across the street, develop a new service line, or compete for the same market segment.

For hospitals, the use of diversion and dissuasion tactics is often difficult. Most hospitals allow the general staff or the executive committee of the medical staff to approve new service offerings. Physicians who participate in these discussions often have staff appointments at two or three hospitals. As a result, information about a new program at one hospital may be quickly available at another hospital, a situation that limits either hospital's ability to use these classic tactics.

As hospitals and physicians consider more joint ventures, problems in the use of diversion and dissuasion are likely to become more widespread. While hospitals and clinics attempt to balance tactical surprise, traditional policy, physician-vested interests, hospital-vested interests, and a competitive environment, they will need to evaluate and develop ways to use these tactics appropriately.

GROWTH IN THE PRESENT MARKET

Many organizations search for new markets, bringing on staff new physicians or more primary care physicians to enhance the referral base. They spend little time, however, increasing the loyalty of current customers. As organizations develop their marketing plans, they must recognize that present buyers are as important as new ones. Furthermore, increasing the loyalty (or usage rate) of current buyers is frequently less costly than attracting those who have never used an organization's services. In the soft-drink industry, for example, the usage figures in the market are as follows:

Soft-Drink Industry Usage Figures

Households	22%	39%	39%
Purchase/usage	0%	10%	90%

Twenty-two percent of the households purchase no soft drinks; 39% of the households purchase 10% of all the soft drinks sold; and 39% purchase 90%. For strategy development, one fact is obvious—the group that purchases 90% of the soft drinks must be maintained. At first, it may appear that because of the potential volume, those who sell soft drinks should focus on the 22% who do not purchase soft drinks. In fact, however, these people may have never tried one, hate soft drinks, or have some other challenging reason for not buying them. Who would be easier to convert: the person who has never had a soft drink, or the person who drinks them occasionally? It may be easier and more profitable to convert the medium user into a heavier user than to convert the person who has never consumed a soft drink into a buyer.

In the healthcare industry, it is similarly important to look for growth in the present market. An analysis done for one specialty group revealed the following referral patterns for primary care doctors:

Referral Patterns for Primary Care Doctors

Primary care doctors	38%	32%	30%
Referrals generated	0%	37%	63%

Thirty-eight percent of the primary care physicians in the service area referred no patients, while a smaller core (30%) accounted for the bulk of the referrals. This specialty group should make no changes in patient procedures without consulting the loyal "heavy users," the 30%. The group should also find a way to increase the loyalty of the 32% of physicians who account for 37% of the referrals. These physicians are either referring patients to more than one healthcare facility, or they are not referring patients in the volume that they might. The issue is not to make these physicians aware of the group's existence, but to generate more volume. Obviously some business can also be received from the group of physicians who account for no referrals. Some of them may not yet be aware of the specialty group, but once they are made aware, they may find the service of value. The vast majority of physicians who do not make referrals to the group, however, have previous commitments or have simply decided not to do so. Conversion of those who have made a conscious decision not to refer is expensive and difficult.

FALL ON YOUR SWORD

Is the medical organization willing or able to live with its own words? If they say they will have the highest quality of care, then are they willing to eliminate clinical privileges for those who do not meet the national standard? If they say they are customer focused, then are they willing to spend significant effort and resources each year to study consumer opinion of their service? An example of this is a remote northern resort hotel that is open in the winter months even though business is slow. The resort's mission is a commitment to couples looking for a romantic weekend. The resort has 20–30% occupancy during slow times and therefore has significant negative cash flow during the winter months. Sports teams who have games scheduled in nearby towns call the resort looking for accommodations for dates during the difficult cash flow periods. The teams could fill the rest of the rooms and generate thousands of dollars of much-needed revenue. But the resort refuses them; it does not want this revenue unless the teams are willing to sign a strict set of guidelines and abide by a prescribed set of rules with significant penalties if the rules are not followed. The resort is willing to "fall on its sword" and keep its promise that, in fact, it is a quiet romantic getaway destination, even if it means saying no to organizations that are not willing to abide by the rules and possible penalty fees.

Some healthcare organizations are willing to keep their promise as stated in their vision, mission, and other strategy statements, while others will grant credentials and privileges to physicians who can bring new volume even though the physicians have had prior issues at other organizations. If a hospital says that it will offer the most efficient, cost-effective service, then an observer would expect to see diligent attempts to reduce waste, including extra tests, procedures, and medical visits. While the marketplace might be competitive, the healthcare community has an ethical and professional responsibility to live its mission statements and to provide for the best interests of its patients.

SUMMARY

Steve Jobs, the founder of Apple, personified the concepts of the Strategic Mindset. In the late 1980s, under pressure, Jobs left Apple, and did not return to the Apple campus until 11 years later in 1997. When he returned, the company was in a shambles, with declining revenue, severe cash flow issues, and a critical loss of customer support. The company was headed toward bankruptcy, as demand for Apple computers nearly vanished. On one of Jobs's first days back to work at Apple, he was astonished to find a dozen different versions of Apple's Macintosh computer and a confusing and disjointed array of products under development. One day he attended a product development meeting and on the board he drew a square and divided it into four quadrants. Above the square, over each of the two columns, he wrote "Consumer" and "Pro." Along the side of the square, he wrote "Desktop" for one row and "Portable" for the next. He then told the horrified engineers that he wanted only one product in each box, and soon 70% of the existing product line was scrapped as the organization was refocused into four product areas.[30] Jobs embodied the use of the Strategic Mindset, including clear vision, absolute focus, attention to customers, and having a champion.

Before starting the planning process, the elements that constitute the Strategic Mindset should be reviewed and discussed to determine if the organization is really ready to move on to the next step. Before moving forward, how well positioned is the company with each of the following Strategic Mindset topics?

1. The company must have a clear vision and focused strategy.
2. Customers, customers, customers—they are the real focus.
3. Services cannot remain static; change is inevitable.
4. There is often a better way, and often a competitor will find it.
5. The marketplace has a decision-making role in directing the future course of a business.
6. A champion must be in place.
7. Tradeoffs among alternative strategies are necessary.
8. Beware of growing and shrinking at the same time—market share is the key.
9. Effort should be focused, and adequate force should be provided.
10. A unique selling proposition is necessary.
11. Barriers to entry should be created, and barriers to exit should be minimized.
12. Diversion and dissuasion need to be utilized.
13. Growth is often most likely with the present market.
14. Be willing to fall on your sword.

Within the framework of this mindset, the remainder of this text addresses the development of a model for creating high-level strategic plans that link to marketing and business plans in healthcare organizations.

QUESTIONS FOR DISCUSSION

1. In a world of federal health reform, how does strategic planning change?
2. Is a champion for an idea more important than the strategy itself?
3. New ideas do not have a history. What is the best way to introduce a new idea into the marketplace?
4. Can organizations grow rapidly and maintain financial margins at the same time?

NOTES

1. Andrews, K. R. (1971). *The concept of corporate strategy*. Burr Ridge, IL: Irwin.
2. Porter, M. (1987, May–June). From competitive advantage to corporate strategy. *Harvard Business Review*, 43–59.
3. Zagotta, R., & Robinson, D. (2002, January–February). Keys to successful strategy execution. *Journal of Business Strategy*, 30–34.
4. Porter, A. (1996, November–December). What is strategy? *Harvard Business Review*, 61–78.
5. Mintzberg, H. (1994, January–February). The fall and rise of strategic planning. *Harvard Business Review*, 107–114.
6. Henderson, B. (1979). *Henderson on corporate strategy*. Cambridge, MA: Abt Books; p. 3.
7. Ibid.; p. 18.
8. Thornhill, S., & White, R. (2007, February). Strategic purity: A multi-industry evaluation of pure vs. hybrid business strategies. *Strategic Management Journal*, 28(5), 553–561.
9. Hamel, G., & Prahalad, C. K. (1994). *Competing for the future*. Boston, MA: Harvard Business School Press.
10. Robert, M. (2006). *The new strategic thinking, pure and simple*. New York: McGraw-Hill.
11. Ibid.
12. Treacy, M., & Wiersema, F. (1995). *The discipline of market leaders*. Reading, MA: Addison-Wesley.
13. Greenley, G. (1983). Where marketing planning fails. *Long Range Planning*, 16(1), 106.
14. Peters, T., & Austin, N. (1985). *A passion for excellence*. New York: Random House.
15. Battle of the Republicans. (1988). *Newsweek*, 21(1), 100.
16. Peters, T., & Austin, N. (1985). *A passion for excellence*. New York: Random House.
17. Ibid.
18. Collins, J., & Porras, J. (1994). *Built to last*. New York: HarperCollins; pp. 115–125.
19. Sheth, J., & Sisodia, R. (2002). *Four's a crowd*. New York: Free Press.
20. Bonoma, T. (1985). *The marketing edge*. New York: Free Press; p. 30.
21. Biggadike, R. (1979, May–June). The risky business of diversification. *Harvard Business Review*, 103.
22. Religious hospitals: St. Joseph's model for diversification. (1986, August). *Modern Healthcare*, 36.
23. Peters, T., & Austin, N. (1985). *A passion for excellence*. New York: Random House.
24. Pahrom, P. (1995, March–April). Competitive strategies for the next generation of managed care. *Healthcare Forum*, 36.

25. Cousins, N. (1986). How patients appraise physicians. *New England Journal of Medicine, 314*, 1317–1319.
26. Buzzell, R. D., & Gale, B. T. (1987). *The PIMS principles: Linking strategy to performance.* New York: Free Press; p. 142.*
27. Michel, R. (1993). *Strategy pure and simple.* New York: McGraw-Hill.
28. Casadesus-Masannell, R., & Ricart, J. E. (2011, January–February). How to design a winning business model. *Harvard Business Review*, 101–107.
29. Henderson, B. (1979). *Henderson on corporate strategy.* Cambridge, MA: Abt Books; p. 3
30. Isaacson, W. (2011). *Steve Jobs.* New York: Simon & Schuster; pp. 337, 359.

---

*These generic strategies are discussed in Porter, M. (1980). *Competitive strategy.* New York: Free Press; ch. 2; and Aaker, D. (1984). *Strategic market management.* New York: Wiley; ch. 12.

CHAPTER 2

UNDERSTANDING THE STRATEGIC, BUSINESS, AND MARKETING PLANNING PROCESS

WHAT YOU WILL LEARN

- The strategic plan and a market-based business plan are different.
- Confusion exists between the role of planning and the role of marketing.
- The differences between a market-based approach and a nonmarket-based approach are subtle.

RESOLVING THE CONFUSION: RELATING THE MARKETING PLAN TO THE BUSINESS PLAN TO THE STRATEGIC PLAN

Planning an organization's activities is a complex process that involves many steps: setting goals, identifying objectives, describing tasks, forecasting demand, setting quotas, monitoring performance, and budgeting. The types of planning activities that are necessary include marketing planning, strategic planning, business planning, and long-range planning. Distinguishing all these activities can be confusing in theory and in practice. As Hamel says, "The essential problem in organizations today is a failure to distinguish planning from strategizing."[1] He goes on to suggest that planning is about programming while strategy is about dreaming and invention. Nevertheless, the planning process involves two plans—a strategic plan and a business plan. The marketing plan is contained within the business plan. In this chapter we look at how the pieces of this puzzle fit together.

STRATEGIC PLAN

The strategic plan is typically a longer term, 5- to 10-year view, with the time frame dependent on the condition of the entity, and the complexity of the proposed vision. Once a new strategic plan has been approved, it will become a "rolling plan," meaning that every year the plan moves forward, it is adjusted as needed and reset. In effect, if the plan is a 10-year strategy, as the organization moves from one year to the next, the strategic plan constantly rolls forward another year. The mission and vision of the business are found within the strategic plan, which is the important differentiation from the business plan. The role of the strategic plan is to address the environment and its changes, to seek or refine competitive advantage, to identify new opportunities, to anticipate change, to set a clear picture for the future, and to determine whether the organization is on course. **Figure 2.1** provides a general idea of what the strategic planning process is all about.

FIGURE 2.1

The Rational Planning Model

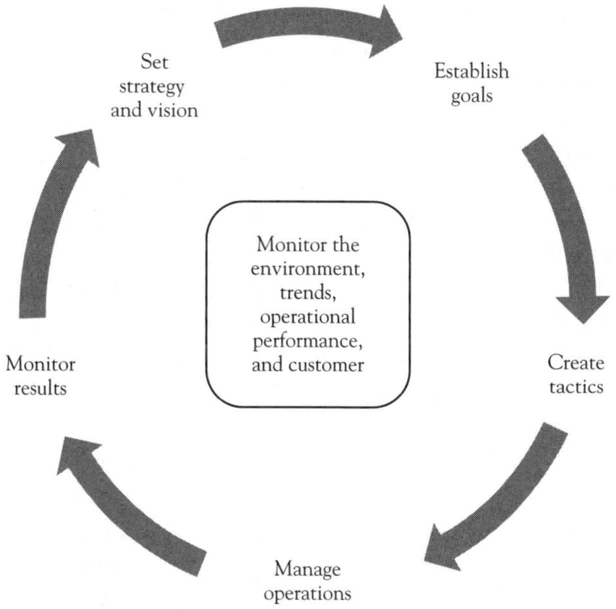

Set strategy and vision

Establish goals

Monitor the environment, trends, operational performance, and customer

Monitor results

Create tactics

Manage operations

FIGURE 2.2

How Strategy Development Really Works

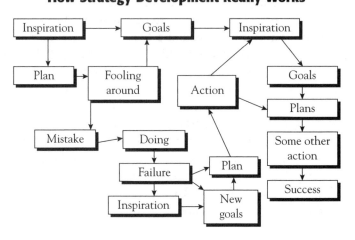

However, developing strategy is not a smooth process. In reality, it often looks like **Figure 2.2**. The strategic process uses much of the data and intelligence from the business plan, and the business plan clearly uses the direction set by the strategic plan. The fundamental difference between the two is the longer term and more visionary nature of the strategic plan versus the shorter term and more tactical nature of the business plan.

When the strategic plan is completed, it will have a list of goals and action steps that will typically be assigned to members of the management team. Many of these goals and steps will have long-term implications and are often not directly related to the day-to-day business of the company. For example, a strategic initiative might be to consummate a merger with another clinical entity, and those discussions might take 2 years. In the meantime, the clinical business must operate day in and day out. The business plan is designed to facilitate the ongoing, successful, and immediate operation of the company, while the strategic plan is designed to be more future oriented. **Figure 2.3** shows the relationship between the strategic plan and the business plan.

At a minimum, the strategic plan provides guidance to the business plan. For example, if the strategic plan suggests that the company will concentrate clinical resources at one site, then the business plan would not spend market research funds looking at creating an owned network of small regional sites. Or, if the strategic plan calls for cutting back on rehabilitation services, then the marketing plan and business plan would not involve opening a new physical therapy center.

FIGURE 2.3

The Relationship Between the Strategic Plan and the Business Plan

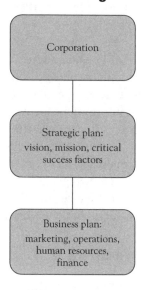

BUSINESS PLAN

A business plan is the year-by-year tactical execution of the overall organizational strategy. Each operating unit of an organization is responsible for producing annually its own distinct business plan, which should incorporate the operational, financial, and marketing needs of the specific unit. These individual business plans, in turn, must fit into an overall plan—the organization's strategic plan. The strategic plan, in turn, is a reflection of the organization's vision of its future—its long-range plan. The business plan coordinates all the organization's functional plans and is developed in light of the current competitive environment. The marketing plan is one chapter (the first one) of the business plan.

An organization's business plan is an integral part of strategy. Before the business plan can be developed, the overall strategy (vision, mission, critical success factors) needs to be established as a future target (**Figure 2.4**). After the vision, mission, and critical success factors have been formed, the first step in the development of the business plan can be taken: to establish the marketing plan. The marketing plan feeds the operational plan, which, in turn, feeds the finance plan. All these items combine to make a business plan. Furthermore, it is not possible to have a business plan without each of these elements mentioned. Within each of these planning elements are goals, objectives, strategies, tasks, forecasts, quotas, budgets, and other appropriate items unique to each functional area. In market-oriented institutions, the marketing plan begins the business planning process as shown in Figure 2.4.

The left column shows the nonmarket-based approach where, in essence, marketing and market considerations come last. This model is common in hospitals where programs are developed and financial assumptions are made without input from the market. What the left column usually means is that after the program, location, and pricing decisions have been made, someone comes to the marketing department asking that advertisements be created. In a market-driven model (the right column), the marketing group would conduct a market analysis, including research, testing of pricing options, and reviewing a host of other factors that would be used to drive operations and finance. In other words, to be customer focused, an organization must first obtain the knowledge of the customers

FIGURE 2.4

Relationship of Strategic Plan to Business Plan to Marketing:
A Hierarchy Model

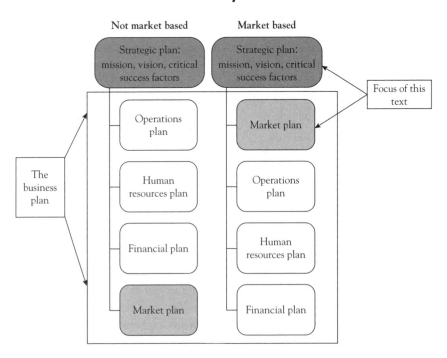

as directly as possible through data and market-research efforts. Step 1 will provide specific ideas on how this is done.

In a multiunit organization, each business should undertake this business planning activity. In a multispecialty clinic or a hospital, planning should take place at the departmental or program level. Each service or program of the business should have its own marketing, operational, and finance plan, which, when combined as a group, are called the business plan (**Figure 2.5**).

Combining the business plans of each department within a hospital or clinic, along with the overall strategy of mission, vision, and critical success factors, creates the strategic plan for the organization. For example, the rehabilitation department of a hospital may have as its marketing plan objective "to act as a feeder for more profitable businesses within the organization." Cardiac may consider one of its objectives to be "providing enough cash and resources for profitability and development of additional hospital services." Both of these clinical areas will have their own business plan, yet taken together, these two clinical areas are part of the same strategic plan; therefore, it is necessary to ensure that each business plan is consistent with the others before the strategic plan is put into action.

A good business plan will have the following characteristics. It will:

1. Be embraced by leadership.
2. Be written and communicated.
3. Be concise.
4. Be doable.
5. Include measurable targets and milestones.
6. Be linked to decision making.

FIGURE 2.5

Integrated Strategic and Business Plan Model—All Business Plans Created in Context of Overall Enterprise Strategic Plan

Enterprise-wide strategic plan (followed by business plan)		
Cardiac business plan	Obstetrics business plan	Rehabilitation business plan
Marketing	Marketing	Marketing
Operations	Operations	Operations
Human resources	Human resources	Human resources
Finance	Finance	Finance

Does a Hospital or Healthcare Organization Need Multiple Business Plans?

If a hospital or clinic has multiple clinical departments, which is the case for most hospitals, then a business plan is needed for each major business line that the hospital chooses to support. Why? Each clinical area has different products and, most importantly, different target markets or customers. Obstetrics, for example, is focused on younger women, while cardiology might be focused on older men. These two different clinical areas have different sets of potential patients with different requirements, and different clinical services are required. Therefore, each clinical area will typically have its own business plan. At the same time, all of these business plans are likely operating within the four walls of the hospital or clinic, and a form of coordination is necessary. A department store is a good example of how coordination works. In a typical department store, one will find children's clothing, a men's department, a perfume area, a home goods section, and others. Each department has its own set of customers, inventory, and methods of paying salespeople. Some departments advertise daily, others, maybe once a month. Each department has a manager who has responsibility for that department, including staffing, revenue targets, and inventory control. Each department also has its own business plan to grow each particular portion of the department store. Yet, from a consumer point of view, the individual department business plans are transparent. The department store looks and feels integrated. The consumers have no reason to sense or think about the fact that 70% of the department store's entire advertising budget is devoted to the women's and perfume portion of the store; or that the perfume staff is on commission while the men's clothing sales staff is on salary. While each department has its own business plan, the job of management is to coordinate those business plans into a package that provides the overall best positioning of the entire store to the marketplace.

MARKETING PLAN

A marketing plan is a section of the business plan. The marketing plan is not the business plan, and the business plan is not the marketing plan. The marketing plan is the first chapter of the business plan, and it is built in light of the business unit and the overall strategies and vision of the company. The marketing section will typically outline the key market and environmental trends, competitive influences and performance, and sales targets and strategies used to accomplish the targets. Those strategies might involve a sales force, new products or services, new locations, and different pricing options.

Planning versus Marketing

There is a great deal of confusion regarding the relationship of planning to marketing. Some authorities have argued that a corporate plan should be established before a marketing plan is developed.[2,3] The problem with this model is that the process may not be market-based because the corporation sets strategies and goals without the input of the market (marketing). The key to a market-based approach is strategy, and the key to the business plan is to obtain market input regardless of how and when the discipline of marketing is involved. Planning is an integrative function in which the interplay between major management functions is constant. For example, the organization establishes its mission within the context of marketplace forces and develops its marketing plan within the context of its mission and goals. Although this is an interactive process, marketing is a crucial first step in that it helps determine which business to enter and provides a foundation for finance and other input areas in formulating these plans.

Planning started as a budgeting role in business and has only recently evolved into a strategic role. The National Professional Organization of Strategic Planners was initially an organization of budgeting experts before it evolved into today's group, the Strategic Leadership Forum. Even more confusion exists regarding planning in the healthcare industry, partly because of the way in which planning was introduced into the healthcare environment. In many healthcare organizations, planning began in the department that handled government regulatory affairs, such as matters that involved systems agencies or regulatory agencies. The first planner in most hospitals helped guide the organization through the regulatory process, but that person often did not participate in the development of the organization's strategic direction.

Over time, the role of the planner was often expanded beyond regulatory activities and into the development of long-range plans and business strategy in general. In the 1980s, healthcare organizations started to put planning, marketing, and communications in the same organizational bucket because it "seemed natural." Healthcare organizations did not realize that the skill sets required of these three professional groups were different.

Today healthcare organizations often have both planners and a marketing staff, and there is sometimes confusion about their separate roles. There need not be any confusion, however, inasmuch as the planner and the marketing person both have valid positions, different responsibilities, and distinct relationships to the organization. The role of the planner is to take a somewhat neutral position and to coordinate the entire business planning process. This role includes balancing the interests not only of the marketing group, but also of the other groups involved in the business plan (i.e., operations, human resources, and finance). For example, a marketing group may be perceived as liberal because it does not hesitate to spend the corporation's money on ideas, whereas the finance department may be perceived as conservative because it invests in 20-year bonds at 3%. The role of the planner is to make sure everyone is focusing on the mission of the corporation, and the planner can be especially useful in providing a balance between marketing and finance interests. Sometimes it is useful to think of the planner as the coach and the components of the business plan (i.e., marketing, human resources, operations, and finance) as the team members. The role of the marketing person, in contrast, is to remain aware of the organization's marketing philosophy and to implement a customer-oriented marketing plan. Regardless of how planning and marketing relate within a given organization, the common element that they both share is an interest in assessment and data.

Everyone now, it seems, has decided to become "market-focused" or "customer-oriented." Nevertheless, when it comes to setting strategy, the customer-oriented theme often is not in evidence. Although the planning process has improved, most healthcare organizations that develop plans do not incorporate a market-based approach. The typical (nonmarket-based model, see Figure 2.4) process often begins with the wants and needs of people who work in the hospital or who own the clinic and their views of the marketplace. These views often become the conventional wisdom because these people sit on the committees or are the leaders of the organization; they have the time to set strategy or are responsible for doing so. But marketing people have always known clearly that the views of the people who are in the business can easily be different from people who use the service or frequent the clinic. Insiders speak of "clinical care," "cost per case," "integration," "ACOs [accountable care organizations]," "quality," and "performance measurement," while patients or plan members speak of "phone call," "billing errors," and "time with the doctor." The market-based approach starts with customer wants and needs, and these become the basis for a program or service to address those needs. Probably the most dangerous marketing judgment we can make is to presume we know what the marketplace wants without actually testing those perceptions.

What Is Market-Based Business Planning?

To accomplish market-based planning effectively, it is necessary to understand what the marketing philosophy is. There is much misinformation about this concept and its implementation. Although the marketing philosophy is quite simple, most healthcare organizations have never been successful in understanding or implementing the concept. Basically, marketing is:

1. The process of listening to consumers and the marketplace
2. The philosophy of organizing to satisfy needs of a group or groups of consumers
3. The satisfaction of these needs in a profitable fashion

The essence of marketing is best highlighted by these points:

1. A philosophy of consumer orientation
2. A system of objective data gathering
3. A road to dynamic business strategy
4. A process of business planning
5. An emphasis on innovation
6. A means of performance evaluation
7. A focus on future opportunities

Good managers understand that planning starts with marketing, and marketing starts with the consumer. Marketing plans are an integrative process of listening to customers and developing strategies and objectives that meet their needs, as well as conforming to the policies of the organization that are realistic within the context of financial and operating parameters. Any other methodology is not market based.

A Market-Based versus a Nonmarket-Based Approach

A marketing plan begins with an analysis of the market. Most healthcare organizations think of their internal needs first and the marketplace second. This is a nonmarket-based approach. A market-oriented manager, however, begins with a determination of external needs and focuses internal actions on those external needs. This is a market-based approach. The two approaches vary in just a few ways, but the difference in the results obtained can be dramatic. **Figure 2.6** shows the nonmarket-based method, and **Figure 2.7** shows the market-based system of planning.

In a nonmarket-based model, the board of directors or physician shareholders of the group establish the goals and objectives for the organization. Then, typically, these individuals set the goals for the coming planning period. At Brighton Hospital, for example, the mission is to provide high-quality care to residents of the immediate community. On the planning committee are two physicians who have had a long-standing

FIGURE 2.6

Nonmarket-Based Approach to Planning

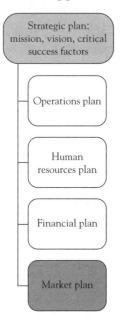

FIGURE 2.7

Market-Based Approach to Business Planning

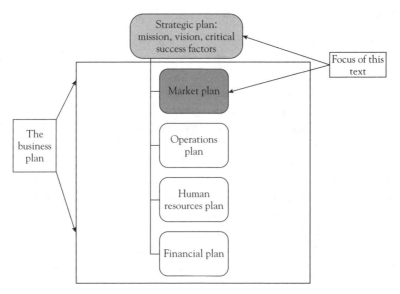

relationship with the hospital and are respected by their peers. Both physicians have served as chiefs of the medical staff. They believe that there is a need for a basic rehabilitation program in their area. Discussions at medical meetings and articles in popular trade journals suggest that such programs are increasingly common. As a result of the political persuasion of these physicians, the hospital allocates resources and space to a full clinic. The public relations department is instructed to build demand through immediate media coverage. Six months after the service becomes available, demand has not met projections.

When a program fails, the organization's executive committee often meets to explore the reasons. The first explanation given may be that the marketing department did not promote the program sufficiently. The action to be taken is clear: Fire the marketing director. Sometimes, the marketing director is ineffective. Other times, a second explanation is posed: The fault lies with the director of the program, who must not be generating enough referrals; therefore, the program director must go. The possibility that the program director is ineffective may also be real. A third explanation is rarely voiced: There was no need for the rehabilitation program, or the program started by this organization had no differential advantage over existing programs.

This scenario changes under a market-based approach. The organization's members still set the mission, but they fulfill this mission with direction from the market. They assess market needs at the start by consulting with potential referral physicians. If these physicians see little need or advantage for a rehabilitation program, for example, yet report referral needs in sports medicine, the organization determines whether a sports-medicine program fits within its mission. If so, such a program is designed, tested, and reviewed by a sample of physicians before full-scale implementation. Hours, costs, and planned patient procedures are described. If this program is not what the referral physicians had in mind, it may have to be reformulated before it is fully implemented. If the program is acceptable, the organization needs to inform the referral physicians that the service is now available in the configuration that they suggested with the desired range of services at an acceptable price.

In this market-based approach, a key ingredient is testing the program before it reaches full-scale implementation. Testing is easier in product-based marketing than in service-based marketing. In testing a product, an organization can create a prototype and offer it to the prospective market. But such testing is expensive and often impossible in health care. A hospital cannot develop a prototype of a rehabilitation program without great cost; staff must be hired, space allocated, and support systems put in place. Instead, a hospital can test a service by developing a detailed description of the program and explaining staff credentials, hours of service, price, and other operational details that the buyer of the service would want to know. This concept description is provided before full-scale commercialization to a sample of the proposed target market for their reactions: likely interest, intention to use, or perceived problems.

A market-based approach is not "right," and the nonmarket-based approach is not "wrong." Yet, as financial resources become increasingly restricted, mistakes (programs that do not meet expectations) are more costly for the organization. A market-based approach helps improve the odds of success. It is easier to listen to buyers and to provide the necessary programs than to attempt to divine what buyers may need.

THE PROCESS OF STARTING A NEW VENTURE—WHAT IT MIGHT LOOK LIKE

If you were starting a new venture, what would a market-based business model look like? The following is an example of how a business could get started following a market-based business model.

Theodore was reading *Time* magazine online when he came across an article about stress therapy. He realized that he had been seeing a number of articles in the popular press about nutrition, stress management, acupuncture, and the like. Wondering whether an opportunity existed to create a business in this area, he decided to investigate.

Theodore began by accessing the Internet to obtain bibliographies on chiropractors, massage, stress, acupuncture, spas, and nutrition. While looking for articles, he noted repeated references to "alternative care" and "complementary care." He probed for information about these topics and read articles on the Internet about these concepts. Next he visited the local library and accessed several publications including *Market Share Reporter, Small Business Sourcebook, Almanac of Business and Industrial Financial Ratios,* and *Statistical Abstract of the United States.* In general, Theodore was looking for information about the size, nature, and scope of alternative and complementary care. Next Theodore went to the *Yellow Pages.* He copied references to alternative medicine. He also accessed services that conduct research in many business categories to see whether they had done any studies on alternative care. He "Googled" alternative care topics and it appeared that no syndicated studies had been completed. Back at his office, he started to call people who had knowledge of the industry. He talked to professional organizations, individual friends who had experienced alternative care, and others who had knowledge about these services.

The next day he started to drive around the community. He wanted to see firsthand where these services were located, what they looked like, and what kind of activity was occurring. He found no particular pattern to location: Therapies were located in professional office buildings, strip malls, and homes. He spent the next several days parked across the street from the entrances to several therapy businesses. During this time he recorded the number of visitors (patients), their demographic characteristics, the hours of the day with the most traffic, the cars they drove, and their license plate numbers. At the same time, using his cell phone, he called for reference and credit checks on the therapy centers he was aware of to get a sense of the size and profitability of the businesses.

Ten days had passed, and Theodore had developed an early sense of the market: He discovered that most visits occurred from 2:00 p.m. to 5:00 p.m.; he noticed that the visitors were about 65% female, appeared to be about 30 to 55 years of age, and tended to drive Hondas or four-wheel-drive Ford Explorer utility vehicles. He called the local Honda and Ford dealerships to inquire about demographics that they might have used to determine store locations. They did have such data, but they were unwilling to share them with Theodore. Beyond this information, Theodore determined that, in this market, alternative care was a fragmented "mom-and-pop" business with no strong entities.

At this point, Theodore developed a preliminary business theory that he decided to explore and test. He wondered whether a business mission could be built around bringing multiple complementary therapies together under one roof, establishing strong ethical principles, mainstreaming the business in the community, and providing a strong brand identity or a national franchise.

In recent years, other industries have grown by bringing a business concept out of the back alley and into the mainstream. The old pawnbroker and flea-market business has not typically been part of mainstream or upscale culture. In this business, people get cash for used (sometimes stolen) merchandise at a pawnshop or a flea market. The pawnshop or flea market resells the used equipment to others at a markup. Within this framework, Grow Biz International (now Winmark Corporation) was formed and became one of the top 10 new start-ups in the mid-1990s. Grow Biz International set up segmented businesses called Play It Again Sports (selling used sports equipment such as skates, skis, and golf clubs), Music Go Round (used musical instruments), Once Upon a Child (used children's toys and clothing), and Plato's Closet (used trendy clothing). These stores were not located in the depressed areas of town or in dingy stores by used-car lots. Rather, they were in upscale neighborhoods within better strip malls; they were patronized by children and adults with significant disposable income and were thought of as respectable retailers within the community. Theodore thought, given what Grow Biz and Pawn America have done to bring backwater business dealing to Main Street, would it also be possible to bring complementary therapies to Main Street with a strong brand that would be respected across the country? Theodore decided to explore the feasibility of this concept.

At this point, Theodore had spent about 2 weeks of his time and $400 to explore the topic. Now it was time to begin to invest additional funds. He contacted a market research firm to design and conduct a study to determine the market size for complementary care and to test his ideas. Because of his interest in a possible national franchise, he decided to gather information on three different markets to see to what extent consumers' thinking and ideas changed from one part of the country to another. He decided to test Phoenix, Arizona; Minneapolis, Minnesota; and Raleigh, North Carolina. The study entailed calling several hundred households in each market to determine what, if any, alternative therapies they had used in the past 2 years, the frequency of use, how the service was paid for, their satisfaction with the service, and demographic characteristics of the user group. Further, Theodore wanted to test the idea of placing multiple therapies in one center to see whether the market was attracted to that concept. The study took about 30 days to complete. It provided data from which a volume forecast could be established along with a demographic profile of the average customer.

With this database in hand, Theodore contracted with a site-location specialist to determine whether a match could be discovered between the demographic profile found in the research and the clustering of similar populations in specific zip codes. Working with a business consultant who was a chiropractor and a friend who was a massage therapist, Theodore found a space with about 4,000 square feet that could work as a location for a prototype for the business idea. With the volume forecast, information about rent, and the cost of utilities, remodeling, and staffing, Theodore was able to profile a preliminary income statement in conjunction with a consulting company. Although work was only preliminary, it appeared that the business would be sound from a financial perspective. Would the market be interested? Theodore decided to do more market research. This time he conducted direct market research through Signe's Research Incorporated (SRI). SRI's task was to determine the market's view of the location, the proposed services, potential names for the business, and pricing. As a result of this test, Theodore was forced to go back to the drawing board because his idea for package pricing was not popular, the market was not interested in spa facilities, and the alternative names did not create enthusiasm. However, the marketplace did find valuable the notion of a "brand" with a board of respected alternative and mainstream leaders who could, in effect, certify quality and ethics without guaranteeing an outcome.

Armed with his data, Theodore contacted a venture-capital firm and continued to explore the possible opportunity. At every important step, he tried to check back with the market to help refine the thinking and the model. Ultimately, the site location, size, and name were modified. The concept was made more upscale and pricey, and physicians were added. The business was launched, and the national rollout proceeded. HMOs from around the country have contacted Theodore to convince him to bring the model to their communities, as they think it can be a useful tool for adding to their membership.

As can be seen from this example, the sequence of the market-based process is relatively simple. It incorporates six steps:

1. Thinking about a vision/idea
2. Performing an external/internal analysis
3. Developing action strategies
4. Testing strategies in the market before launch
5. Creating a plan that is financially responsible and contains accountability
6. Providing appropriate control procedures, feedback, and integration of all plans into a united effort

WHEN THE CUSTOMER VIEW IS DIFFERENT FROM YOUR VIEW

Organizations that consider themselves knowledgeable about their customers are often surprised when they find out what their customers really want. For example, a firm that specialized in services for the elderly was planning to build a large retirement center for the frail elderly. The management team, planners, and marketing staff had years of experience working with these people, and they went about designing apartments that would be attractive to them. They knew that 90% of the people in this project would be women who were age 85 and older, and they theorized that these women would have long-standing interests in caring for their homes, cooking, and taking part in traditional family activities. Therefore, these experts planned to construct one- and two-bedroom apartments with convenient and spacious modern kitchens. There were to be 12 units on each floor.

After much discussion, the marketing department of the hospital that was sponsoring the project persuaded the firm to conduct group discussions with these elderly consumers. The focus groups confirmed that the women did, in fact, have a commitment to traditional values, but they did not want large kitchens because they were basically cooking for themselves. One of them suggested that each apartment have a small galley kitchen and that each floor have a single large kitchen to be shared by the residents of all 12 apartments. Such an arrangement would make it necessary for residents to interact with their neighbors, do things together, develop a feeling of community, and, thus, reduce their loneliness. The person who came up with this idea had probably never developed a strategic plan or done environmental assessment for elderly people, but the other members of the focus group immediately agreed with her idea.

Clearly, an institution's view of a desired service may be different from what customers are seeking. The example of Physicians Computer Network (PCN) is a perfect illustration.[4] Wouldn't a doctor love to have a free multi-station IBM computer, with full practice-management and online medical record software, and professional education that includes interactive online teaching? In 1988, PCN thought so and went about attempting to provide this package to doctors. In exchange, PCN would be able to automatically collect data about pharmacy ordering patterns without the doctors' having to fill out any forms, and the doctors had to be willing to look at a few drug company ads sent via the computer. The business lost $44 million. Why? Postmortem market research indicated that even though the computers were "free," the doctors felt uncomfortable with the drug companies' gaining information from them. Since that time, PCN has changed the arrangement: no more free computers, no requirements for doctors to look at ads, and no sharing information with drug companies. Instead, PCN charges for the software, access to databases, and leasing of the computers. What seemed like a great idea initially was flawed because it did not connect with the needs or wants of the physician marketplace.

This market-based orientation requires healthcare professionals to accept the fact that the marketplace should have an impact on decision making. For example, the growth of a clinic may depend on the establishment of new office hours based on expressed consumer need, or a clinic's relationship with a healthcare system and how successful that overall integrated system is in attracting patients in the market relative to the competition. Many professionals find it difficult to engage consumers in these discussions or to allow them to participate in decisions.

In the mid-1990s, Andy Grove, then-president of Intel Corporation, described in *Fortune* magazine his attempt to get answers and to coordinate information when he was diagnosed with prostate cancer.[5] When doctors told Grove that he had cancer and recommended a course of action, Grove went on the Internet and found vast amounts of information and data. Some of the data conflicted. Nevertheless, Grove learned about options that his doctors never told him about. Grove, in essence, became the manager and decision maker of his own situation, and he chose a path that was different from the one his doctors suggested. Doctors at Dartmouth Medical School have studied diseases like prostate cancer and have concluded that when patients are given options, they will often not choose surgery when no difference in mortality or morbidity is demonstrated.[6] More and more patients are questioning conventional wisdom and are willing to press for options. Professionals who have felt a need to control the options in the past will be at odds with the market-based approach.

THE OVERALL STRATEGIC AND MARKETING MODEL

The integration process involves the coordination of marketing plans with finance, human resources, operations, and resource allocation. Also included are the development of the organization's entire product or service portfolio as well as the sharing and coordination of plans with the other services within the organization.

Many organizations have a reasonably good system for determining and controlling expenses, but then, mistakenly, consider it a planning or marketing planning process. Other companies confuse budgeting with planning. Although budgeting and forecasting are important in the development of marketing plans, they are not the sole ingredients. When completed, a marketing plan contains answers to the questions in **Exhibit 2.1**. Answering these questions in sequence is the foundation for most marketing strategy sessions.

The complete strategy and market-planning model is shown in **Figure 2.8**. Once all the steps shown in the figure are completed, the company can finish the business plan with the completion of the operations and financial plan. The steps in this process are sequential and interconnected. A complete business plan requires a marketing plan, and a marketing plan requires knowledge of the strategic vision of the company. Step 1 will explore the essential elements of an internal/external assessment. In Step 2, a deeper understanding of corporate strategy will be examined along with the tools necessary to have the strategic conversation. In Step 3 and beyond, a framework for

EXHIBIT 2.1

Marketing Planning Questions

Who is the market?

Where is the market?

What are the needs and demands?

Where are you now?

- As an institution?
- As a department?
- As an individual?
- With respect to the environment and competition?
- With respect to capabilities and opportunities?

Where do you want to go?

- Assumptions/potentials
- Objectives and goals

How do you want to get there?

- Policies and procedures/levels of initiative
- Strategies and programs

When do you want to arrive?

- Priorities and schedules

Who is responsible?

- Organization and delegation

How much will it cost?

- Budgets and resource allocations

How will you know if you did it?

- Feedback and review sessions
- Continuous monitoring

---

creating tactics will be explored, along with the tools to monitor and evaluate results.

To establish an effective marketing plan, and therefore a market-based business plan, it is necessary to understand an important premise. Market-based thinking is the process of determining customer wants and needs and then, to the extent possible, designing appropriate programs and services to meet those wants and needs in a timely, cost-effective,

FIGURE 2.8

The Overall Strategic and Marketing Model*

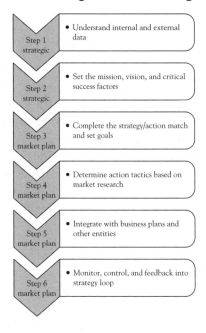

Step 1
strategic
- Understand internal and external data

Step 2
strategic
- Set the mission, vision, and critical success factors

Step 3
market plan
- Complete the strategy/action match and set goals

Step 4
market plan
- Determine action tactics based on market research

Step 5
market plan
- Integrate with business plans and other entities

Step 6
market plan
- Monitor, control, and feedback into strategy loop

*Note: Not the complete business plan model.

and competitive fashion. It is the process of molding the organization to the customers rather than convincing customers that the organization (for example, a clinic) provides what they need.

SUMMARY

This chapter concerns understanding how and where the strategy and business plan fit alongside marketing. Essentially, strategic planning is designed at the top levels of the company and involves the board. A specific business plan is at the operating level, or product line of the company, and marketing is a component of the business plan. Strategic planning is about corporate direction, and business planning is about the day-to-day execution of tactics to reach corporate objectives. Strategy and business planning are important and both exist side by side in successful organizations:

1. Top management must be committed to the process.
2. The CEO is the chief strategist, but the board sets the vision.

3. Marketing planning must be a way of life, not an activity that occurs during a certain time within the business year.
4. The approach must be balanced and integrative.
5. There must be detailed goals.
6. There must be an action plan.
7. The action plan must be result oriented.

However, the execution of the marketing and business plans is not straightforward, and therefore it is necessary to obtain organizational understanding of the planning process as early as possible. Step 1 will evaluate the importance of understanding the environment, and the tools that are used to assess opportunities will be examined. Step 2 will focus on the strategic planning process, including methods to come to an agreement on a mission, a vision, and critical success factors. Step 3 will concentrate on determining a marketing strategy, and Steps 4–6 will look at tactics to use in a marketing strategy and, in turn, how to manage and evaluate marketing strategy.

QUESTIONS FOR DISCUSSION

1. What is more important, a strong strategic plan or a strong business plan?
2. Why is it difficult to achieve the strategic plan?
3. Should the CEO be evaluated on the vision, the mission, or the annual profitability?
4. In health care, is it ethical to have a strategic plan that, in essence, would cause a competitor to go out of business?
5. Why is there often confusion regarding the differences between a business plan, a marketing plan, and a strategic plan?

NOTES

1. Hamel, G. (1996, July–August). Strategy as revolution. *Harvard Business Review*, p. 71.
2. Higgins, C. (1980). *Strategic and operational systems*. Upper Saddle River, NJ: Prentice Hall.
3. Hussey, D. E. (1989). *Corporate planning*. New York: Pergamon Press.
4. Rescue Team. (1996, April 22). *Forbes*, p. 100.
5. Grove, A. (1996, May 13). Taking on prostate cancer. *Fortune*.
6. The Dartmouth Working Group. (2009). *The Dartmouth Atlas of Health Care 2008*. Lebanon, NH: The Dartmouth Institute for Health Policy and Clinical Practice.

CHAPTER 3

THE CHALLENGE OF A COMPETITIVE
MARKETPLACE

WHAT YOU WILL LEARN

- The external environment affects a healthcare organization's strategy.
- An environmental scan must include demographic, regulatory, technological, competitive, and market shifts.
- No one environmental factor drives strategy.

THE EXTERNAL ENVIRONMENT

Marketing strategies must be developed in light of major changes, events, or trends in the marketplace. Consequently, many organizations have as an ongoing part of their marketing activities an environmental scanning process. An environmental scan tracks and monitors local, national, and global trends that may affect the organization's strategy.

Environmental trends often have five basic sources: demographic shifts, regulatory changes, technological advances, competitive shifts, and changes in the corporate area. For example, an obvious trend in the United States is the rapid aging of the large Baby Boomer population; people in this group are now beginning to enter their retirement years. The implications for healthcare use and for interactions with the healthcare system will be dramatic. Boomers came of age in the 1960s, and they have been more interested in alternative medicine and other non-Western approaches to maintaining their health than previous generations. An environmental scan of this trend might suggest the obvious need for many traditional healthcare providers to extend their product lines.

ENVIRONMENTAL TRENDS

Some of the major environmental trends that healthcare marketers must consider when developing their strategies are presented here.

Changing Demographics

The demographic complexion of the United States is changing in many ways. Two major trends are increases in ethnic and racial diversity and the aging of the population.

Increasing Ethnic and Racial Diversity

The U.S. population grew from 248.7 million people in 1990 to an expected 310 million in 2010.[1] The most interesting part of this growth for marketers is the increase in racial and ethnic diversity. Because of the greater detail provided in more recent censuses than in previous counts, it is difficult to compare racial and ethnic breakdowns and composition to previous census data. For example, the 2000 census included 36 different categories for Native Americans and 28 for Latinos (or Hispanics). This change in census methodology causes problems for marketers. The United States, however, is expected to see significant increases in racial and ethnic diversity, except among non-Hispanic whites, who are projected to have a slight decline in population over the next 4 decades to the year 2050.[2] The growing diversity of the "average American" is becoming important for marketers to recognize.

One significant change in the composition of the U.S. population is the need to have a multicultural perspective in marketing to reflect this shift. Certain subgroups are experiencing significant population increases. One in five Americans is African American, Asian American, Native American, or a member of another minority group. The minority population in the United States grew to 34% in 2008 from 31% in 2001.[3] In 2007, 15% of the population claimed Hispanic heritage.[4] In 2006, nearly one-quarter of all births in the United States were to Hispanic women.[5]

Latinos in the United States are significantly shaping the face of the marketplace. Between 1980 and 2009, the U.S. population grew by 9%, while the Latino population grew by four times that amount—37%. Latinos now make up almost one-sixth of the U.S. population.[6] Outside of one Northeast state, New York, the map in **Figure 3.1** shows the 12 states with the largest Latino populations. Fifty percent of all Hispanics live in metropolitan areas.[7] The median age of the Hispanic population is almost 10 years younger than the median age of the U.S. population as a whole.

FIGURE 3.1

States with the Largest Latino Populations

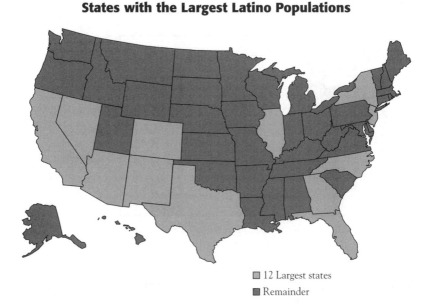

□ 12 Largest states
■ Remainder

Source: Population bulletin update: Latinos in the United States 2010.
Population Reference Bureau. Retrieved February 15, 2012, from: http://
www.prb.org/Publications/PopulationBulletins/2010/latinosupdate1.aspx

The black population increased significantly more than the population as a whole over the same decade. While the population as a whole increased by less than 10%, the black population increased to 13.6% of the total population, up from 12.9% in 2000.[8] One implication of the change in the composition of the U.S. population is the need to have a multicultural perspective in marketing. Attention to subcultural differences is important. For example, 53% of Hispanics say they think more positively about, and remember, companies that advertise in Spanish than those that do not. Forty-six percent of Hispanics say they are more loyal to these companies.[9] However, healthcare organizations must also be sensitive to some other key factors in terms of ethnic differences. **Figure 3.2** shows that Internet use is significantly lower among Hispanics and blacks compared to whites, a factor that must be considered in terms of social media strategy.

Healthcare organizations will need to reflect these changes in their promotional strategy, signage, and employee sensitivity.[10] One of the differences between groups is evident in **Figure 3.3**. As can be seen in this graph, the percentage of African Americans and Hispanics who have

FIGURE 3.2

Ethnic Differences in Internet Use

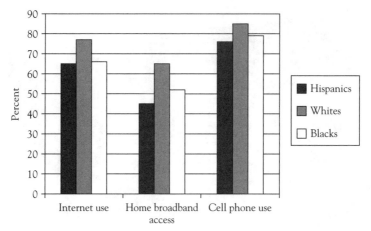

Source: Pew Hispanic Center. (2011). *Latinos and digital technology, 2010.* Washington, DC: Pew Research Center. Retrieved February 15, 2012, from: http://pewhispanic.org/files/reports/134.pdf

their own physician has been significantly lower than the percentage of Caucasians who do. The characteristics people value in a physician also vary by ethnic and racial profile. For example, in one survey 27% of African Americans wanted a physician who showed concern for their emotional as well as their physical well-being, compared with 25% of Latinos and 22% of Asians. Only 17% of Caucasians listed this characteristic as a major quality. A similar percentage of African Americans wanted a physician who was courteous and respectful, versus 24% of Latinos and 22% of Asians. Again, Caucasians valued this attribute less (15%). Asians also required a higher standard of expertise in their doctors: 87% strongly agreed with the statement, "recovery from illness requires good medical care more than anything else," compared with 78% of African Americans and Latinos. Only 60% of Caucasians strongly agreed with this statement.[11]

Aging of the Population

The graying of the United States is one of the most dramatic shifts in the population. In 1960, only 9% of the population was older than the age of 65, compared with more than 12.9% in 2009. The aging of America is

FIGURE 3.3

Who Has Their Own Physician?

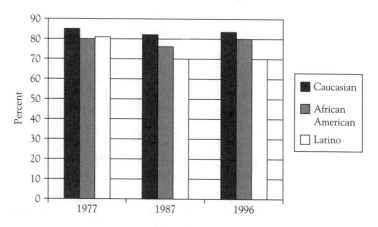

Source: Adapted from the Henry J. Kaiser Family Foundation. (1999). *Key facts: Race, ethnicity, medical care*; p. 21.

startling in many ways, in that by 2010, 29% of Americans were age 40 or older.[12] In 2000, people over the age of 65 represented 12.4% of the U.S. population; by 2030, there will be 72.1 million older than the age of 65, more than twice the 2000 number. **Figure 3.4** shows a continued rise in U.S. population over the age of 65 that will rapidly increase over the next 2 decades. For health care, the greatest change may be the substantial growth in percent of the population over the age of 65 (the Medicare-eligible population), as seen in **Figure 3.5**. Over the next 6 decades, the U.S. population is actually expected to experience a slight decrease in its rate of growth from the 1.10 growth rate experienced between 1990 and 1995 to 0.54 between 2040 and 2050. This decline is due to the aging population.[13]

The elderly are living longer, healthier lives. Life expectancy for a person age 65 has increased more in the last 30 years than the entire period from 1750 to 1950. A person age 65 today might expect to live another 15 years, while a man age 75 has a 50% chance of reaching 84 years of age and a woman age 86. Mortality rates have declined greatly as major causes of death have dropped in significant disease categories: influenza and pneumonia (down 8.4%), heart disease (6.5%), stroke (4.6%), diabetes (3.9%), hypertension (2.7%), cancer (1.8%).[14]

FIGURE 3.4

Continued Growth in the Graying Market Segment

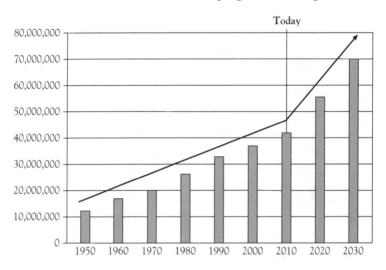

Source: Reproduced from Pirkl, J. J. (2009). The demographics of aging. *Transgenerational Design Matters.* Retrieved October 4, 2011, from: http://transgenerational.org/aging/demographics.htm. Used with permission.

FIGURE 3.5

Changing Composition of the U.S. Population

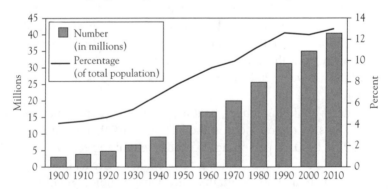

Source: Reproduced from U.S. Census Bureau. (2011). *The Older Population, 2010 Census Brief.* Retrieved February 3, 2012, from: http://www.census.gov/prod/cen2010/briefs/c2010br-09.pdf

The Baby Boomers heading to Medicare are a staggering number. By 2010, when the first Boomers started to reach Medicare age, almost one in four Americans, 40 million in all, were over age 65 (as seen in Figure 3.5). With the large number of Boomers moving to Medicare, hospitals in the state of Massachusetts proposed in 2011 that the age limits for eligibility be raised by 2 years. Representatives of AARP were opposed, saying this was a strategy to keep Boomers in higher paying private insurance plans.[15] In either case, it demonstrates the future stress that will occur in health care as the graying of the marketplace continues. There will be costs and significant marketplace opportunity for which strategic plans will have to be formulated. The concern of healthcare costs among Boomers is looming large.

Healthcare organizations face vast marketing opportunities within the increasingly older population. A 2011 survey conducted by Merrill Lynch (as shown in **Figure 3.6**) found that even the affluent Boomers are concerned about the rising costs of health care as they head into retirement. As this active Boomer segment ages, retirement communities that still have an active lifestyle of golfing and tennis also have medical facilities onsite for the access

FIGURE 3.6

The Looming Cost of Health Care

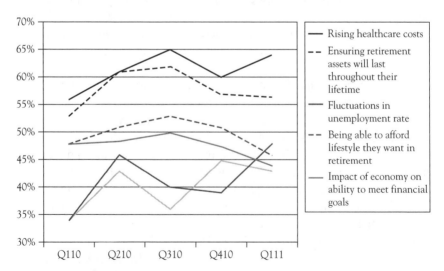

Source: Sarasohn-Kahn, J. (2011). Affluent boomers worry about health care costs in retirement. *Health Populi*. Retrieved October 4, 2011, from: http://healthpopuli.com/2011/02/02/boomers-worry-about-health-costs-in-retirement/

advantage for doctors—for example, Passavant Retirement Community in Zelienople, Pennsylvania. Countries such as Costa Rica, which is investing in its retirement community as medical tourism continues to grow, are recognizing the potential of this segment. A retirement project called the Sun Ranch Project is building an 18-hole Robert Trent Jones golf course, a $40 million dollar Clinica Biblica hospital onsite, and retirement homes in one of Costa Rica's prime tourist areas (see www.sunranchcostarica.com).

Regulatory Changes

Monitoring the regulatory environment is essential in the formation of any marketing plans or activities. Changes in regulations, whether they are state or federal, can affect a host of marketing strategies. Healthcare organizations face new challenges because of changes in federal laws as well as continued scrutiny from the Department of Justice and the Federal Trade Commission.

The HIPAA Challenge

The Health Insurance Portability and Accountability Act (HIPAA) was signed into law on August 21, 1996 and went into effect in April 2003. HIPAA requires all healthcare providers to have patient consent for access to their medical records or information. In the individual physician's office, this law entails logistical as well as operational changes. For example, a doctor who uses an outside vendor for cleaning the facility after hours needs to ensure that all medical records are locked. A physician who sends out information on a patient needs to obtain prior approval for such a transmittal.

Marketers must ensure that all their actions comply with HIPAA regulations. This regulation might have the greatest impact on programs for managing databases. Data need to be aggregated so that medical information cannot be attached to the names and addresses of individual patients.[16] Because patient-identifiable information cannot be used to send patients' marketing materials, organizations must create systems that allow patients to opt out of marketing activities tied to their personal information.

HIPAA does allow for certain marketing activities in which the healthcare organization can use patient data without the person's prior approval. One of the interesting implications of HIPAA is the use of patient data for marketing and fundraising activities. In 2009, under President Obama's $787 billion American Recovery and Reinvestment Act, many additional provisions were included to further strengthen the HIPAA provisions. Of note were provisions that pertained to the marketing and release of patient information. Hospitals, particularly, must be far more careful in terms of not marketing to patients who opt out of hospital fundraising lists. According to section 13406 of this Reinvestment Act, healthcare organizations may not communicate about a product or service that encourages people to purchase or use a product or service; nor may they communicate with consumers if the hospital receives or has received direct or indirect payment in exchange for making such communication.[17]

In these cases, healthcare organizations and institutionally related foundations (foundations that qualify as nonprofit charitable foundations under section 501[c][3] of the Internal Revenue Code and that have in their charter statement of charitable purposes an explicit link to the healthcare organization) may use or disclose an individual's demographic information and the dates on which the individual received treatment without obtaining written authorization. These uses and disclosures are permissible as long as:

1. The covered entity's notice of privacy practices states that individuals may be contacted for the purpose of raising funds.
2. Any and all fundraising materials include instructions on how to opt out of future communications.
3. The covered entity makes reasonable efforts to ensure those individuals' opt-out requests are honored.

The use or disclosure of patient health information for marketing purposes is permissible without an authorization in three instances:

1. When marketing information is communicated in face-to-face encounters. These communications may include discussion of any services or products, including the services or products of a third party.
2. When marketing communications involve products or services of nominal value. This exclusion allows for the distribution of calendars, pens, and other merchandise generally considered to be of a promotional nature.
3. When marketing communications are about health-related products or services of the healthcare organization, if the communication (a) identifies the covered entity as the party making the communication, (b) discloses any direct or indirect remuneration received by the covered entity for making the communication, (c) contains instructions on how to opt out of similar future communications, and (d) explains why the individual has been targeted for the communication when the communication is based on the individual's health status or condition.

The third type of marketing communication is restricted to uses by covered entities or disclosures to their business associates pursuant to an agreement with them.[18]

Under HIPAA, marketing professionals and providers must recognize that patients have certain basic rights:

1. The right to written notice of the information practices of healthcare plans and providers
2. The right to inspect and copy their protected health information
3. The right to request an amendment or correction
4. The right to an accounting of disclosures for purposes other than treatment, payment, or healthcare operations

Healthcare organizations are allowed to maintain communication relationships with patients using protected health information without patient consent unless it falls within the definition of marketing as defined by the revisions of HIPAA. Any marketing communication requires prior authorization. With certain stated exclusions, marketing is defined by HIPAA as follows:

- "To make a communication about a product or service that encourages recipients of the communication to purchase or use the product or service."
- "An arrangement between a covered entity and any other entity whereby the covered entity discloses [PHI] to the other entity, in exchange for direct or indirect remuneration, for the other entity or its affiliate to make a communication about its own product or service that encourages recipients of the communication to purchase or use that product or service."[19]

The following three types of communications were exempted from the definition of marketing:

- Communications describing a health-related product or service that is offered by the provider or included in its plan of benefits
- Communications describing the individual's treatment
- Communications for case management or care coordination for the individual or directions/recommendations for alternative treatments, providers, or settings of care[20]

Stark and Its Limitations[21]

Because so much of strategy within health care often involves physicians, it is important to review another federal law that provides guidelines as to the appropriate boundaries in terms of areas between relationships. Within health care, there is a separate set of regulations pertaining to the issue of patient referrals. In 1991, the Health Care Financing Administration (now known as Centers for Medicare and Medicaid Services [CMS]) published regulations for the Ethics in Patient Referrals Act, referred to as "Stark I" (for the Congressman who sponsored the legislation). This law prohibited physician referrals to entities in which they held a financial interest. This law was broadened in the Omnibus Budget Reconciliation Act of 1993. The new law, known as Stark II, also prohibits physician referrals to entities in which they hold a financial interest and applies to both Medicare and Medicaid. Effective January 1, 1995, no physician or physician family member who has a financial interest in an entity may refer a patient to that entity for health services. This law puts restrictions not only on the physician, but also on the entity to which the patient is referred. That organization cannot present a claim or a bill to any individual or third party for reimbursement. While there are degrees of interpretation and exceptions to this legislation, it greatly determines the strategies used to control the channel of distribution for patient referrals.[22]

On July 26, 2004, some technical corrections went into effect regarding Stark II. The details of these changes are subtle, but pertain to the following sections of the Stark rule:

- Methods for establishing physician compensation that will be deemed to be consistent with fair market value
- An accommodation for percentage and other formula-based physician compensation methodologies
- CMS's decision to adopt a very narrow interpretation of the statutory exception for "hospital remuneration unrelated to designated health services"
- A new bright-line definition of "same building" for purposes of the in-office ancillary services exception
- A physician-recruitment incentives exception that permits certain incentives to residents and interns already practicing in the hospital's service area, and incentives to physicians recruited to existing medical practices
- A new physician retention incentive exception
- A new exception for unavoidable and temporary lapses in compliance[23]

In December of 2007, phase III of the Stark III regulations became effective. These changes are further clarifications and modifications of Stark I and II. The complete listings of these changes were published in the *Federal Register* of September 5, 2007, titled "Stark III: Refinement Not Revolution."

The list of changes is fairly extensive, but for marketing individuals or managers of practices several aspects are notable in these changes:

- Permits group practices to impose certain practice restrictions on recruited physicians
- Expands geographical area in which a rural hospital can recruit a physician
- Clarifies that a hospital can list a doctor on its website or in advertisements as a medical staff incidental benefit, but physician payment for referral services must be both within an exception and an anti-kickback safe harbor[24]

Ongoing Federal Monitoring

Beyond the HIPAA challenges, the Department of Justice and the Federal Trade Commission have six areas in which they provide rather close supervision of the healthcare industry. These pertain to (1) mergers, (2) hospital joint ventures involving high technology, (3) physicians' provision of information to purchasers of healthcare services, (4) hospital participation in exchanges of price and cost information, (5) healthcare providers' joint purchasing arrangements, and (6) physician network joint ventures. In regard to mergers, the Federal Trade Commission has stated that it will not challenge any merger between two general, acute-care hospitals where one of the hospitals (1) has had an average of fewer than 100 licensed beds over the 3 most recent years, and (2) has had an average daily inpatient census of fewer than 40 patients over the 3 most recent years, absent extraordinary circumstances. This antitrust safety zone does not apply if that hospital is less than 5 years old. Rules and concerns about joint ventures are extremely detailed and entail definitions of the relevant market and the technology under consideration.[25]

THE GROWING USE OF TECHNOLOGY

Health care has always been an industry in which technology has had a significant impact. Historically, this effect has been seen in clinical procedures. To a large extent, this impact is continuing. A related technological effect has direct marketing significance: the increasing use of the Internet to communicate and interact with patients.

The Internet's Impact on Health Care

The impact of the Internet on health care has been dramatic. Healthcare institutions have shifted their promotional platforms to increasingly use the web and supporting social media to communicate with stakeholders;

patients go online in increasingly large numbers and across a broader array of demographics in search of health information; and physicians have adopted this technology within their offices and as part of their strategy in terms of referrals.

The change among hospitals has been dramatic in recent years. **Figure 3.7** shows the number of hospitals that have a social media presence as of October 2011. In the same regard, consumers have turned to the Internet and are also utilizing social media in greater number for health care. Pew Internet Research has found that one in five Internet users have gone online to find someone who might have similar health concerns to theirs; one in four with those with chronic disease.[26] There are now sites like PatientsLikeMe, Inspire, and CureTogether that have evolved in light of this changing behavior of patients and caregivers in this Web 2.0 world. This change in patient behavior is a direct result of the widespread use of the Internet. As of 2010, 79% of all adults over the age of 18 utilized this technology. In another Pew Internet study, 61% of all adults report getting health information online, 60% said it affected a decision about how to treat a condition or problem, and 53% said it led them to ask a doctor a new question or seek a second opinion.[27]

Interestingly, the rate of Internet use is fairly similar among Caucasians and Hispanics at 79% and 78%, respectively, while blacks' (non-Hispanics) Internet use is at 67% according to a May 2011 Pew Internet study.[28]

FIGURE 3.7

Hospitals with Social Media Accounts

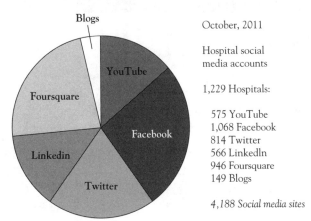

October, 2011

Hospital social media accounts

1,229 Hospitals:

575 YouTube
1,068 Facebook
814 Twitter
566 LinkedIn
946 Foursquare
149 Blogs

4,188 Social media sites

Source: Hospital Social Network List. (2011, October). Retrieved January 23, 2012, from: Ebennett.org/hsn/

Physician practices have also moved into this arena as a way to link with patients. At the primary care level, there are practices like Kids Plus Pediatrics in Pittsburgh, which has one of the more advanced websites (www.kidspluspgh.com) and provides a patient portal where parents can print out many of their children's records and information, as shown in **Figure 3.8**. Parents and other interested potential parents can learn about the group through various social media sites; the website is also integrated into staff recruiting and much more.

Increasingly, medical groups are recognizing that the Internet can potentially be a barrier to exit for customers and protect them from the competition if it is used strategically. A well-designed website can insulate the customer from competition by providing a resource that makes the group accessible and easy for the customer (a referral physician) or patient to interact with the physician. For example, the Gastroenterology Care Center in Miami, one of the more progressive, larger GI practices in the United States, has an online referral page for doctors as one alternative by which they can conveniently access the expertise available within the group for patients in need of a Gastroenterology Care Center physician.

FIGURE 3.8

A Progressive Pediatric Care Group with a Highly Developed Web Presence

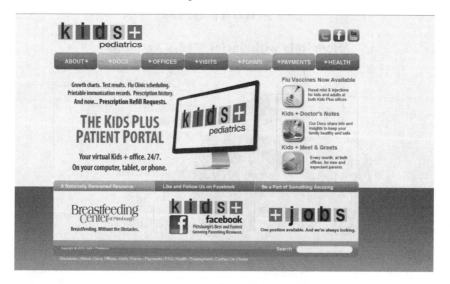

Source: Kids Plus Pediatrics. (2010). Retrieved December 14, 2011, from: http://kidspluspgh.com/

Clinical Impact

Technology has increasingly become a basis of competition in health care. Helicopter services, for example, have by themselves been money-losing operations in nearly every instance, but bring high visibility on the marketing side and can ideally attract profitable patients depending on reimbursement models to other parts of the hospital.[29]

The most significant change now has been the integration of information technology (IT) within physician practices and hospitals as well as health systems. According to a survey by the Centers for Disease Control and Prevention (CDC), slightly more than half of all physicians (50.7%) now use the electronic medical record (EMR) within their offices (double the level from 2005). This has occurred as older physicians retire, more doctors become comfortable with the technology, and there is greater integration between hospitals and their medical staffs.[30]

THE INCREASE IN COMPETITION

Developing effective marketing plans and the strategies to implement these plans must be done with a view of the competitive landscape. Monitoring competitive changes is critical. Three factors are affecting the competitive landscape: industry consolidation, global competition, and transparency of price and quality data.

Consolidation Within the Industry

An important change in the competitive climate in health care is the mergers occurring among hospitals and insurance companies. Among hospitals, the number of beds that were involved in the mergers during the decade from 2000 to 2010 ranged from single facilities with as few as 9 beds to the largest merger deal that accounted for a chain comprised of 176 hospitals, 92 outpatient surgery centers, and affiliated services, with a total of 41,850 beds. Two of the larger hospital mergers were at the proprietary system level when a private equity consortium acquired HCA, Inc. in 2006. Then, in 2007, Community Health Systems acquired Triad Hospitals, which had posted $5.4 billion on a 12-month basis.[31]

For health insurers, the mergers have also created a significant shift in the competitive landscape that must be considered as strategic plans are formulated. In 2000, the two largest health insurers, Aetna and United Healthcare, had a combined total membership of 32 million lives. As a result of mergers over the succeeding decade, these two large insurers, now WellPoint and United Healthcare, each have a total of 34 million and 33 million subscribers, respectively. Combined, they control slightly less than 70% of the total commercial health insurance marketplace.[32] The result is that much of the competition today among providers is large organization against large organization.

Global Competition

As strategic plans are developed, the focus of competition must be broadened to consider not only immediate competitors within the service area, but also a more concerted need exists today to take a broader geographical scope both regionally and globally.

This growing trend of patients seeking care abroad has been referred to as medical tourism. Mercer found that procedures in Thailand and Malaysia cost only 20% to 25% of comparable ones in the United States; and hospitals in India are even less expensive.[33] In a 2011 study by the Deloitte Center for Health Solutions, they reported that almost 25% of people would consider traveling outside the United States for elective surgery, and that a similar number would consider going abroad for necessary procedures.[34] **Figure 3.9**

FIGURE 3.9

Willingness to Seek Elective Surgery Overseas

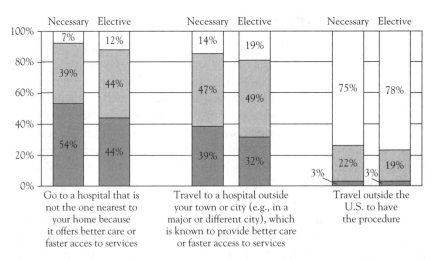

Source: Deloitte Center for Health Solutions. (2011). *2011 survey of health care consumers in the United States: Key findings, strategic implications.* Retrieved February 9, 2012, from: http://www.deloitte.com/assets/Dcom-UnitedStates/Local%20Assets/Documents/US_CHS_2011ConsumerSurveyGlobal_062111.pdf

shows a demographic breakdown of the strong response to support the trend toward medical tourism and the competitors who are acting on this attitude.

Hospitals around the world are beginning to change their strategy in response to this growing trend. In Asia and Mexico as well as Europe, there is a strong positioning of healthcare organizations to demonstrate quality. Hospitals are touting that they have received Joint Commission accreditation, or are noting that there is research actively occurring at their institutions. As is happening here within the United States, there is a vigorous presence in social media to market to prospective U.S. patients for elective procedures.

In Mexico City, there are private hospitals that have been aggressively seeking to attract patients from the United States with the notation that the Joint Commission accredits the institutions. For example, the American British Cowdray Medical Center in Mexico City has it prominently displayed on the homepage of its website, along with its affiliation to Methodist Hospital in Houston, Texas.[35]

Thailand's Bumrungrad International Hospital, which has received significant media attention, has one of the most interesting approaches to describing its pricing. It too is a Joint Commission–accredited institution. Labeled their "REALCOST" approach, the institution's website shows the potential patient the median, low cost, and high cost; and if Bumrungrad offers a package price for a procedure, it also provides the consumer with that information (see www.bumrungrad.com/realcost/index.aspx). Additionally, it has posted multiple videos on YouTube touting the 1 million patients who visit each year, elective surgery, and the many amenities at Bumrungrad. All these efforts are in an attempt to capitalize on the medical tourism interest abroad.

External Outcome Data Sources for Consumer Search and Transparency

A significant change in health care in the first decade of the 21st century is related to the growing increase in transparency of data quality and price as well as the information sources that are available on providers and hospitals on these attributes. Some of this change is regulatory, some is self-motivated and done for competitive reasons, and some is third-party driven as a way to provide consumers with information. Regardless of the provider of the information, the accessibility to information, coupled with the ease of access via the Internet, means there is greater likelihood that consumers will engage in a different level of "shopping" behavior and evaluation of healthcare alternatives in the coming years; organizations must be cognizant of this in the formation of strategic responses.

Regulatory Transparency

In recent years, there has been a growing requirement for data for users of different segments of the healthcare system from both federal and state regulators. CMS has required hospitals to publish outcome data on a list of defined areas such as percentage of patients who were given an antibiotic at the right time (1 hour before surgery) to help prevent an infection (there are seven surgical care improvement process measures), percentage of heart attack patients given aspirin at arrival (there are seven heart attack care measures), percentage of patients given oxygenation assessment (there are seven pneumonia process care measures), and percentage of heart failure patients given discharge instructions (there are four heart failure process measures). There are other distinct measures for children's asthma process care, hospital death rates, hospital readmission rates, and 10 items assessing patient experiences. The Department of Health and Human Services has a website that allows anyone in the United States to conduct a comparison of hospitals in their state on these multiple measures of performance in a general search, on a specific medical condition, or on a surgical procedure search (www.hospitalcompare.hhs.gov/Hospital/Search/SelectDRG.asp).

Continuing with government, at the state level, there are many interesting approaches to transparency. Most states have now moved to have price information with regard to charges posted on a website for consumers.

Self-Motivated Transparency

In this era where consumers are increasingly utilizing the Internet and economics are a greater factor in terms of health care, many organizations have become more transparent independent of any regulatory requirements. This trend is seen most clearly outside of the hospital segment of health care. Nationally and internationally, one can find examples of organizations that have recognized transparency as a valuable strategy within the healthcare market. In Michigan, Oakwood Healthcare has both their quality metrics and the hospital's prices on one easily accessible page of the institution's website for consumers who are searching for information (see **Figure 3.10**).

International facilities, as noted earlier, are providing price data to consumers, often with aggressive discount promotions. In terms of quality metrics, institutions will usually note that they have Joint Commission international accreditation certification (when this is true for the facility). Clinical outcome metrics are rarely presented.

Third-Party Transparency

There is another aspect of transparency or evaluative approaches that have also appeared in the marketplace for consumers. These might be

FIGURE 3.10

Demonstrating the Price-Value Relationship to a Self-Motivated Consumer Search

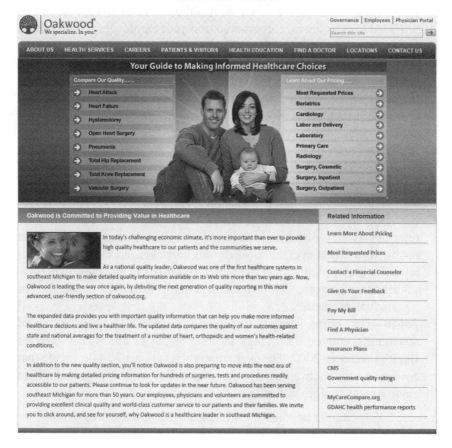

Source: Oakwood Healthcare. (2012). Retrieved October 4, 2011, from: http://www.oakwood.org/value/

termed as third-party or proprietary rating services. They may also be viewed as a point on the continuum of legitimacy or accuracy in terms of transparency of information sources. Some of these evaluative services that grade providers have been in existence for several years, while others are relatively recent and are being developed in recognition of the fact that because of the lack of sufficient transparency of quality data or the ease by which consumers might still understand and use the information, there are opportunities for others to provide a service. **Exhibit 3.1** provides a brief overview of some of these third-party evaluative services.

EXHIBIT 3.1

Third-Party Evaluative Services

- HealthGrades—A NASDAQ-traded company that rates hospitals, physicians, and nursing homes (www.healthgrades.com). This service is provided to consumers, corporations and their employees, and hospitals and physicians.
- Angie's List—This rating service originally started for consumers to help provide a reference for home repair services. Consumers pay a membership fee and rate providers, whether they are a dentist, ophthalmologist, primary care physician, sports medicine provider, or pediatrician (www.angieslist.com).
- RateMDs.com—This site was founded by the same individual who began RateMyTeachers.com. Individuals input information about their doctor experience. In early 2012, there were more than 1.3 million ratings on this site (www.ratemds.com).
- Best Doctors—This service is less of an evaluation site and more of a referral service (www.bestdoctors.com). It states it is a way to connect people to the best specialist. There are, however, no ratings or evaluations of the specialist, just the belief that this site has their names by asking other doctors, "Who would you get to treat your loved one for a particular problem?"
- Zagat—This rating service, historically known for its evaluation of restaurants, entered the ratings service for physicians with WellPoint Health Insurer in 2007. The evaluation is based on a 30-point scale that covers factors such as trust, communication, availability, and office environment. It does not assess clinical expertise.

Source: Reprinted from Berkowitz, E. N. (2011). *Essentials of health care marketing* (3rd ed.). Burlington, MA: Jones & Bartlett Learning.

Factors That Affect Competition

In conducting an environmental scan of the competitive climate, it is important to consider the factors that drive or affect the intensity of competition. These factors are the barriers to entry, the power of buyers and suppliers, and the existing competitors and possible alternatives.

Many barriers to entry can be created or have to be faced by a new competitor. Historically, in health care, many states had a certificate-of-need or determination-of-need requirement: Approval by the state regulatory body was required before a healthcare organization could make a capital expenditure for a particular technology or program. In essence, the organization that received approval was given a license (or almost a franchise) to operate. Popular through much of the 1970s, such regulations began to give way to a more free-market approach in health care. Thus, a barrier to entry began to disappear, and as a result, healthcare providers had to develop a more competitive approach.

A second strong barrier to entry is a pure marketing advantage, a strong brand identity. In health care, this advantage has been acquired within a local market. For many decades, there were only a few national brand identities among healthcare providers and organizations like the Mayo Clinic or Memorial Sloan-Kettering Cancer Center. Now, in each region of the United States, many organizations have focused heavily on the creation of a brand identity to create a preferred position among consumers. Geisinger Health System, Scott and White Healthcare, Scripps Health, Sentara Healthcare, and Joslin Diabetes Center are but a few of the names known and valued in their respective parts of the country. The barrier of brand identity is a psychological one that translates into a financial cost for a competitor. In the Northeast, a competing diabetes-management program would have to commit significant promotional dollars to establishing a brand identity to match Joslin in the minds of consumers.

A third valuable barrier to entry is distribution access. Outside of health care, for example, Walmart has so many outlets and such broad geographical dispersion that it has affected many other large retailers like Kmart that, at one time, had dominated the scene. In health care, as hospitals began to merge, physician practice structures also began to change. Between 1996–1997 and 2004–2005, physicians with an ownership stake in their own practice dropped from 61.6% to 54.4% as doctors moved increasingly to an employment model within larger systems. Additionally, the trend was also away from solo and two-physician practices toward mid-sized groups of 6 to 50 physicians.[36]

Capital requirements are a fourth useful barrier to entry. Initiating expensive products or services creates a business environment into which only those with money can enter. These capital requirements, in and of themselves, serve as a major barrier.

A fifth useful barrier to entry is switching costs. To a large extent this is the barrier that Microsoft has created for its system. To switch from Microsoft to some other platform may well require too much learning and too many infrastructure changes to make it worthwhile for users of computer software or computer manufacturers. Manufacturers of healthcare devices often find advantages in the barrier of switching costs as clinicians become used to their particular equipment. For patients, historically, the costs involved have been more psychological than monetary, because switching involves leaving their physicians. Now, however, technology has been able to bring a more value-driven switching cost to consumers with the development of patient portals that enable consumers to access their medical records, integrate other services into their care, and interact with the doctor or provider. Since they can efficiently set up appointments, view lab results, manage their child's health care, and the like, a potential barrier is that patients may not want or be inclined to switch to another provider as easily as in the past. The Marshfield Clinic (www.marshfieldclinic.org/mymarshfieldclinic/?page=loginhome) is one of many groups—similar to Geisinger Health System with their MyGeisinger.org portal (https://mygeisinger.geisinger.org/mygeisinger/login.cfm) or Dean Health Systems in Madison, Wisconsin (www.deancare.com/deanconnect/)—with a portal for patients, employers, providers, or agents. All of these are now bringing in technology to raise the switching costs.

A second major factor that drives competition is the power of buyers and suppliers. A competitive analysis and scan must consider this component in the marketing strategy and plans. Powerful buyers have emerged in health care. The Leapfrog group, discussed in the next section, began in 1998 to focus on quality, safety, and affordability in health care. Beginning in 2001 by collecting hospital data, it presently operates in 38 regions, covering over half of the U.S. population and 62% of all hospital beds. Thirteen hundred hospitals participate in Leapfrog surveys.[37] For example, the Colorado Business Group on Health began in 1995 and has more than 250,000 employees represented by participating organizations, including GlaxoSmithKline, Pfizer, the University of Colorado, and TIAA-CREF. The mission of the coalition is to "engage the healthcare marketplace through leadership and active participation, driving positive changes to address quality and realize savings."[38] The Pacific Group on Health has 50 large members who spend $12 billion annually to cover 3 million employees and retirees in California alone.[39] The Pacific Group on Health has four key strategies: Engage consumers to choose the right care at the right price; ensure providers are rewarded for quality and efficiency; support the healthcare system to achieve improved outcomes at a better price; and help policymakers create public policies that improve care and reduce costs. Similar coalitions exist in Massachusetts, New York, Louisiana, and metropolitan areas like Memphis, Dallas, Houston, and Savannah. Because of the large number of employees and families they represent, these coalitions can engage in powerful negotiations over prices, contracts, and standards of care. Suppliers are a powerful factor when they provide a critical component for the delivery of a service. In health care, the competitive tension between buyers and suppliers has often been described in the context of a hospital and its medical staff. Physicians who establish their own freestanding surgical facilities become a significant competitive factor.

A third consideration in examining the competitive environment is the existing competitors and possible substitutes. In most areas, local competitors are closely monitored and their strategies are assessed. However, as mentioned previously, in health care, competition is increasingly waged on a regional scale. The University of Michigan Health System has primary care facilities and specialty centers throughout the state of Michigan, while the Cleveland Clinic, for example, has satellite facilities in Fort Lauderdale and Naples, Florida. Similarly, it has purchased medical groups in part of central Ohio, as well as establishing international relationships in the Middle East and Asia. The Mayo Clinic offers access in Florida, Arizona, and Minnesota and has 7 clinics in Iowa as well as 24 in Wisconsin. For many years, medical providers in Wisconsin knew and referred to the Mayo Clinic, but now find they compete directly with this organization in their own immediate market areas of Eau Claire, Menomonie, and Chippewa Falls, among others.

Substitutable services are also a factor that affects competition. The most recent trend in health care, for example, is the use of the term *doctor* by health professionals other than physicians. Nurses, pharmacists, and physical therapists are claiming the right to this title. In 2004, pharmacists were required to obtain a doctorate to practice. Prior to that year, all that was necessary was a bachelor's degree. A similar change will go into effect for physical therapists in 2015. And a similar change has occurred within the nursing profession. In 2004, four schools awarded the Doctor of Nursing Practice; in 2009, the number of degrees was 7,037 awarded from 170 nursing schools. Some physicians fear it may lead to some of these groups seeking prescribing authority. In 2011, a bill was proposed in the New York State Senate that would bar nurses from using the title of doctor no matter what their degree.[40]

SHIFTS IN THE CORPORATE MARKET

Health care is dramatically affected by changes in the reimbursement and insurance policies of companies and the government, which have borne the bulk of healthcare costs. For many firms, increasing costs are requiring an aggressive approach to their containment. In 2011, companies expected their healthcare costs to rise by 9% over the 7% experienced in 2010. The changes that employers are making to combat this increase have been most felt by their employees. From 2005 to 2010, while overall premiums have risen by 27% for health insurance, workers' premium payments have increased 47% (wages have increased by a far more modest 18% during this same time period). From 2006 to 2010, the percentage of employees with single coverage who are subject to a $1,000 deductible has also risen from 10% to 27%; while for those who work for a small firm (defined as between 3 and 199 workers), the percentage increase is from 16% to 46%. The result in a large study conducted by RAND of over 800,000 households from 53 large employers (28 of whom offered high-deductible health plans) was that spending was lower among those enrolled in such plans. Individuals in high-deductible plans cut back on childhood vaccination, mammography, cervical cancer screening, and colorectal screenings.[41] In 1999, the average insurance cost per employee was $3,779 for a firm of 10 to 49 employees, and $4,357 for a firm with more than 1,000 employees.[42] The cost of employer-sponsored health plans increased 11% in 2001, the largest 1-year jump since 1992. In 2009, the average corporate health benefit expenditure was $9,660 per employee, which was a 33% increase since 2004.[43]

With the economy slowing to a snail's pace and sales significantly down in many industries, rising premiums may force many businesses to drastically change their coverage. The pendulum has begun to shift from traditional managed care to high-deductible health plans. As of 2010, more than 10 million people are enrolled in these plans, up from 6 million in 2008. **Figure 3.11** shows the steady growth of these plans since the spring of 2005. Under this arrangement, companies provide their employees with a set amount of money each year in a health savings account. The company also offers a plan that usually pays for annual physicals and other wellness programs. The employee can then choose a high-deductible plan with pre-tax dollars and the incentive is then on the employee to shop for the "best value."[44]

Employees who select a higher-cost plan pay the difference from their own pockets. This approach allows companies to try to control increases in healthcare costs by passing them on to the end user, the consumer.

To a large degree, health care will return to being a retail market in which Internet-based middlemen may be the store where consumers shop to decide where they want to spend their healthcare dollars.

Another major effect of corporations on health care has been an increased focus on quality. The largest corporate group in this area, as noted previously, is Leapfrog, which has a growing membership of companies such as Carlson Companies, Daimler-Benz Chrysler, IBM, PepsiCo, General Mills, and TRW, Inc. Employers in the Leapfrog group buy health care for more than 28 million people. This group has established three standards that hospitals must meet in order to get members' business: (1) implement a computerized system for physician orders, (2) meet threshold volumes for certain complex medical procedures, and (3) hire intensivists. Although some healthcare organizations may not believe

FIGURE 3.11

Growth of High-Deductible Health Plans

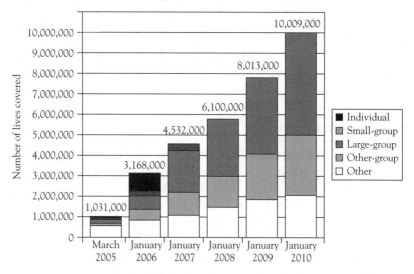

Note: For 2010, the minimum annual deductible for self-only HSA/HDHP coverage was $1,200, and the maximum out-of-pocket limit was $5,950. For family HSA/HDHP coverage, the minimum deductible was $2,400, and the maximum out-of-pocket was $11,900. These amounts are indexed annually for inflation.

Source: AHIP Center for Policy and Research. (2010, May). *January 2010 census shows 10 million people covered by HAS/high-deductible health plans*; p. 3. Retrieved October 4, 2011, from: http://www.ahipresearch.org/pdfs/HSA2010.pdf

that these three criteria should be the keystones to the Leapfrog program, the initiative does underscore the importance of monitoring the corporate environment as a major market.[45] Leapfrog members like Verizon, a telecommunications company, are making Leapfrog quality data available on websites for their employees. Leapfrog reports on hospital safety issues on their website (www.leapfroggroup.org/for_consumers). Empire Blue Cross Blue Shield of New York, an insurer of 4 million people, is awarding hospitals financially for meeting Leapfrog standards.[46] The Leapfrog group has also teamed with HealthGrades to publish combined reports on hospitals.

SUMMARY

Environmental scanning is essential in the development of marketing plans and actions. Ongoing monitoring of the shifts that occur in each of the five areas discussed in this chapter must be an integral part of planning activities. Although demographic shifts are generally long term, changes in regulations and competition can occur in a matter of months. Technological shifts can be so disruptive that they eliminate major business lines or open unforeseen opportunities. Monitoring technological changes is difficult, but necessary in health care given the amount of research and development being directed not only at devices, but also at biotechnological advances.

QUESTIONS FOR DISCUSSION

1. A medical group scanned its past patient records to assess who has not visited its primary care medical practice in the past 18 months. The group has one major clinical site and four satellite facilities. The physicians want to send these individuals some promotional material as well as a small premium such as an emergency medical kit for their automobiles. Outline for the doctors whether this is appropriate and what are the boundaries that are allowed.

2. From an industry perspective, competition in health care has been affected by multiple factors. Identify three critical elements that are shifting the landscape of the competitive environment on a macro level.

3. Your orthopedic group has developed a pediatric sports medicine program. It is the first such specialized program in the metropolitan area. You have recently heard that your largest competitor is thinking of entering the market with a similar offering. Suggest three possible barriers to entry that you might be able to create to make it a challenge for new competitive entries.

4. In many states, the medical societies are fighting back efforts by advanced practice nurses and other clinicians from having authority to prescribe medications. Pharmacists are now able to provide flu shots. Explain this movement to deny prescribing privileges in terms of the factors that affect competition.

NOTES

1. United States Census (2010). Resident Population Data. Retrieved March 21, 2012, from: http://2010.census.gov/2010census/data/apportionment -pop-text.php.
2. Ortman, J., & Guarneri, C. E. (2009). United States population projections: 2000 to 2050. Retrieved February 15, 2012, from: http://www.census.gov/population/www/projections/analytical-document09.pdf.

3. Christie, L. (2009, May 14). Hispanic population boom fuels rising U.S. diversity. *CNN U.S.* Retrieved February 15, 2012, from: http://articles.cnn.com/ 2009-05-14/us/money.census.diversity_1_hispanic-population-latinos -and-other-minority-pew-hispanic-center?_s=PM:US.

4. Minckler, D. (2008, May 14). U.S. minority population continues to grow. *American.Gov Archive.* Retrieved February 15, 2012, from: http:// www.america.gov/st/diversity-english/2008/May/20080513175840zjsre dna0.1815607.html.

5. Associated Press. (2008, January 15). Baby boomlet pushes U.S. birth rates to 45-year high. *Fox News.* Retrieved February 15, 2012, from: http:// www.foxnews.com/story/0,2933,323028,00.html.

6. Saenz, R. Population bulletin update: Latinos in the United States 2010. Population Reference Bureau. Retrieved February 15, 2012, from: http:// www.prb.org/Publications/PopulationBulletins/2010/latinosupdate1.aspx.

7. U.S. Census Bureau. (2000, March). The Hispanic population in the United States; p. 2.

8. Bass, F. (2011, September 29). U.S. Population is less white, more black, census figures show. *Bloomberg.* Retrieved February 15, 2012, from: http://www.bloomberg.com/news/2011-09-29/u-s-population-is-less-white -more-black-census-figures-show.html.

9. Raymond, J. (2002, March). ¿Tienen Numeros? *American Demographics, 24*(3), 22–25.

10. Noonan, M. D., & Savolaine, R. (2001, Winter). The new childbearing family. *Marketing Health Services,* 45–47.

11. Gardyn, R. (2000, May). Paging Marcus Welby. *American Demographics, 22*(5), 12–13.

12. Flat Rock Population Pyramid. (2010, July 31). The boom moves along. Retrieved February 15, 2012, from: http://flatrock.org.nz/topics/money _politics_law/boom_moves_along.htm.

13. U.S. Census Bureau. (2010). Population profile of the United States. Retrieved February 15, 2012, from: http://www.census.gov/population/ www/pop-profile/natproj.html.

14. Transgenerational Design Matters. (2009). The demographics of aging. Retrieved February 15, 2012, from: http://transgenerational.org/aging/ demographics.htm.

15. Jan, T. (2011, September 30). Hospital executives push hike for age in Medicare. *Boston Globe.* Retrieved February 15, 2012, from: http://www.boston.com/news/nation/washington/articles/2011/09/30/ hospital_executives_lobby_to_raise_medicare_eligibility_age/?page=2.

16. Paddison, N., & Hallick, J. (2001, November). HIPAA privacy regulations can guide, strengthen marketing efforts. *Healthcare Marketing Report, 19*(11), 16–19.

17. Lisa, A. (2009, February 24). Stimulus package dramatically alters HIPAA privacy and security. *WTN News.* Retrieved March 21, 2012, from: http:// wtnnews.com/articles/5558/.

18. Hall, Render, Killian, Heath, & Lyman. (2009, May 28). Changes to fundraising, marketing, and other restrictions on disclosure. *Impact Series.* Retrieved March 21, 2012, from: http://www.hallrender.com/library/seminarTopics/Marketing.pdf.

19. Ibid.

20. U.S. Department of Health and Human Services. (2003, April 3). Health information privacy: Marketing. Retrieved March 21, 2012, from: http://www.hhs.gov/ocr/privacy/hipaa/understanding/coveredentities/marketing.html.

21. This section is from Berkowitz, E. N. (2011). *Essentials of health care marketing* (3rd ed.). Burlington, MA: Jones & Bartlett Learning; ch. 3.

22. Swibel, H. J., & Zaremski, M. J. (1995). Surfing Stark II: Prohibition against self-referrals. *Physician Executive, 21*(2), 11–15.

23. McDermett, W., & McDermett, E. (2004, April 19). Phase II of the final Stark II regulations. Retrieved February 15, 2012, from: http://www.mwe.com/index.cfm/fuseaction/publications.nldetail/object_id/081a59b2-7f74-4bc9-aaf5-7012b8110bfc.cfm.

24. American Academy of Family Physicians. (2009). What is Stark III? Retrieved February 15, 2012, from: http://www.aafp.org/online/en/home/practicemgt/specialtopics/regulatory-compliance/faqsstarkcompliance/whatisstarkiii.html.

25. Department of Justice and the Federal Trade Commission. (2009). *Statements of Antitrust Enforcement Policy in Health Care.* Retrieved February 15, 2012, from: http://www.ftc.gov/reports/hlth3s.htm.

26. Fox, S. (2011, September 18). Medicine 2.0: Peer-to-peer healthcare. Pew Internet. Retrieved February 15, 2012, from: http://www.pewinternet.org/Reports/2011/Medicine-20/Part-1.aspx.

27. Rainie, L. (2011, May 5). The rise of the e-patient: Understanding social networks and online health information seeking. Retrieved February 15, 2012, from: http://www.pewinternet.org/Presentations/2011/May/Institute-for-Healthcare-Advancement.aspx.

28. PewInternet. (2011, May). Demographics of Internet users. Retrieved February 15, 2012, from: http://pewinternet.org/Static-Pages/Trend-Data/Whos-Online.aspx.

29. Anderson, H. J. (1990). Survey identifies trends in equipment acquisitions. *Hospitals, 64*, 30–35.

30. Cook, B. (2010, January 1). Physician EMR use passes 50% as incentives outweigh resistance. Retrieved February 15, 2012, from: http://www.ama-assn.org/amednews/2011/01/10/bil10110.htm.

31. Steever, S. B. (Ed.). (2010). Largest hospital mergers and acquisitions for the 10-year period ended December 31, 2009 revealed by DealSearchOnline.com. Retrieved February 15, 2012, from: http://www.levinassociates.com/pr2010/pr1003hospital.

32. American Medical Association. (2007). Competition in health insurance: A comprehensive study of U.S. markets, 2007 update. Retrieved February 15, 2012, from: http://www.ama-assn.org/ama1/pub/upload/mm/368/compstudy_52006.pdf.

33. Kher, U. (2006). Outsourcing your heart. *Time.com.* Retrieved February 15, 2012, from: http://www.time.com/time/magazine/article/ 0,9171,1196429,00.html.

34. Deloitte Center for Health Solutions. (2011). *2011 survey of health care consumers in the United States: Key findings, strategic implications.* Retrieved February 15, 2012, from: http://www.deloitte.com/assets/ Dcom-UnitedStates/Local%20Assets/Documents/us_chs _MedicalTourismStudy(3).pdf.

35. Higgins, L. A., Medical tourism takes off, but not without debate. *Managed Care Magazine.* Retrieved February 15, 2012, from: http://www .managedcaremag.com/archives/0704/0704.travel.html.

36. Liebhaber, A., & Grossman, J. M. (2007, August). Physicians moving to mid-sized, single-specialty practices. Center for Studying Health System Change. Retrieved February 15, 2012, from: http://hschange.org/ CONTENT/941/941.pdf.

37. The Leapfrog Group. (2011). Factsheet. Retrieved February 15, 2012, from: http://www.leapfroggroup.org/about_us/leapfrog-factsheet.

38. Colorado Business Group on Health. (2012). About. Retrieved February 15, 2012, from: http://coloradohealthonline.org/cbgh/index.cfm/about/.

39. Pacific Business Group on Health. (2012). About. Retrieved February 15, 2012, from: http://www.pbgh.org/about.

40. Harris, G. (2011, October 1). When the nurse wants to be called "doctor." *New York Times.* Retrieved February 15, 2012, from: http://www.nytimes.com/2011/10/02/health/policy/02docs .html?pagewanted=1&_r=1&emc=eta1.

41. Beeuwkes Buntin, M., Haviland, A. M., McDevitt, R., & Sood, N. (2011, March). Healthcare spending in high-deductible and consumer directed health plans. *The American Journal of Managed Care, 17*(3), 222–230.

42. Haugh, R. (2000, October). Son of HMO. *Hospitals and Health Networks, 74*(10), 65–68.

43. Towers Watson. (2008, September 24). Towers Perrin health care cost survey shows average annual per-employee cost of $9,660 in 2009—And the health affordability gap widens. Retrieved February 15, 2012, from: http:// www.towersperrin.com/tp/showdctmdoc.jsp?url=master_brand_2/usa/ press_releases/2008/20080924/2008_09_24b.htm&country=.

44. Konrad, W. (2010, August 27). High-deductible plans grow, but not everyone should get on board. *New York Times.* Retrieved February 15, 2012, from: http://www.nytimes.com/2010/08/28/health/28patient.html.

45. Sarudi, D. (2001, May). The Leapfrog effect. *Hospitals and Health Networks, 75*(5), 32–36.

46. Lovern, E. (2002, January 21). Wave of the future. *Modern Healthcare, 32*(3), 4–6.

CHAPTER 4

STEP 1: CONDUCTING THE INTERNAL/EXTERNAL ASSESSMENT

WHAT YOU WILL LEARN

- Both internal views and views from the outside environment are important.
- Detailed secondary data are readily available at a detailed level.
- Primary market research is an important tool.

THE ASSESSMENT PROCESS

Competitive strategic, business, and market plans are based on a detailed internal/external analysis, which includes an assessment of the environment, an evaluation of competitors, an internal analysis, an evaluation of the market, and a review of marketing activities (**Figure 4.1**).

Accomplishing Step 1 in the most appropriate fashion requires keeping corporate purposes and missions in mind, but setting goals in relation to the marketplace. In other words, business must be designed around the environment and consumer. This is a strategy used by successful companies and is "one of the best-kept secrets in American business," according to Peters and Waterman.[1]

The detail required in Step 1 and the importance of this step to the overall planning process cannot be overestimated. The specific targets that the organization will move toward over the years depend on information from the internal/external analysis. Therefore, this analysis, although time consuming, is critical in the development of strategic and marketing plans. It may uncover numerous opportunities for the organization that fit its mission and provide substantial rewards.

FIGURE 4.1

Conducting the Internal/External Assessment

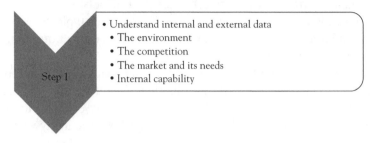

- Understand internal and external data
- The environment
- The competition
- The market and its needs
- Internal capability

Step 1

Because the internal/external analysis provides the assumptions on which the entire plan is built, the plan will suffer if the analysis is inadequate, incomplete, or untruthful. Many organizations assume that they know all the necessary information, have adequate data, and need not spend much time on this step. To many who have never undertaken an internal/external analysis, the process may seem elementary. Some managers mistakenly think that their experience makes the internal/external analysis unnecessary. Although this process often requires a month or more of staff time and some intraorganizational stress, the thought-provoking inquiry usually reveals valuable opportunities and insights. In fact, the internal/external analysis is the foundation of the marketing approach—that is, to listen, to inquire, to study, and to ask questions. The purpose of the analysis is to uncover marketing opportunities and threats. The internal strengths and weaknesses of the firm are examined, as are external opportunities. Several questions must be addressed within each component of the analysis. This chapter examines those questions that are most important in conducting the internal/external analysis. The analysis and situation review encompass five major areas: the environment, the market and its needs, the competition, internal capabilities, and marketing activities.

Many organizations are able to conduct the analysis internally. In these cases, the internal/external analysis is typically the responsibility of one individual who, with the support of others on the staff, gathers the necessary information. It is possible to conduct an internal/external analysis for an entire organization. As the organization grows larger, however, the analysis becomes more meaningful if it is done on a departmental or service-by-service basis. In other words, a small clinic of three to five practitioners can effectively conduct a single internal/external analysis, but a hospital with 400 beds gets the most value from an analysis conducted on a department-by-department or product-line basis. Large, complex organizations often find it necessary to use outside consultants to conduct the internal/external analysis, but the questions typically asked are similar. Often an outside facilitator can ensure that critical questions are answered, regardless of political sensitivity.

Sometimes group culture is so intimidating that it is uncomfortable to feel free to challenge the current thinking. Therefore, the first step in creating new views is to review the conventional way of doing things. A good example is how medical treatment changes. Not too many years ago, the conventional wisdom was that when a person had a heart attack, the patient should stay in a hospital bed for days, or often weeks in order to recover. Challenges to that thinking through clinical research resulted in a completely different treatment protocol that now indicates that clinicians should get patients up, moving, and exercising the heart muscle more quickly.

Not-for-profit organizations can have a tendency to be like a close family or community and may surround themselves with like-minded people. The board may be made up of people with similar lifestyles, values, and norms who will tend to agree with the common point of view. There is often not much dissent, which may be viewed as a positive climate, but healthcare entities would be wise to elicit a contrarian viewpoint. Ask a staff member to pretend to be a competitor. What would a competitor do? Ask a board member to do the same. Actively seek out other points of view as a way to test the thinking of the organization. Elicit the opinions of people who are older and younger and of different genders, religions, or ethnic backgrounds. Organizations will find insights into current operations and ideas for new approaches through these kinds of discussions. The following tools are intended to help organizations consider balanced, honest, and fresh thoughts as a first step in the strategic process.

It Is Uncomfortable to Challenge What We Think We Know

It is often uncomfortable to challenge long-held beliefs. Sometimes the challenge to long-held thinking is viewed as criticism. Obviously this is not the intent. The intent of challenging and stretching your thinking is to get you into a position to provide the best possible service and products to your customers in an attempt to reach your vision. Challenging your thinking propels you forward, unplugging you from the past and allowing you to plug into the future.

Get an Outsider's View

Too often boards and management teams tend to pat themselves on the back and tell each other how wonderful they are. Or, they tend to view the world through their own eyes, but not the eyes of the community. The enormously successful medical device company, Medtronic, has a view of the world, yet they are not bashful about bringing into the company former patients from every walk of life to let them tell their medical stories to the scientists, executives, and employees of the company. It is the outsiders, or the customers, who often provide the words of wisdom that a company needs to reexamine its vision or to focus more diligently. So it is for a medical group, hospital, or evolving accountable care organization (ACO).

When Data Are Not Data: Looking at the SWOT Analysis Method

Sometimes the assumptions clinical groups may be using about their not-for-profit organizations are backed by data that are not really data. There is a tendency to confuse or disguise internal opinion as data. For example, a favorite strategic planning tool of many organizations is the SWOT analysis. SWOT is a process where the organization identifies its Strengths, Weaknesses, Opportunities, and Threats (SWOT). The process works like this: A group of leaders from the hospital work as a team, and each person identifies and transfers onto a flip chart as many items as possible for each of the following categories: strengths, weaknesses, opportunities, and threats. When these lists are completed, the group will vote on the top five to six strengths, five to six weaknesses, five to six opportunities, and five to six threats. Inevitably, this process is then used as "data" from which a plan is built. Unfortunately, more often than not, this process does not provide data, it provides opinion—opinion from the executive suite that is steeped in history and often unchallenged assumptions said enough times that they start to become believed and begin to filter into the organization as data. Here are some typical statements that one will often find in a SWOT analysis exercise:

- We have great people.
- We are recognized as the caring organization.
- The market is declining.
- Our staff is committed to us.
- Our outcomes are the best.

Maybe these statements are true, or maybe they are not. But in reality, the following could represent the gap that is often seen between organizational opinion and real marketplace data:

Gap Between Opinion and Actual Data

Leadership Team Opinion	Versus	Actual Data
We have great people.		No data exist to verify claim.
We are a caring organization.		Community survey says "average."
The market is declining.		This organization is declining, but total citywide volume is increasing.
Our staff is committed.		Employee survey says that average manager sees this job as temporary.
Our outcomes are the best.		Statewide outcomes study confirms.

A SWOT analysis often does not provide data—it provides opinion, and that opinion is provided by insiders. A study in 2009 of 700 hospital board chairmen demonstrates the point.[2] In this survey, board chairmen were given a list of possible issues and the chairmen were asked to name the top issues that were pertinent to their hospital. In those hospitals that Medicare data suggest are among the worst in the country, 58% of those hospital board chairmen said they thought their hospital was above average! More surprising, not one hospital said that their performance was below average. As this example points out, it would be helpful for the organization to have the actual data so that improvements could be made, versus depending on an opinion that may be off base.[3]

If organizations make assumptions about what their customers think, companies need to remember they are only assumptions. The assumptions could be right—or they could be wrong. In order to develop strategic plans, organizations need firsthand viewpoints from customers. What the hospital thinks about how customers make decisions is patently invalid, unless the hospital actually has customer data. Further, self-congratulatory statements also need to be challenged. When a hospital says it is the "#1 cancer program in the city," it needs to ask the question: "Where are the specific data that support this claim?" Is it an internal view of employed doctors, or is it a real, not wishful, marketplace view?

Using the Five Forces Model

Most master of business administration (MBA) programs have rejected the SWOT method and now use the Porter Five Forces model (see **Figure 4.2**) as a tool when creating business strategy.[4] This model is more objective and data based and provides a way for organizations to better understand their risks and opportunities. This model assumes that there are five forces that determine competitive power or likelihood of being secure in a given clinical line. The model asks five questions:

1. *How easy is it for suppliers to drive up prices?*
   When we think of suppliers, we often think of suppliers of goods such as inventory and raw materials. But in health care, very important suppliers are the professional service providers. Emergency room physicians under contract to a hospital, or pathology services or radiology coverage are examples of suppliers of services to the hospital. What options does the hospital have if the current supplier of emergency room treatment decides to raise its hourly rate by 50%? Is the hospital

FIGURE 4.2

Porter's Five Forces Model

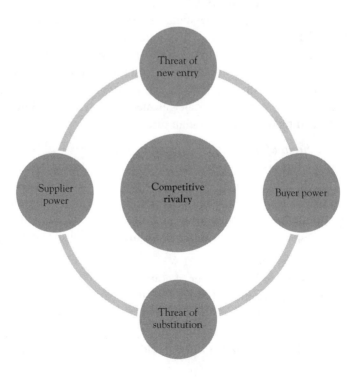

vulnerable or are other options available? Another example is a medical doctor or other specialty provider who comes to hospital or clinic management with an idea to start a new program in spine surgery or radiation therapy. A 58-year-old physician proposes that she will be the supplier of technical services and the hospital is expected to invest in staffing and equipment. In this example, the equipment cost alone could exceed $1 million. The issue facing the hospital is the dependency the hospital would have on this supplier. What would happen if the supplier were to raise the proposed contract terms or retire, or if it were determined that there are quality issues? In these types of situations, does the hospital have alternative supplier options available to provide care and protect the investment of the organization?

2. *How easy is it for buyers to drive down prices?*
   The answer to this question is driven by the number of buyers—usually patients—and the ability and likelihood of those buyers switching to some other provider of care. In a rural community with limited options for care, it might be difficult for patients to drive to another community to switch providers, but in an urban area, switching providers might be easy as price information becomes more available.

3. *Is there a threat of substitution?*
   Imagine building a new free-standing pediatric clinic only to see a Walgreens drugstore open a convenience clinic across the street with prices at $29 and the ability to see 50% of the pediatric clinic's volume. This is an example of competitive substitution. Substitution activities are currently underway in places like drugstores, supermarkets, and on the Internet, where a patient can get medical advice and information without needing to see a physician directly.

4. *Is there a threat of new entry by a similar provider?*
   If Watson Clinic is contemplating an outpatient radiation center, what would be the likelihood and impact of a duplicate center opening three blocks away? Too often, when providers look at new programs, they fail to think about and model the potential for new competition. This question forces providers to think about the potential for new entry.

5. *How much competitive rivalry exists?*
   This is a function of the number of competitors in the area and the likelihood of even more in the future. This item is critical, which is why it is in the center of the circle in Figure 4.2. If the Watson Clinic is the only offering in an area, then patients and suppliers do not have many options and their leverage is limited. However, if the doctor's office is

one of a multitude of offerings, then what is the likelihood that buyers such as patients and insurance companies would seek alternatives to the clinic? If the clinic is considered average in the community, with no special features, the insurance company can easily drop the clinic and concentrate on sending patients to other locations. As insurance companies seek to control cost, they will often tend to limit their network of providers. If a zip code has, for example, eight clinics, an insurance company might only need six clinics to cover its subscribers. Because it has leverage due to the number of provider clinics available, the insurance company will be able to negotiate better rates from the doctors and tighter standards. Usually, the insurance company will seek to retain those clinics with the highest market share in the zip code and likewise tend to reject those with the smallest market share. If the Watson Clinic only has a 10% zip code market share, the clinic could be vulnerable to losing insurance company (supplier) participation.

Porter's model is an outside-to-inside way of thinking. The Porter model and the strategic planning and marketing model described in this text require critical thinking and actual data, with a large portion of the data focused on external factors. The following sections provide insight into the types of questions typically found in a strategic and marketing analysis.

THE ENVIRONMENT

The first component of the internal/external analysis is an understanding of the macro-environment. Information from a variety of sources is gathered in order to make judgments regarding opportunities, threats, and future business outlook. This information is eventually matched to an assessment of the organization's capabilities and weaknesses.

Market Share as Baseline Information

Understanding market share is a key requirement to understanding opportunity and performance. Market share is a better indicator than actual volume or patient revenue as to whether or not the clinic is growing or dying relative to the competition. Therefore, it is a very useful tool to assist in the strategic Five Forces analysis and the marketing model strategy action match.

Figure 4.3 shows examples of the many ways an organization can look at market share. Assume in column 1 the chief executive officer (CEO) selected the total hospital option, and in column 2 she selected immediate zip code. Selecting only these two variables will give the CEO's hospital's market share versus all other hospitals in its immediate zip code. If, for

FIGURE 4.3

Understanding Market Share

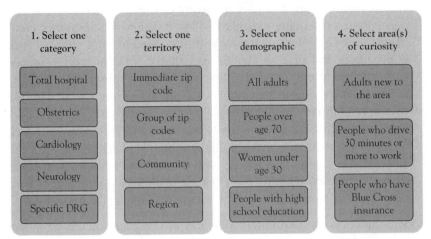

example, there were 100 total admissions from the immediate zip code to several different hospitals, and Wilson Hospital acquired 40 of the total admissions, the market share for Wilson Hospital would be 40%. If the CEO decided to study women under age 30 in column 3 and people who have Blue Cross insurance from column 4, we would now be able to look at hospital usage of women under age 30 with Blue Cross who live in the immediate zip code. If there are 100 women from the immediate zip code who fit this profile, and 32 of them went to Wilson Hospital and the other 68 went to other hospitals, she would know that the Wilson Hospital market share for that particular group was 32%. For the purpose of illustration, Figure 4.3 has been limited to only a few variables. But as one can see, even in this limited example, there are a host of possible interesting options that are valuable to analyze.

How are these data captured? The data in columns 1 and 2 can often be gathered by looking at data collected by state agencies that monitor hospital discharge data. Usually, a request is made to the agency that generates the data and fees are paid for the reports.

Data in all four categories can be captured through primary market research by talking with a representative sample of households. Using primary market research will not only tell you how well you are doing relative to the competition, but it can also give valuable insight into how well the organization is doing in capturing people new to the area, or those who commute to work, or other variables that determine if people will choose hospital A or hospital B for care. Later in this chapter, an overview of market research is reviewed so managers can see how these tools can be used to help find answers to consumer opinion, why customers like or do not like a hospital service, what an organization's market share is, and other marketplace questions.

An external marketplace assessment should be conducted on a program or service basis if you are creating a marketing plan, or at a corporate level if you are creating an organization-wide strategic plan (**Exhibit 4.1**). The object of this exercise is to ensure that the hospital or clinic has considered the major factors that could have an impact on the future of the program. Included within this assessment are several global questions pertaining to the marketplace. Competitive factors must also be addressed, along with factors that may change the nature of competition, such as technology, financial concerns, and reimbursement.

For each program, the manager must provide some indication of market attractiveness and make judgments about present conditions and likely conditions over the next 3 years. These judgments are rated from low to high with a designation for attractive or positive. The organization needs to define the scale points at the beginning of the process, because operating scale will vary for an acute-care hospital, a tertiary facility, or a 10-person multispecialty clinic, for example. A 3% predicted growth in the market may not be attractive to a clinic operating at near capacity, but 3% may be highly attractive to a group needing revenue flow. Therefore, one clinic might place 3% growth in the negative category, while another clinic might place it in a neutral or positive category.

Because this review is suggested as a first-cut evaluation of multiple programs, data should be gathered from existing sources. Furthermore, because the regulatory environment affects the healthcare industry to a greater extent than many other industries, this environmental factor must always be monitored. Regulations often vary by program, and several specific regulatory questions should be posed for the major service areas:

1. What kinds of external controls affect the organization? Local? State? Federal? Self-regulation?
2. What are the trends in recent regulatory rulings?
3. Does (can) this program meet minimum case volumes for accreditation? Do competitors meet minimum case volumes?

State and national professional associations, congressional staff members, and planning agency documents should all be used in making this assessment. This procedure should be conducted at least yearly for each existing program within the facility.

EXHIBIT 4.1

External Marketplace Assessment

Service Line _____	Market Attractiveness					
	Current			Three Years Forward		
	High	Med	Low	High	Med	Low
Size of market						
Growth rate						
Stage of lifecycle						
Price stability						
Distribution requirements						
Service requirements						
Level of technology						
Potential for substitute product or service substitution						
Captive patients						
Customer concentration						
Degree of competition						
Attitude: Passive? Aggressive?						
Number of competitors						
Strength of leader						
Service profitability						
Leverage potential (e.g., economies of scale)						
Service intensity						
Utilization of service capacity						
Social attitudes/trends						
Reimbursement climate						
Regulatory exposure/vulnerability						
Overall market attractiveness						
Positive score						
Negative score						
Net score						
Conclusion:						

THE MARKET AND ITS NEEDS

The role of any marketing plan is to define the major markets and their respective needs. Completing this analysis helps identify the major markets and appropriate segments (**Exhibit 4.2**). The identified markets are both internal and external. Organizations that have established foundations supporting their medical research may consider donors of high current importance. Another group may consider this segment to be of high future importance, as their clinic or hospital moves into research activities. For a Catholic hospital, the board of directors, which may have strong church ties, may be of both high current and high future importance.

Exhibit 4.2 lists some, but not all potential markets. Some hospitals may prefer to identify their markets by race or geographical location. The purpose of this exercise is to encourage the management team to state explicitly the relevant markets and the existing attitude (or support) of those markets to the service offered.

The second part of Exhibit 4.2 requires consideration of the organization's key market segments. Forecasting the future size of these segments is essential. Common problems for many organizations are identifying a key segment and forecasting its future decline. The second part of Exhibit 4.2 also forces managers to examine the key segments from a marketing perspective by considering what the likely needs for these groups are. Lack of knowledge of future needs highlights an information gap for market research to fill. In this second part, as with all aspects of the analysis, it is important to remember that the opinion of the management team might not match the perception of the customers or of the overall market. Market research can validate assumptions and answer questions management cannot answer.

Data to complete the form can be obtained from several sources. Opinions of staff members are valuable. In addition, it is useful to examine billing files, medical records, and physician reports. Often this analysis reveals that the markets served by the group differ from those its members perceive that it serves.

In the provision of health care, little can be done without the physician, the primary provider of services. Because of the significance of this market to a hospital trying to attract (or retain) medical staff or to a group practice needing productive members, a separate review is necessary. Data on several dimensions are required, as indicated in **Exhibit 4.3**.

For the hospital, a staff review identifies the major producers. Moreover, it identifies individuals whose practices are developing or who are beginning to shift their caseloads to another facility. Typically, a small group of physicians accounts for a disproportionate share of the volume.

EXHIBIT 4.2

Identification of Major Markets and Needs

Part I—Identifying markets. A market or market segment consists of a group of people who have common demographic, specialty, or social characteristics; it is large enough for the organization to concentrate resources on.

Markets (partial list of examples)	Potential Importance		Current Attitude Toward Organization		
	Current	Future	Favorable	Neutral	Not Favorable
General medicine					
Surgeons					
Other MDs					
Inpatients (by specialty)					
Outpatients					
Community at large					
Insurance companies					
Regulators					
Business/industry (specify)					
HMO patients					
Females					
Over-65 market					

Part II—Based on the analysis discovered in Part I, indicate key markets, potential volume, and key needs/requirements related to the markets selected.

Top Market Segment Opportunity	Potential Revenue/ Volume	Market Needs/ Requirements
1.		
2.		
3.		
4.		
5.		

EXHIBIT 4.3

Analysis of Physician Staff

Physician Name	Age	Specialty	Location of Practice	Practice Type	Years on Staff	Overall Comment	Activity This Year		Projected Activity 5 Years From Now		
							Revenue Generated	Share of Hospital Procedures	Revenue Generated	Share of Hospital Procedures	Percent Change Expected

Identify those who provide 80% of activity (or billed revenue) for further analysis.

Name	Age	Specialty	Revenue Generated This Year	Key Issues/Strategies to Retain, Grow, or Replace

Conclusion:

1. Where are we vulnerable?
2. What specialty area needs more focus?
3. What is our core medical strength that we should focus on?

This group must be identified and its loyalty maintained. Likewise, the age of this group may reveal recruiting needs of varying levels of immediacy.

Following are several questions that management should consider in its market determination:

1. What are the main developments with respect to demography, the economy, technology, government, and culture that will affect the organization's future?

Overall changes like these, which are beyond the control of the organization, must be considered. In answering question 1, many organizations have found that the demographics of their communities have necessitated changes in the specialty composition of their group or the program offered by their hospital.

2. How large is the realistic service area covered by the market?
3. What are the major segments (e.g., men, over age 70, new to the community) in each market?
4. What are the present and expected future profits and characteristics of each market or market segment?
5. What is the expected rate of growth of each segment?
6. How fast and far have markets expanded?
7. Where do the patients come from geographically?

Most of the questions outlined above can be answered through direct market research. Answering the preceding questions requires determining the market the organization serves. One tertiary facility wanted to determine the area in which its patients lived (questions 2 and 7). Although the hospital had always believed that it drew its patients from three states, answering this question resulted in a different perspective: 75% of the patients were found to come from eight counties around the hospital (all in the same state). This finding led to a different focus for promotion efforts, as well as a new program for physician outreach and off-site clinic investment.

The remaining 11 questions pertain to why the various market segments buy or use the organization's services. And again, direct market research is useful in gathering the answers. For example, what characteristic encourages people to use a certain clinic (question 8)? Is it technical skill or accessibility? If accessibility, how might your competition eliminate this advantage? Or, consider the impact of question 11—requirements for market success. If your market is patients who need after-hours care, what is required? Physician coverage may mean a new medical recruitment effort. A safe environment for the clinic is a necessity for night care. Where is the facility located?

8. What are the benefits (e.g., economy, better performance, displaceable cost) that customers in different segments derive from the product?
9. What are the reasons (e.g., product features, awareness, price, advertising, location of the clinic) different market segments buy the product?
10. What is the organization's market standing with established customers in each segment (e.g., market share, pattern of repeat business, expansion of customers' product use)?
11. What are the requirements for success in each market?
12. What are the customer attitudes (e.g., brand awareness, brand image) in different segments?
13. What is the overall reputation of the product in each segment?
14. What reinforces the customer's faith in the company and product?
15. What circumstances force customers to turn elsewhere for help in using the product?
16. What is the lifecycle of the product?
17. What product research and improvements are planned?
18. Are there deficiencies in servicing or assisting customers in using the product?

It may not be possible to answer all questions because of personnel constraints or, more often, lack of knowledge. The value of this process is to identify where the organization needs to gather more data before specifying marketing actions.

THE COMPETITION

A third component of the internal/external analysis is an examination of existing and future competition. Organizations must realize that having a good product may not be enough if their competitors also have one. A thorough evaluation of competitors' strengths and weaknesses can help lead to a product or service design that most competitively positions a clinic or hospital. It is important to develop an understanding not only of competitors' strengths and weaknesses, but also of their organizational capabilities and likely future thrusts. Once a thorough situation analysis has been completed, reasonable objectives can be specified for action in these areas.

A detailed analysis of competitors should be undertaken from an external view. Key issues to be addressed are who the competitors are, which competitors are likely to emerge, and where competitors are most vulnerable. A detailed profile should be compiled for each major competitor (**Exhibit 4.4**).

EXHIBIT 4.4

Competitor Profile: Clinic Example

Part I—Develop a profile sheet on each relevant competitor.

A. Overview
   Name of competitor: _____ Revenue: _____
   Net income: _____ Return on investment: _____
   Market share this year: _____
   Market share 3 years ago: _____

B. Nature of organization/operation (size, physician mix, type of organization):

C. Competitive strength:

D. Competitive weakness:

E. Likely key competitive moves:

F. Likely key long-range vision:

G. Top clinicians by revenue produced for the competitor:

	Name	Revenue	Age	Notes
1.				
2.				
3.				
4.				
5.				
6.				

Overall Competitive Assessment of Individual Competitor:

Unlike market identification (Exhibit 4.2), which is based on the opinions of internal personnel, this competitive analysis should be based on as much objective external data as are available. Several sources may be helpful in completing this review:

- State certification-of-need agency
- American Hospital Association
- Health-related professional associations
- American Medical Association
- Other planning agencies
- Regional transit authority

- Chamber of Commerce
- Commercial research firms (such as Dun & Bradstreet, Thomson Reuters, or National Research Corporation Health Care Market Guide)
- U.S. Census Bureau
- Drug/pharmaceutical companies
- Business/industrial organizations
- City and county directories
- Registration/licensure agencies
- Other government agencies/publications

The first part of the competitor profile contains overview information. The second part focuses on market-share data. Often, planning data can provide the necessary market-share data. Ignoring the organization's market share relative to the competition can have serious consequences. Most healthcare groups evaluate their own absolute performance by patient days, gross revenue, or patient visits. This approach ignores the relative issue. A clinic's absolute number of patient visits could be increasing in family practice, but its growth could be at a lower rate than that of the competition. Thus, the group is not attracting its proportion (or share) of new family-practice business. Over time, the group may find itself with little impact in the market.

There are real competitors and there are potential competitors. Real competitors are those that can be observed, while potential competitors are those who may or may not be in the same business. Other potential competitors might be "outsiders" who decide to enter the business. Examples of competitive substitutions in health care include CVS drugstores, who decided to enter the pediatric care business; the Mayo Clinic, who moved into Florida, which was a completely new market; or even books published by the American Medical Association (AMA) that provide consumers with algorithms that, in essence, can help consumers avoid a medical visit. Another competitive substitution could be an online physician site that offers opinion and medical advice via email for a fixed fee, and therefore is competing with the stand-alone medical clinic. Porter's Five Forces model is helpful in this regard because it forces organizations to explore the risk of competitive product substitution or entry by seemingly unlikely competitors.

The objective of a relative assessment is to provide an internal perspective on the organization's relative competitive position in comparison to your organization (**Exhibit 4.5**). Several key personnel should complete the form independently. Before an organization begins to develop plans and allocate resources to actions, there should be some similarity of views on the external competition. Otherwise, conflict often occurs

EXHIBIT 4.5

Relative Competitive Assessment

Relative to Our Organization: _____ Date:_____

Competitor (specify): _____

Are we:

Much Worse	Somewhat Worse			About the Same	Somewhat Better			Much Better
−4	−3	−2	−1	0	+1	+2	+3	+4

1. Medical care ____
   A. Emergency ____
   B. Surgery ____
   C. General medical ____
   D. Special care ____
   E. Other ____
2. Nursing care ____
3. Market share ____
4. Facility: capacity/attractiveness ____
5. Community reputation ____
6. Image (overall) ____
7. Location ____
8. Convenience ____
9. Equipment: capability/technology ____
10. Other ____

Conclusion and Score:

Special Note: Be careful that the above evaluation is not made based on an internal opinion of the competitor. What do the actual data suggest?

---

because members perceive other groups or hospitals in different ways. In the SWOT analysis discussion, it was noted that organization bias without data can be an issue. The same is true when using Exhibit 4.5. The personal biases revealed in completing this form are its strength and its weakness. Varying views on competitive position must be resolved early in the planning process. The second part of the relative competitive assessment focuses on how competitive other organizations are and the basis for the competition.

It is important to overcome an organization's tendency to be myopic with regard to competition. Any clinic's competitive environment is dynamic. For-profit systems might move into a market area and dramatically change the nature of competition. Recognition of their potential competitive threat is critical, as is devising ways to discourage market entry by a potential competitor.

The following questions provide direction in addressing the issue of competitive intensity and focusing on the basis of competition:

1. How many competitors are in the industry? How are competitors defined? Has the number increased or decreased in the previous 4 years?
2. What is the organization's position (size and strength) in the market relative to competitors?
3. Who are the organization's major competitors?
4. What trends can be foreseen in competition?
5. Are other companies likely to be enticed to serve the organization's customers or markets? What conglomerates or diversified companies may be attracted by the growth, size, or profitability of these markets?
6. What about companies on the periphery—those that serve the same customers with different, but related products, including related pieces of equipment? (It is impossible to list all related items, but those closest should be included.)

A major difficulty in the healthcare industry is the impact of technology. New technological developments can cause a new threat to appear or a hospital's competitive advantage to be eliminated. Two additional questions focus thinking on this factor:

7. What other products or services provide the same or similar functions? What percentage of total market sales does each substitute product have?
8. What product innovations could replace or reduce sales of the organization's products? When will these products be commercially feasible? (Information about potentially competitive products can be found by searching the records of the U.S. Patent Office and foreign patent offices.)

Existing competition must always be considered. Of particular concern is the basis for competition. It is important to understand the competitive thrust of others and their potential impact on market share.

9. What are the choices afforded patients? In services? In payment?
10. Is competition on a price or nonprice basis?
11. How do competitors (segment/price) advertise?

Finally, the organization's sensitivity to geographical susceptibility should always be maintained, and the diversification strategies of those who are familiar with the industry should always be monitored.

12. Might competitors in other geographical regions or other segments who do not currently compete in the organization's markets or segments decide to?
13. Who are the customers served by the industry?
14. Who are the suppliers to the industry? Are they changing strategies? Why?

Competitor data are difficult to obtain, although healthcare regulations often require public notification of plans—a requirement that often makes competitive monitoring much easier. Managers in an organization must recognize that whenever a competitor changes its strategy, the organization must change its strategy. The competitor has possibly restructured the basis for competition or the perception of the market. Too often, healthcare providers ignore competition, but no market plan should be developed without addressing competitive issues.

INTERNAL CAPABILITY

The fourth component of the internal/external assessment is the analysis of internal capabilities. The objective of this review is to obtain a general understanding of the workings of the organization from key participants. As a first step, each participant should independently evaluate the program or clinic with a form such as **Exhibit 4.6**.

Completed forms should be compared for consistency among group members. Areas of low satisfaction or inconsistency should be explored. Recognized weak points may be obvious to competitors as places where they can establish dominance. It is important to realize, however, that this tool is for internal assessment and does not necessarily reflect accurately the opinions that outside physicians, consumers, and other important users have regarding the organization.

In addition, a comprehensive review should include examination of several other issues:

1. What has the historical purpose of the organization been?
2. How has the organization changed over the past decade?
3. When and how was it organized?
4. What has the nature of its growth been?
5. What is the basic policy of the organization? Is it health care or profit?

Answering these questions requires examining the original purpose of the organization. This investigation can lead to a reexamination of the appropriateness of the original mission in light of the competitive factors addressed in the internal/external analysis.

EXHIBIT 4.6

Overall Internal Assessment: Hospital Example

	Evaluation Today			Evaluation 3 Years Ago		
	High	Medium	Low	High	Medium	Low
Outpatient utilization						
Inpatient census						
Age of medical staff						
Medical staff relations						
Quality of service rankings in the community						
Relationships with key regulatory agencies (e.g., rate commission)						
Community support ("This is my hospital or clinic.")						
Level of community awareness						
Share of market served						
Breadth of product line						
Compensation structure for employees						
Financial position of organization						
Technological capability						
Efficiency of organization in service delivery						
Investment intensity						
Vertical integration						
Other: _____						

Conclusion:

Next Step:

Any marketing actions contemplated by a healthcare organization will be affected by finances. A review of this functional area is a necessity. Here are some questions to ask:

6. What has the financial history of the organization been?
7. How has it been capitalized?
8. Have there been any problems with accounts receivable?
9. What is the return on investment?
10. How successful has the organization been with the various services it has promoted?
11. Is the total volume (gross revenue, utilization) increasing or decreasing?
12. Have there been any fluctuations in revenue? If so, what caused them?

The following questions require an honest and challenging investigation of the organization's strengths and weaknesses. A reputation as a major teaching hospital with excellent research capacity may not be a strength in establishing a primary care clinic. Consumers may perceive the teaching hospital as appropriate only for "serious" illnesses, not for primary care.

13. What are the organization's present strengths and weaknesses in management capabilities? Medical staff? Technical facilities? Reputation? Financial capabilities? Image? Medical facilities?

MARKETING ACTIVITIES

The final component in the internal/external analysis is the marketing activities of the clinic or hospital. Important in this assessment is a determination of whether the organization has adopted and implemented the marketing concept. The answers to the following questions will indicate whether the organization has a marketing perspective:

1. Does the marketing department have a key role in the planning activities of the organization?
2. Do the manager and other key personnel have marketing experience?
3. Are there specialized training programs for key personnel that emphasize the marketing concept?

Along with the concern about the adoption of the marketing perspective, an internal analysis should assess whether the organization has, in fact, implemented the marketing concept.

4. Does the person with marketing responsibility report directly to the CEO or top administrator?
5. Is market research appreciated as an ongoing task necessary for the development of effective marketing plans?
6. Are policies and procedures in place to coordinate the marketing activities with the other ongoing activities of the organization?[5]
7. Does the organization have a high-level marketing officer to analyze, plan, and implement its marketing work?
8. Are the other persons who are directly involved in marketing activities competent? Do they need more training, incentives, or supervision?
9. Are the marketing responsibilities optimally structured to serve the needs of different activities, products, markets, and territories?

These questions make it possible to determine whether the functional arrangement of the marketing activity is appropriate. Implementation of action strategies requires control by an individual with responsibility and authority.

As any manager familiar with marketing knows, service, price, promotion, and distribution decisions are the core aspects of the marketing mix. Although inspection of each element in isolation is a part of the internal/external analysis, it is also necessary to review the overall marketing program:

10. What is the organization's core strategy for achieving its objectives, and is it likely to succeed?
11. Is the organization allocating enough resources (or too many) to accomplish its marketing tasks?
12. Are the marketing resources allocated optimally to the various markets, territories, and products of the organization?
13. Are the marketing resources allocated optimally to the major elements of the marketing mix (i.e., product quality, pricing, promotion, and distribution)?

The preceding questions focus on the organization's strategy and the resource allocation necessary to implement this strategy. Related consideration must be given to the implementation of the marketing program:

14. Does the organization develop an annual marketing plan? Is the planning procedure effective?
15. Does the organization implement control procedures (e.g., monthly, quarterly) to ensure that its annual objectives are being achieved?
16. Does the organization carry out periodic studies to determine the contribution and effectiveness of various marketing activities?

17. Does the organization have an adequate marketing information system to meet the needs of managers in planning and controlling various markets?

The remaining areas of the marketing analysis pertain to specific mix elements. Much of the data needed to complete the remaining portions of this task are contained in the internal records of the group or in the collected judgments of managers.

Products and Services

As marketing actions are prepared for the next planning period, a reanalysis of existing service strategies is warranted:

1. What are the organization's products and services, both current and proposed?
2. What are the general outstanding characteristics of each product or service?
3. How are the organization's products or services superior to or distinct from those of competing organizations? What are their weaknesses? Should any product be phased out? Should any product be added?
4. What is the total cost per service (in use)? Is the service over- or underutilized?
5. Which services are most heavily used? Why? Are there distinct groups of users? What is the profile of patients/physicians who use the services?
6. What are the organization's policies regarding number and types of services to offer? Regarding needs assessment for service addition/ deletion?
7. What is the history of the organization's major products and services?

   - How many did the organization originally have?
   - How many have been added or dropped?
   - What important changes have taken place in services during the previous 10 years?
   - Has demand for the services increased or decreased?
   - What are the most common complaints about the services?
   - What services could be added to make the organization more attractive to patients, medical staff, and nonmedical personnel?
   - What are the strongest points of the services to patients, medical staff, and nonmedical personnel?

8. Does the organization have any other features that individualize its services or give it an advantage over competitors?

It is important for members of the analysis team to maintain a marketing perspective as they proceed through the questions: They must consider the advantages of a program from the buyer's view, not from the internal perspective of the clinic or hospital.

Pricing Strategy

The importance of pricing need not be reviewed here. Changing reimbursement structures and competitive trends mandate a close reexamination of historical pricing practices. Internally, the rationale for existing prices should be reviewed in the context of external price trends.

1. What is the pricing strategy of the organization? Cost plus? Return on investment? Stabilization? Demand?
2. How are prices for services determined? How often are prices reviewed? What factors contribute to a price increase or decrease?
3. What have the price trends been for the past 5 years?

In addition, the organization must take into account market perceptions of price, as well as price elasticity. Although the common view is that prices must be reduced, one group practice discovered in a proprietary study on its market's price sensitivity that area consumers expected to pay more for an office visit than the group's present price.

4. How are the organization's pricing policies viewed by patients? Physicians? Third-party payers? Competitors? Regulators? Managed-care organizations?
5. How are price promotions used?
6. How would a higher or lower price affect demand?

Promotional Strategy

An organization's promotional strategy consists of personal selling, advertising, and public relations. Multispecialty clinics often have salespeople to aid outreach efforts, and hospitals may have them for industrial healthcare programs. Compensation, size of the sales force, and account allocation should be periodically reexamined:

1. Is the sales force large enough to accomplish the organization's objectives?
2. Is the sales force organized along the proper principles of specialization (e.g., territory, market, product)?
3. Does the sales force show high morale, ability, and effort? Is it sufficiently trained and motivated?
4. Are the procedures adequate for setting quotas and evaluating performance?

Healthcare organizations are increasingly paying attention to the advertising component of promotion. Central to a review of advertising is campaign focus:

5. What is the purpose of the organization's present promotional activities (including advertising)? Protection? Education? Search for new markets? Development of all markets? Establishment of a new service?
6. Has this purpose undergone any change in recent years?
7. To whom has advertising been largely directed? Donors? Patients? Former? Current? Prospective? Physicians? On staff? Potential?

Media strategy should also be evaluated periodically:

8. Is the cost per thousand viewers, listeners, or readers still favorable?
9. Are the media delivering to the desired audience?
10. What media have been used?
11. How effective is the organization's website and what do the data say in terms of page visits?
12. How current is the website in terms of offering appointments, medical advice, and pricing information?

Further concerns cover strategy for and periodic evaluation of advertising:

13. Are the objectives (reviewed in question 5) being met?
14. What company advertising and Internet copy has had the most favorable response?
15. What methods have been used for measuring company advertising and Internet effectiveness, including social media such as Facebook and Twitter?

Public relations is a common promotional tool for healthcare providers. Yet, this activity also requires a periodic reanalysis in order to retain its value:

16. What is the role of public relations? Is it a separate function/department? What is the scope of its responsibilities?
17. Has the public relations effort led to regular coverage?
18. Are the public relations objectives integrated with the overall promotional plan?

Question 18 is of particular importance. Because advertising and public relations are often the responsibilities of different people within a hospital, a structure must be established to integrate their objectives and coordinate their activities.

A final question pertains to the assessment of effectiveness:

19. Are procedures established and used to measure the results from the public relations program?

Distribution Strategy

The final component of the marketing mix that must be examined is distribution—the way in which services are delivered or provided to the market, including location of facilities, and application of strategies to connect services of the organization with customers.

1. What are the distribution trends in the industry? What services are being performed on an outpatient basis? What services are being performed on an at-home basis? Are satellite facilities being used?
2. What factors are considered in location decisions?
3. How important is distribution in establishing a competitive advantage for a particular service?
4. Where does the hospital or clinic stand on this component?[6]

Visual Tools

The sample forms and lists provided in this section are useful tools for conducting an internal/external analysis. Sometimes, however, visual tools can help managers examine data from several sources at one time. For example, **Figure 4.4** illustrates in one place the profit margins, revenue, and relative size (reflected by the size of the circle) of various programs in a hospital.

MARKET RESEARCH

A market-based planning approach is not based solely on the beliefs, assumptions, or feelings of those inside the organization. Market research is essential in the development of effective marketing strategies. The price that a hospital should charge for a service is not an internal issue, for example, except for the fact that the comptroller must inform the planning committee of the cost structure; the key question is the price that the market will bear. Similarly, although it may be valuable to hear how individuals who work in a clinic perceive that clinic, the patients' perceptions are more critical in reinforcing, changing, or repositioning the business.

The greatest difference between the healthcare industry and other industries is probably in the conduct of market research. In today's marketplace, few companies in the traditional industries do not engage in ongoing market research. Too often in health care, however, market

FIGURE 4.4

Typical Bubble Map Showing Health Services Profit Margin and Magnitude of Clinical Revenue

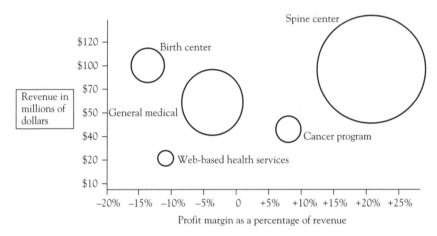

research is a one-time or sporadic activity; furthermore, healthcare organizations rely on or refer back to the results of such research for several years, even as marketplace conditions change.

It is impossible to say how much an organization should spend on market research. The guiding principle should be not to spend more on researching a new program idea than can be lost if the new venture should fail. Concomitantly, the more complicated the project, the more complicated and expensive the research should be because of the multiple constituencies involved (e.g., patients, referring physicians, and third-party payers).

There are two broad classifications of market research data: primary and secondary. Secondary data are collected by third parties, often for a range of purposes. In the healthcare industry, a great deal of secondary market data have become available. Primary data are gathered by an organization on a specific topic.

Secondary Data

An organization should always begin with secondary data, which may save time and money. A user must answer several questions in evaluating secondary data, however:

1. How timely is the information?
2. How large and representative is the sample relative to the population of concern?

3. How free of bias do the data appear to be?
4. Are the classifications of the data appropriate for the topic being researched?

Asking these questions does not imply that secondary data are not useful. Rather, like information from any other external source, the data must be carefully evaluated for validity and relevance.

There are several possible sources of secondary data. The U.S. Census Bureau, along with companies such as Urban Decision Systems, USA-DATA, and Thomson Reuters, offer simplified ways of examining a variety of *census data*. For example, these organizations can provide a census analysis, both historical and forecasted, to a hospital that is considering opening a clinic in a particular location. This analysis can be done on a variety of parameters, including a 1-mile and 5-mile radius of the location (**Table 4.1**) and by zip code. As Table 4.1 indicates, at this particular proposed clinic site, a gain is projected in the population; however, a decline of young children is predicted. This information provides insight into the economic mix that a new clinic may expect: Obviously, adding more pediatric staff would not be a good tactic. Through the use of web-based market research service data providers, this information is available on an instantaneous basis from the sponsor, often for less than $100.

Other industries have benefited from *syndicated market information* for years, but hospitals were forced to reinvent the wheel each year in order to receive baseline market information. Each hospital spent large portions of its limited market-research budget to obtain basic benchmark information and had no additional money available to probe for special needs and opportunities. With syndicated research, healthcare marketers can now build a market database without asking the same questions over and over again on a customized basis.

Several types of syndicated research projects on the market are specific to health care. The National Research Corporation's Healthcare Market Guide, for example, is based on an annual survey of 100,000 households in the top 100 markets of the United States. Individual reports are made available to a variety of purchasers, including hospitals and clinics, within each of these markets. National, state, and regional summaries, as well as special reports, are part of the package. This kind of program gives a hospital or a clinic inexpensive benchmark data on an annual basis; the marketing staff can then spend other market-research dollars on special needs and interests. This type of program does not, however, include customized questions. Furthermore, anyone, including competitors, can purchase the information. The Healthcare Market Guide contains several sections, as seen in

TABLE 4.1 EXAMPLE OF CUSTOMIZED SECONDARY DEMOGRAPHIC DATA
AVAILABLE TO PURCHASE

224 General Street **Anywhere City, State**	Total Zip Code		Project Proposed Site	
	2012	2020 Est.	1-Mile Radius	5-Mile Radius
Total Population	34,500	38,200	8,500	28,000
Median Age	43	46.5	39	45
Age 65+	22%	27%	23%	30%
Female	53%	55%	51%	54%
Male	47%	45%	49%	46%
Household Size 1	30%	34%	38%	35%
Household Size 2	35%	33%	32%	40%
Household Size 3–4	29%	30%	28%	24%
Household Size 5+	6%	3%	2%	1%
Rents Home	32%	29%	38%	39%
Owns Home	68%	71%	62%	61%
HH Income Above $75,000	21%	24%	31%	23%
HH Income $35–74,999	55%	57%	54%	49%
HH Income Below $34,999	24%	19%	15%	28%
College Graduate	19.0%	20.0%	24%	16%
High School Graduate	71.0%	69.0%	68%	74%
Not High School Graduate	10%	12%	8%	10%

Note: This example provides data projected forward for a zip code in a community, and it
provides data for a radius around a possible project within a portion of the same zip code.

Table 4.2. This sample report shows a sample of marketplace-based data.
Multiple views of quality and utilization by different demographic variables
are available.

Other data provide an overview of consumer usage of services by competitor, customer satisfaction information, and other data that would help
an organization understand its market.

TABLE 4.2 Houston MSA Quality by Age

Houston MSA, 2011
HEALTHCARE SYSTEM
Quality/Image Profile
Best Overall Quality by Decision-Maker Age

	Total	Average Age	18–34	35–44	45–64	65+
Total	**3,677**	**46**	**873**	**819**	**1,497**	**488**
Memorial Hermann-Texas Medical Center	11.81%	44.49	13.33%	11.71%	12.18%	8.14%
The Methodist Hospital System	7.70%	50.72	4.61%	7.40%	8.17%	12.25%
St Luke's Episcopal Hospital	5.19%	52.03	2.53%	4.55%	5.58%	9.83%
St Luke's The Woodlands Hospital	3.39%	48.44	2.06%	3.39%	3.96%	4.04%
North Cypress Medical Center	0.79%	52.18	0.23%	0.81%	0.90%	1.40%
Veterans Affairs Medical Center	0.57%	59.03		0.22%	0.94%	1.02%
Other Facilities	8.57%	43.18	11.70%	8.79%	6.98%	7.47%

Source: Reprinted with permission from the National Research Corporation (2011).

Another syndicated service provides use-rate information at today's volume, and the data can be predicted 5 years into the future at the ICD-9 procedure level by purchasing another report. Data provided by organizations such as Thomson Reuters can provide valuable information on projected doctor visits, hospital admissions by product line, and demand for specific outpatient services. **Table 4.3** is an example. All these data are available by zip code and include a breakdown of Medicare and commercial-pay patients.

All these services are reasonably comprehensive and, on an annual basis, provide the marketing person with cost-efficient syndicated market research that is considered secondary, but fills many needs of the health-care marketing manager.

TABLE 4.3   PROJECTED MARKET OUTPATIENT PROCEDURES BY ICD-9 PROCEDURE PRODUCT LINE

Area: ABC Sample
Selected Age Group: All Ages
Ranked on Total Market Change Count (Descending)

	ICD-9 Procedure Product Line	Total Market				Hospital-Based 2016 Projected Procedures	Physician Office 2016 Procedures	Other Sites 2016 Procedures
		2011	2016					
Code	Description	Procedures		Count	Change %			
39	Office Visit or Consult Claim	1,103,068	1,286,197	183,129	16.6%	246,804	1,005,298	34,095
37	Physical Medicine and Rehab	743,567	874,707	131,140	17.6%	125,143	616,811	132,753
42	Other Medical Services	659,106	781,506	122,400	18.6%	159,090	534,736	87,680
18	Radiology	237,797	276,134	38,338	16.1%	88,214	100,162	87,759
41	Pathology and Laboratory	224,281	258,490	34,209	15.3%	98,086	78,938	81,466
31	Behavioral Medicine	188,807	213,108	24,301	12.9%	23,142	160,565	29,401
9	Surgery—Integumentary System	95,137	116,605	21,468	22.6%	16,179	99,174	1,253
16	Diagnostic Ultrasound	100,165	115,233	15,068	15.0%	39,222	75,486	525
24	Electrocardiogram	51,167	62,480	11,313	22.1%	22,240	39,787	453
15	Computerized Axial Tomog (CAT)	36,899	44,096	7,197	19.5%	31,410	12,580	106

Note: Sample data of some ICD-9 codes.

Source of Market Outpatient Data: Thomson Procedure Outpatient Rates.

Source of ICD-9 Procedure Data: Thomson Procedure Product Line (2011).

Reprinted with permission from Thomson Reuters Healthcare. (2011). All rights reserved.

Primary Data

Sometimes secondary data are not enough. More insight is often required to answer specific questions such as those in **Exhibit 4.7**. One goal of primary research is to get a better understanding of what key customers are thinking and how they decide which provider they want to use. In the Twin Cities of Minneapolis and St. Paul, the Hmong ethnic group represents a large and prosperous community. By studying and listening to this market segment, Hennepin County Medical Center learned about Hmong expectations, based on tradition, after the birth of a baby. As a result, the hospital created a rooftop garden for rare herbs that could be used in the traditional post-birth meal. By adding this feature, the popularity of the hospital grew and more Hmong people decided to have their children delivered at the hospital.

When organizations need to have a deeper understanding of purchase behavior and opinions in general, managers turn to primary market research. Two issues are critical in primary market research: sample and methodology.

Sample

No decision is more critical to the usefulness of market research than the *definition of a sample*. The more specific the sample, the more precise the research results. For example, an organization that wants to open a women's clinic must decide whether to research the needs of all women or only those in their child-bearing years, women in the entire community or women who live in the northern suburbs. Too often, however, healthcare institutions leave this vital decision to an external consultant or firm. The question of whom to study is a management issue. The appropriate people to sample are those who look like the target market for the program or service under study. The more defined the profile of the target market provided to the researcher, the greater the confidence the healthcare institution can have in the final results of the research efforts.

A second key issue in selecting a sample is the *size of the sample*. There are a host of formulas and tables for sample size that require assumptions about the population and the issue under study. The National Committee for Citizens in Education published one of the quickest and most useful of such tables: All that is required is an estimate of the size of the target market, or population; from that figure, an appropriate sample size is given at both the 90% and 95% confidence level (**Table 4.4**). Thus, for a 95% degree of accuracy, according to this table, the sample must be 351 for a community of 50,000 people; the sample needs to be only 384 for a city of 1 million. Some statisticians may argue that this guideline

EXHIBIT 4.7

Typical Questions Used in Conducting Primary Market Research

Example 1: A Study to Select a Site for a New Clinic
Areas probed should include at least the following questions:
- Does respondent have a doctor?
- How often is the doctor visited?
- Does the entire family use the same doctor?
- How satisfied is respondent with:
    o Doctor?
    o Cost?
    o Waiting time?
- Does respondent know where proposed new clinic site is located?
- Is this new site convenient?
- What is the likelihood of visiting a new medical group at this site?
- What services should be available in a doctor's office?
- How much would respondent expect to pay for a routine visit?

Example 2: A Study to Determine Consumer Satisfaction with a Hospital
Areas probed should include at least the following questions:
- Does respondent have a hospital preference?
- Rank this hospital against all other competitors for specific service areas.
- What do you like best about this hospital?
- What do you like least about this hospital?
- If your doctor told you to use this hospital, what would you do?
- Have you been a patient or visitor at this hospital?

Example 3: A study of Physicians' Attitudes Toward a Specific Hospital Department
Areas probed should include at least the following questions:
- Rank order this department (and competitors) for each of the following:
    o Quality:
    o Attitude:
    o Modern technology:
    o Price to patient:
    o Convenience:
- What do you like best about the department?
- What do you like least about the department?
- In the next 2 years, what new services should the department offer?
- If these services were offered, how many more patients would you bring to the hospital?

is too simplistic to reflect sampling variations. Their concern may be legitimate in some market research. For example, if a hospital in Boston is conducting a study of men and women over 21 years of age, there are two populations. Ideally, a sample of approximately 350 men and 350 women must be drawn. Although the statistician may raise some concerns, management may believe it necessary to reduce the sample size from this ideal range of 700 to a more affordable, yet still large number.

The way in which the data will be analyzed may affect the sample size needed. In some instances, it is necessary to increase a sample size because of anticipated breakdowns in market segments. For example, a medical group wants to do a study among primary care physicians in their primary and secondary referral areas to determine whether the attitude of family practitioners about referring differs from that of internists, pediatricians, and obstetrician-gynecologists. In this instance, the sample size must be large enough within each one of these subspecialties to provide some degree of confidence in the results. Therefore, the total sample size must be increased to a level that will provide reasonable confidence.

One final decision in designing a sample is the *type of sample* that should be selected. There are several variations.

Often in conducting market research, someone suggests that a *random sample* be selected. Something about the "randomness" of such a sample

TABLE 4.4 SIZE OF SAMPLE NEEDED TO BE CONFIDENT OF ACCURACY

Population	Sample Size That Will Provide 95% Confidence Level	Sample Size That Will Provide 90% Confidence Level
Infinity	384	271
100,000	384	271
50,000	381	269
10,000	370	263
5,000	357	257
3,000	341	248
2,000	322	238
1,000	278	213
500	217	176
100	80	73

Note: Error margin held constant at ±5 percentage points.

Source: Adapted from PACE Manual with permission of Phi Delta Kappa, © 1984.

makes many people believe in its reliability and validity. In drawing a random sample, a person may take every 10th person from the telephone directory, for example. In these types of samples, everyone has an equal chance of being selected. In market research, however, random sampling is rarely done, primarily because the organization wants to learn about a target market or market segments. In these instances, a judgment sample or a quota sample is more appropriate.

Individuals are selected for *judgment samples* based on what management or the researcher thinks they will contribute to answering the question at hand. For example, in the design of an industrial medicine program, benefits officers and medical directors employed at corporations with more than 500 employees may be selected.

A variation of the judgment sample, the *quota sample*, includes individuals who have been selected because of some particular characteristics. The example of the medical group involved a quota sample; the important characteristic was the subspecialty area of the primary care physicians, and a quota was taken from each group. In most marketing-research studies, as data are subsequently broken down into segments for analysis (e.g., 40 years of age or younger, 41 to 64 years of age, 65 years of age or older), it is important to consider these characteristics in developing the final quota sample.

Methodology

After the sample has been selected, the method must be selected. Various techniques are available to market researchers (**Table 4.5**).

Potentially the most expensive of data-gathering approaches is the *personal interview.* The primary reason for the high cost is the need for trained interviewers. Because the personal interviewer cannot be monitored while conducting the interview, the interviewer must be well trained to ensure that questions are asked correctly and in the same way each time. It is difficult to collect negative or sensitive information in a personal interview; because of the lack of anonymity, the individual being interviewed may be inhibited in expressing opinions.

The personal interview does, however, have the advantage of flexibility. Interviewers can probe respondents on their answers. Also, if respondents must complete forms, the interviewer can assist them. In addition, personal interviews permit some control over respondent selection; the personal interviewer knows who is answering, whereas in a mail survey any household member may complete the form.

Another strength of the personal interview is that the interviewer can be certain to obtain a complete sample. If an organization needs the opinions of five specific company executives regarding preferred-provider

TABLE 4.5 ALTERNATIVE MARKET RESEARCH METHODS

Criterion	Personal Interview	Telephone Survey	Mail or Internet Survey	Focus Groups
Economy	Most expensive	Avoids interviewer travel Relatively expensive Trained interviewers needed	Potentially lowest costs (if response rate is sufficient)	Relatively expensive
Interviewer bias	High likelihood of bias • Trust • Appearance	Less than personal interviewer No face-to-face contact Suspicion of phone call	Interview bias eliminated Anonymity provided	Need trained moderator
Flexibility	Most flexible method • Responses can be probed • Assistance can be provided in completing forms • Observations can be made	Cannot make observations Probing possible to a degree	Least flexible method	Very flexible
Sampling and respondent cooperation	Most complete sample possible, with sufficient call-back strategy	Limited to people with telephone No answers. Refusals are common	Mailing list problem Internet access issues Nonresponse a major problem	Need close selection

organizations, for example, the interviewer will eventually have a session with all five people (although doing so may require repeated call-back visits and some persistence). The other methods do not ensure sample completion.

The expense of the *telephone interview* is less than that of the personal interview, because the interviewer need not travel, and to some extent there is greater anonymity in the telephone interview. Most companies that conduct telephone interviews monitor their interviewers to determine whether they are asking questions appropriately and recording data correctly. Consumers are not always happy to be interrupted by an unsolicited call, however, and they are often suspicious about who is calling and the real purpose of the call. It is easy for them to terminate a telephone interview at any point just by hanging up the receiver.

Telephone interviews are a good way to collect information quickly. For example, if a clinic runs an advertisement in the Wednesday newspaper for its after-hours clinic, it may conduct telephone interviews Thursday morning to determine how many people noticed the advertisement. Data can be obtained quickly, and appropriate decisions can be made in a timely fashion. Of course, the speed of data collection is a function of the number of telephone interviewers.

Telephone surveys offer an opportunity for extensive and sophisticated analysis. Because large and reliable sample sizes can be generated, rich data tables can be created. **Table 4.6** is an example of data generated from a professional telephone survey.

Almost all consumers are familiar with *mail or Internet surveys* in one form or another. Online services such as Zoomerang or Survey Monkey offer inexpensive survey administration and data reporting. Because there is no need for trained interviewers and the cost of postage is relatively low or nonexistent in the case of an Internet survey, these can be the most inexpensive methods of collecting data. The problem with this approach is the response rate. Rarely do all people who receive a survey return a completed form, and those who do return the form may be different from those who do not. Maybe people who have nothing else to do will return the survey or send back an Internet survey form. These people may be less likely to represent the community at large. Therefore, the data may not present a true picture of the real views of a market. If there is a desire to determine the opinions of a specific zip code regarding physician preference, it is important to obtain survey results that reflect the demographic characteristics of the community. Online surveys do not automatically provide for this requirement.

In a survey of a healthcare organization's patient population, the demographic characteristics of survey respondents can be compared with those

TABLE 4.6 Austin Market Survey: What Respondents Have Heard About the Austin Clinic

| Insured | | Key Age/Sex/Income Data | | | | Respondents Primary Clinic | | Have Used Austin Medical | | |
	TOTAL	+65	F 30-45	+$75K	New to Town	Austin	All Others	Yes	No	BX
Base	402 100.0% (A)	150 100.0% 37.3% (B)	100 100.0% 24.9% (C)	100 100.0% 24.9% (D)	52 100.0% 12.9% (E)	228 100.0% 56.7% (F)	170 100.0% 42.3% (G)	311 100.0% 77.4% (H)	87 100.0% 21.6% (I)	211 100.0% 52.5%
Have not heard of problems/okay/pleased	72 17.9%	35 23.3% 48.6%	16 16.0% 22.2%	13 13.0% 18.1%	8 15.4% 11.1%	56 24.6% 77.8%	16 9.4% 22.2%	61 19.6% 84.7%	11 12.6% 15.3%	54 25.6% 75.0%
Good doctors	68 16.9%	35 23.3% 51.5%	10 10.0% 14.7%	16 16.0% 23.5%	7 13.5% 10.3%	52 22.8% 76.5%	16 9.4% 23.5%	62 19.9% 91.2%	6 6.9% 8.8%	51 24.2% 75.0%
Doctors do not care	35 8.7%	15 10.0% 42.9%	8 8.0% 22.9%	9 9.0% 25.7%	3 5.8% 8.6%	25 11.0% 71.4%	10 5.9% 28.6%	30 9.6% 85.7%	5 5.7% 14.3%	24 11.4% 68.6%
Wrong treatment/misdiagnosis	34 8.5%	8 5.3% 23.5%	9 9.0% 26.5%	10 10.0% 29.4%	7 13.5% 20.6%	17 7.5% 50.0%	17 10.0% 50.0%	31 10.0% 91.2%	2 2.3% 5.9%	14 6.6% 41.2%
Rude doctors	31 7.7%	7 4.7% 22.6%	12 12.0% 38.7%	6 6.0% 19.4%	6 11.5% 19.4%	10 4.4% 32.3%	20 11.8% 64.5%	24 7.7% 77.4%	7 8.0% 22.6%	5 2.4% 16.1%

of the organization's patient population to determine whether the survey respondents are representative. In a general community survey, respondents' profiles may be compared with those in the community census. When the organization knows who responded and who did not, nonrespondents' opinions can be sought through an alternative method and compared with those of respondents.

There are alternative strategies for improving response rates on mail surveys. Follow-up calls with an additional mailing of the survey form often help. Each successive follow-up wave improves the response rate. Many organizations have used incentives to encourage survey responses. Depending on who is being surveyed and the value of the information, the incentive may be a direct monetary payment, a premium (e.g., a pen, gift certificate), or the chance to win a prize. Response rates also improve as the form becomes easier to complete.

Mail surveys are the most limited approach in flexibility, a factor that is both a weakness and a strength. A weakness is that respondents cannot be probed on their responses. An advantage is that once the question is printed on the form, it cannot be altered or sequentially changed. The organization can be assured that all people will read the same question. Interviewers may inadvertently change the wording or imply a different meaning through voice intonation. The anonymity of a mail survey may be one of its strongest advantages. Sensitive information and negative evaluations may be most easily obtained with this data-gathering method.

Internet surveys can be modified easily as the sponsor begins to see the data coming in. If the response to a question is unclear or more information is needed, the survey can be reexamined, changed, and sent out again to continue the study. However, many people are concerned about anonymity when they respond to these kinds of surveys. Therefore, response rates can be low.

An approach gaining increasing popularity in healthcare research is the use of *focus groups*. In this process, a trained interviewer uses a limited number of probing questions in a group interview. Usually 8 to 12 people participate in the interview. As an example, the following four questions were presented to consumers to obtain their impressions of hospitals:

1. When people are new to a city, one of the first things they might consider is where they would go for a doctor or hospital. When you are thinking about hospitals, what things are most important to you?
2. Sometime during the past several months, you may have been inside a hospital. In walking around a hospital and speaking with people who work or practice there, what things stood out in your mind to tell you that the hospital was "OK"?

3. People often have some negative impressions of hospitals. What things do you look for in hospitals that tell you to never come back?
4. Cost and quality are important to everyone. When you are thinking about hospital reputations for quality, what things are most important in building that reputation?

The expense involved in a focus group is the cost of the trained moderator. This person must have the skills to probe and lead a group without dominating the discussion. Occasionally, people receive a nominal fee to participate in the sessions, which usually last from an hour and a half to 2 hours.

The focus group allows for maximum probing in a group setting. Depending on the topic, the participants may have to be as homogeneous as possible. In a focus group of physicians discussing ways to improve a hospital, for example, it may be best to have physicians from similar specialties. Physicians from different specialties may raise issues that do not pertain to all participants. Thus, rather than being a group discussion, the focus group might become a series of individual interviews in a group setting. Members of a focus group should have similar experiences to allow maximum participation.

Running a focus group is often helpful at the beginning of a research study. It may reveal the issues that should be explored in a structured mail or telephone survey. Many organizations have found the information obtained from a focus group sufficient for certain decisions, however. It is often valuable to conduct more than one focus group on an issue to ensure that responses received in one session are not unique to the group's composition or dynamics. A note of caution is required: This method is only directional; the sample is not large enough to predict that the results of these limited interviews are accurate. Therefore, the interviews should not be used to create a predictive model of activity or volume.

SUMMARY

The internal/external analysis requires introspection regarding management's views and the organization's position. Both large and small organizations should attempt some level of environmental analysis. Although a small group practice cannot implement the detailed analysis that has been discussed, it can perform a brief overview analysis. When an organization uses an abbreviated form (**Exhibit 4.8**), the questions posed in the more detailed analysis can be used as guidelines.

At several points in such an analysis, information gaps become apparent. For example, an organization may not have real measures of its image

EXHIBIT 4.8

Review of Internal/External Assessment

I. Review of market environment

   A. Markets: Who are your major markets and publics (i.e., whom are you serving now)? List in order of importance and indicate the percentage of your total business that each market represents. How will this list look 5 years from now?

   B. Customer satisfaction and needs: What is your position in your markets (i.e., physicians, patients)? List positives and negatives in short phrases.

   C. Competition: List major competitors in order of significance to you. What advantages do they have?

   D. External environment: What trends or developments are currently taking place that will affect (positively and negatively) your ability to market your products?

II. Review of marketing system

   A. Program objectives

      1. State your program objectives with expected outcomes and methods of measurement.

      2. If you were required to reduce your financial resources by 30%, how would you allocate your resources?

   B. Marketing mix

      1. What is the basic strategy for achieving the program's current objective (e.g., diversify, specialize, increase medical staff, encourage more physician participation, attract different kinds of employees)?

      2. How would you be affected by changes in the following:

         a. Pricing?

         b. Promotion?

         c. Distribution?

         d. Products?

III. Review of marketing activity

   A. Products: What needs do they meet? What is your competitive advantage?

   B. Price: How are prices set? Describe current pricing policy. Please comment on the following factors: relationship to cost, impact of competition, reimbursement implications, physician relationships.

   C. Distribution: What alternatives exist?

   D. Promotion: What is your competitive strategy?

in various markets. Market research may be required to obtain the needed data. Completing the internal/external analysis should clarify the organization's existing market position and the way in which it was achieved, however, so that strategy formulation becomes possible.[7]

QUESTIONS FOR DISCUSSION

1. If only five pieces of data were available for the planning process, what would they be?
2. Are physicians practicing at a hospital considered internal or external data?
3. What are the key differences between a SWOT and a Five Forces analysis?
4. Should board members who do not participate in conversations around the strategy be replaced?
5. Does the nominal group process encourage new ideas or does the process suppress critical thinking?
6. What are the difficulties with telephone-based market research methods?
7. Why is market share a critical data point?

NOTES

1. Peters, T., & Waterman, R. (1982). *In search of excellence.* New York: HarperCollins; p. 157.
2. Jha, A., & Epstein, A. (2020). Hospital governance and the quality of care. *Health Affairs, 29*(1), 182–187.
3. Leonhardt, D. (2009, November 8). Making health care better. *New York Times.*
4. Porter, M. (1979, March–April). How competitive forces shape strategy. *Harvard Business Review, 57,* 86–93.
5. Arnold, D. R., Capella, L. M., & Sumrall, D. A. (1987, March). Organization culture and the marketing concept. *Journal of Healthcare Marketing, 7,* 18–28.
6. Ibid.
7. Berkowitz, E. N., & Flexner, W. A. (1978, Fall). The marketing audit: A tool for health service organizations. *Health Care Management Review, 3,* 51–57; Enis, B. M., & Garfein, S. J. (1992, December). The computer-driven marketing audit. *Journal of Management Inquiry,* 306–318; King, W. R., & Cleland, D. L. (1974, October). Environment information systems for strategic marketing planning. *Journal of Marketing, 38,* 35–40; Kotler, P., Gregor, W., & Rodgers, W. (1989, Winter). The marketing audit comes of age. *Sloan Management Review,* 49–62.

CHAPTER 5

STEP 2: CREATING THE MISSION, VISION, AND CRITICAL SUCCESS FACTORS

WHAT YOU WILL LEARN

- Both the vision and mission statements are critical in business planning—and they are different.
- Based on data, visions are created through strategic conversations.
- Mission statements are about what the profession is doing today; vision statements are about what the profession dreams of doing tomorrow.

ESTABLISHING THE CONTEXT

Two 20th-century presidents of the United States provide an excellent instructional case study from which we can understand the role of a vision and a mission in any enterprise. After seeing the Soviet Union make major strides in space exploration, President John F. Kennedy focused the country with a clear vision: "We will be the first to put a man on the moon."[1] This vision was precise, simple to understand, and clear, but at the same time, it was difficult, if not, as some thought, impossible to achieve. President George H. W. Bush, more than 25 years later, had trouble with what he called "the vision thing" and was quickly criticized for a lack of focus and platform. In short, Bush did not have a vision for leading the country. He lost his bid for reelection.

A board of trustees has three principal responsibilities: select a vision, select management, and monitor operating results. The vision should be a robust, interesting, and engaging conversation; it will be one of the most critical and important conversations a board can have. This chapter examines how the strategic plan of an organization comes together and relates

FIGURE 5.1

Step 2: Creating the Mission, Vision, and Critical Success Factors

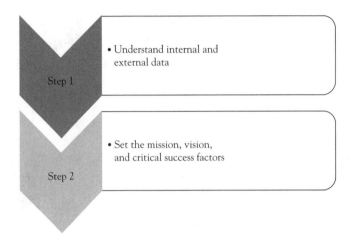

to the various clinical business lines of the organization. Specifically, this chapter explores tools and guidelines on creating meaningful mission and vision statements.

The marketing tools provided in Step 1 serve as a backdrop for the conversations that will be explored in this chapter. Each aspect of the strategic planning process will be based on the availability of robust and meaningful data from which leadership can make insightful decisions. Step 2 (**Figure 5.1**) shows the three key initial elements of a strategic plan built by the senior leadership team.

CONSTITUENT PARTICIPATION

To arrive at a vision and mission statement for a healthcare organization, it is valuable to have input from the various constituencies of the hospital or clinic (**Figure 5.2**).

A difficulty in developing market-based plans in health care is the number of constituencies whose opinions and input must be assessed. These views often differ in direction and intent. Further, some board members will tend to dominate the conversation, while other board members will be reluctant to participate because they do not understand enough about the medical business or they are intimidated by the professional staff. Other board members might not fully understand the importance of the conversation while

FIGURE 5.2

Constituents Who Influence the Planning Process

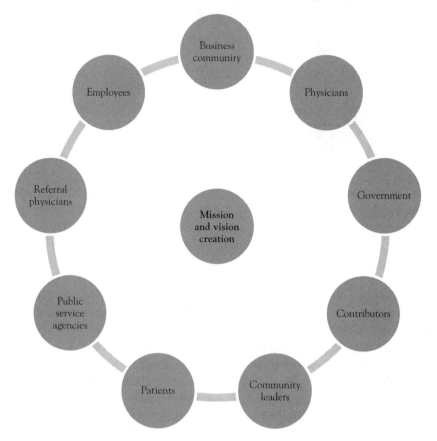

still others might sit on the sidelines early only to disrupt the conversations later on at a critical stage when the plans are at the point of being finalized. Bryson claims that it is important to develop support among key stakeholders and legitimacy for strategic planning before the process begins. He goes on to say, "Every strategic planning effort is in effect a drama that must have a correct setting, themes, plot and sub-plots, actors."[2] Because of the importance of the decisions and the drama that often surrounds the discussion, getting the group to accept responsibility for the task and to take it seriously is an important first step. Allison and Kaye also discuss how critical it is to have identified in advance the reasons for strategic planning.[3] Before the conversations can begin, it is important to make sure that the board understands the importance of the process and that board members are willing to diligently participate. How do we get this to happen?

The first step is to discuss with the participants that setting the vision of the company is one of the most important conversations that the board can ever have and that the decision around the vision will guide business strategy from this point on. Next, it is important to make sure that every board member or executive team member understands that they are expected to participate. If a board member chooses to not participate at all, or chooses to not voice a view, then it is legitimate to ask why that person is a board member at all. Third, it is important to get out in the open the idea that all views are to be respected. This is particularly important when there is a board of community members and medical professionals, as sometimes the community members might feel intimidated to speak. Fourth, discuss rules of engagement for the conversations around expected participation, showing respect for various opinions, and the notion of seeking congruence of thought. It has often been said that "culture eats strategy." If the culture or behavioral environment of the entity is out of balance, it is unlikely that the vision conversation will be maximized.

Finally, in advance of formal strategy conversations, each member should be asked to spend some private time thinking about the following questions in order that he/she begin to appreciate the nature of the strategic conversations that are about to take place:

1. What "business" are we in?
2. What is the likely future of the external environment?
3. What is our most important product/service?
4. Who are our clients/customers?
5. How have we changed in the past 5 years?
6. What are our unique strengths and major weaknesses?
7. What should be the dream of the organization?

The answers to these questions can be both engaging and perplexing, and it will help prepare the board for the conversations they can expect as the process moves forward.

UNDERSTANDING THE DIFFERENCE BETWEEN VISION AND MISSION

Many managers and board members are confused about the vision and mission. Some feel that the two are redundant. But, in fact, they are not redundant at all, and each has a different and clarifying function. The mission is about what an organization does today, and vision is about what an organization will become in the future.

The mission is a statement about why the organization exists now. Campbell and Yeung described it best by saying mission is, "an organization's character, identity, and reason for existence. . . . It provides a rationale for action."[4] Others suggest that there are six important components for a hospital's mission statement, although not all need to be included in a mission statement:

• Target customers and markets
• The principal services delivered
• The geographical area serviced
• The organization's philosophy/values
• The hospital's preferred self-image (or distinctive competence or strength)
• The organization's desired public image[5]

In one study among Canadian hospitals, however, it has been found that mission statements in which specific mention was made to "distinctive competence/strength," "unique identity," and "concern for satisfying customers [patients]," correlated positively with seven outcome measures of financial performance.[6] For example, assume that the core business is the ownership of a community homecare agency. The agency's stated mission is to assist its clients in becoming self-sufficient. That is what the agency does today; it is their mission. But what would the board like the community homecare agency to look like in 10 years? The answer to that question equals the vision of the organization. The vision is an exciting look forward into the future; it attempts to answer the question: What is it that we want to look like or accomplish 5, 10, or 15 years out? For example, a homecare agency's vision for the future might be that no one should ever have to enter a nursing home. That is a future view or vision statement. The difference between the vision and the mission is that the vision is an idealized dream, while the mission is an honest statement of fact about what the agency does today. The mission is set first, and then the vision is established. The next task is to develop specific success factors to help the organization reach the vision. Often the vision will lack any meaningful direction, making it impossible to connect goals to the vision. When this happens, constituents have a difficult time seeing how all the pieces fit together, and they tend to see the visions as just a bunch of words rather than as a road map.

Think about the following vision example. Assume a worldwide food relief organization is called Feed Our Children (FOC) and that every day of the year FOC works on providing food to children in war-ravaged countries. That is their mission, and it is clear. But regarding its vision for the future, there could be several different vision options and each would have different operational implications. For example, FOC's vision could be to see a world free of hunger, or another option could be children free of hunger, or Africa free of hunger, or even America free of hunger. Each of these visions is different, and therefore, each requires different strategies and operational tactics. But on a day-to-day basis, FOC's mission is to feed starving children in war-torn countries—not any specific country, not any specific hunger problem, but simply hunger related to children in countries at war. FOC's vision for the future, however, offers many options including continuing on the same path or moving in other directions as outlined above. Nevertheless, the mission for today is clear, and once they choose a vision for the future, that will also need to be clear. Therefore, reflect back on the first possible vision described above; a *world* free of hunger. While that example might be something we would all love to see, it is probably an unlikely scenario and therefore too big and too broad to help provide the organization with direction. To have an impact, FOC has realized they need to focus. Should FOC have a vision around children in countries at war, or children in Africa, or children in general? What should its vision be? This is an example of the art of strategic thinking and conversation.

How do the mission and vision fit within a company? A one-product company will have one vision and mission that is shared by all employees. In a multi-product clinic, the enterprise will have one vision and mission that encompass the entire organization. But in addition to that, each operating unit will have a mission that indicates exactly what that operating unit is about on a day-to-day basis.

Do the words really make a difference? Most clinics have never discussed what business they are in, why they exist, or what their most important service is. Because they have not had these conversations as a group, it is understandable why so many physicians feel like they are sharing office space, but do not feel like they are really part of a group. Yet, while every member of the medical group has an individual vision of what the group could be, finding the common theme or thread that they can gel around is often a long and difficult process. Although everyone might have his/her own vision, there is not often a clinic-wide vision. To demonstrate that visioning is not just an exercise of words, look at the following examples of vision statements and notice that they are all very different and that they lead an organization in different directions. All are viable, and there is no right or wrong answer:

1. We will be the largest single-site, internal medicine practice in the state.
2. We will be the top-ranked internal medicine practice for quality care.
3. We will have a national reputation for internal medicine research.
4. We will have a 70% market share for all internal medicine patients within our zip code.

Every vision possibility listed above is different and everyone takes the practice in a different direction, making it unlikely that all four options can be achieved. The value in a group-wide vision statement is clarity of direction and the opportunity to get everyone moving in the same direction, versus one person wishing that the group would do more research while someone else thinks that the key is to grow, grow, and grow more.

The difference between mission and vision statements should be very clear: Mission is about what an entity does today, and vision is a clear statement about where it wishes to go in the future.

SHOULD WE CREATE BROAD OR NARROW STRATEGY?

One of the first articles master of business administration (MBA) students are asked to read is about the mission of a business. The article is a classic around which more lectures, case studies, and board presentations have been made than have probably been discussed on any other singular *management* topic. The article, entitled "Marketing Myopia," is by Professor Theodore Levitt; it was first published in the *Harvard Business Review* in 1960 and has been reprinted many times since.[7] This article is as fresh today as when it was first published. It asks the simple question: What business are you in? The article discusses examples of business organizations that defined themselves too narrowly and therefore missed opportunities as the needs of the marketplace changed. Levitt's major example is the railroad industry. He argues that railroads thought of themselves as being in the railroad business and not in the transportation business. Just think of what might have happened to the railroads if their mission had been about transportation—not just railroads (see **Figure 5.3**). Maybe it would

FIGURE 5.3

Railroads versus Transportation—Thinking Narrow or Broad

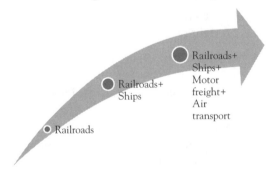

have been Penn Central Transportation Company leading us to the moon or delivering packages anywhere, anytime, within 24 hours guaranteed!

So it is with health care. Some health organizations have created a rather narrow approach to their business, while others have created strategies that are very broad, including clinics, hospitals, research, and the management of device patents (see **Figure 5.4**).

Some hospitals, clinics, and nursing homes, for example, can be myopic in their thinking about their mission, believing that they are in the business of only operating an inpatient setting for sick people, or just a medical clinic. In reality, most of these organizations are providing broader services, such as home visits, disease-specific counseling, and family-support systems. **Figure 5.5** shows a typical example of a narrow versus broad strategy concept using pediatrics as the narrow clinical service.

Along with a limited mission comes myopic thinking regarding future options for the organization. As a business matures, a narrow mission can restrict the examination of opportunities for growth. For example, banks cannot afford to be in banking; they must be in financial services in order to grow in their complex marketplace. Medtronic is not in the pacemaker business; it is in the medical device business. But by the same token, Medtronic is not so broad as to say they are in the "healthcare business" or "hospital-supply business." In other words, while Medtronic has a reasonably broad business line, it is still a line of business within the healthcare

FIGURE 5.4

Examples of Range of Healthcare Strategies

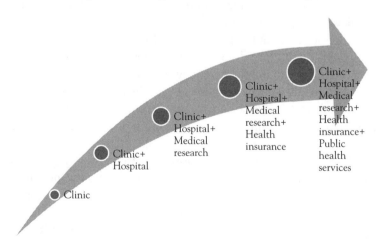

FIGURE 5.5

Narrow to Broad Strategy

Narrow strategy
We provide pediatric
service to our community.

Broad strategy
We provide health and
wellness to the region.

device sector. Additionally, within the device sector, it has grown not only in the cardiac area, but also in neuroscience, and it is working in areas such as Alzheimer's and Parkinson's disease.[8]

Nevertheless, since Levitt wrote "Marketing Myopia" in 1960, management research and thinking have evolved.[9] While the question of "what business are you in?" is important, one should not interpret Levitt's work as a license to create an unrealistic, improbable, or less-than-honest view of what the organization actually does or could do in the future. Most prominent management thinkers would suggest that successful companies have a focused capability or driving force. Porter argues that successful firms concentrate on a very narrow set of differentiating factors that become critical to the organization's success. Raynor calls this the concept of strategic purity.[10] Simply stated, the more focused or pure the strategy, the greater the likelihood of success. Hospitals, for example, are generally good at providing patient care, but not as skilled at developing public health policy, managing community health issues, or creating new medical devices. Therefore, when stating a clinic's strategy, the balance is around being honest about what the clinic does: having enough flexibility to move in new directions without being so broad that the organization has no sense of reality and no clear, driving, focused skill.

We have already stated that clinics or railroads, for example, might have a strategy that is either narrow or broad or somewhere in between. Levitt argued that it would have been in the best interest of the railroad industry to have a broader view and to have a strategy that said it was in transportation, not just railroads. A hospital strategy that is about health care provides many possible options, as Figure 5.4 shows. Indicating, via the mission statement, that the organization is only in the pediatric business narrows its options. However, focusing operations in pediatric care and, therefore, the hospital's clinical care, usually gives pediatric hospitals

FIGURE 5.6

Narrow to Broad Strategy—Range of Service Options

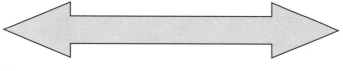

Narrow strategy

We provide pediatric
service to our community.

Broad strategy

We provide health and
wellness to the region.

Narrow services

Pediatric sports medicine
Pediatric chemical dependency
Pediatric surgical care

Broad services

Pediatric medicine
Pediatric chemical dependency
Pediatric sports medicine
Sports medicine
Emergency care
International care
Health classes

a competitive advantage over other hospitals in the area that seem to want to do everything but are known for nothing in particular.

The major rationale for a broad strategy is that the marketplace is always changing and the organization has to be flexible and make room for change. The case for a narrow strategy is that it allows for focus and likely clear clinical dominance in the market. The decision to have a narrow or broad strategy will help decide what product opportunities are available, as visualized in **Figure 5.6**.

But the decision goes deeper than that. As **Figure 5.7** shows, an organization's decisions at the top reflect down to products offered, which indicates customer focus. The less focused the strategy is at the leadership level of the organization, the more the operating units within the organization are left to make tactical and sometimes conflicting decisions.

Strategy is important in deciding whether the vision and mission of the business, the marketing goals, the target market, and the tactics used will be narrow or broad. As indicated early in this chapter, Levitt argued for broad strategy, while more recent observers argue for a narrowed and more precise strategy. As an example, Levitt's article would support being the broad retail business, much like the strategy that Sears has selected. Sears sells electronics, washing machines, and baby clothing. Porter, on the other hand, would suggest a more focused model such as the Best Buy model. Best Buy is in the electronics business, and it is difficult for

FIGURE 5.7

Narrow to Broad Strategy–Target Markets

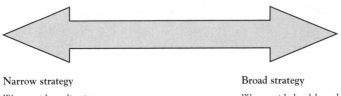

Narrow strategy

We provide pediatric
service to our community.

Broad strategy

We provide health and
wellness to the region.

Narrow services

Pediatric sports medicine
Pediatric chemical dependency
Pediatric surgical care

Broad services

Pediatric medicine
Pediatric chemical dependency
Pediatric sports medicine
Sports medicine
Emergency care
International care
Health classes

Narrow target market

Children under age 16

Broad target market

Children and adults

Sears to sell televisions against Best Buy's focused strategy and perceived greater expertise in service and electronics advice.

The notion of broad versus narrow strategy is something with which organizations constantly wrestle. Regardless of the choice, the core of this issue in health care must be the question of how to deliver value with the strategic option chosen. The provider organization in health care today must provide a leap in value, whether using a broad or niche strategy, to be successful in today's era of transparency. Southwest Airlines was successful to a large degree, not so much in that it was a niche player, but in that it provided a service that made flying almost as inexpensive as driving for many destinations for consumers. In today's strategic framework, some strategists are increasingly referring to this as a "Blue Ocean" perspective.[11] The core of the strategy focus, whether it is niche or mass market, is around value innovation in terms of utility, cost, and price—the three critical drivers in health care today.

Some experts argue that it is best to leave your strategy broad, while others suggest that broad strategy provides little direction, little focus, and little opportunity to carve out a unique niche. With the issue of narrow versus broad strategy ever present in the background, it is time to begin the strategic planning process. The following discussion is based on the assumption that the health organization management team has gathered data (Step 1) and has provided an analysis of that data to the constituencies who will be involved in the strategic conversation(s).

STATING THE MISSION

Placing the mission on a piece of paper should be straightforward—if the management team is willing to be honest about reality. The mission is the first formal starting point, and it is a statement of what the organization does. The mission statement is not about a dream, and it is not a set of feel-good platitudes. It is a statement of current daily reality. One way to check to see if the healthcare organization's board members are being honest with themselves is to see if the mission statement matches the income and expense statement. If, for example, a hospital has a mission statement that says, "We are the catalyst for health and health education," one would expect to see substantial expenditures on the income statement for health education services. However, if the income statement shows that 95% of total expenditures are related to hospital inpatient services, and health education is not even a line item on the income statement, then the mission statement is not accurate.

A mission is simply a statement of fact of what the organization is currently committed to. It is therefore important for a healthcare organization to define as appropriately as possible its general mission without overstating reality. For example, two hospitals may be in the healthcare business, but their missions might be very different. One hospital's mission statement may be rather narrow: to provide health care in an urban setting, operating within a religious framework. The second hospital may have a broader mission statement: to provide healthcare services. These mission statements should reflect a different reality for each entity. As a result of these mission statements, when the first hospital looks at opportunities, it considers only traditional programs in a geographically constrained area. The second hospital's broad mission means that it looks at a range of healthcare services that can be provided in various locations: It uses some space on the hospital grounds for an indoor running track. In addition, after 5:00 p.m., the pool used during the day for physical therapy is available for open swimming. The hospital also hopes to offer a health and exercise program in which its nutritionists provide assistance in dietary planning. The hospital is discussing the possibility of contracting with corporations, as well as with the police and fire departments, to offer this program to their employees. For an additional charge, a physical examination would be included. The hospital also plans to provide support to four primary care physicians who want to open a satellite office in a community where residents expressed a desire for increased accessibility to routine medical care. The two different mission statements point the hospitals in different directions. Both mission statements are honest, and though one is broader than the other, both are within realistic parameters and can be observed and reflected in income and expense statements.

Examples of Different Mission Statement Ideas

The following mission statements are typically not appropriate for hospitals and clinics. This list likely does not reflect the reality of the business for most clinics—unless a clinic is a true community-based organization or wellness clinic—and these statements are also broader than the scope of the core capability of a typical healthcare hospital or clinic:

"We are the leader in community health."
"We exist to help people achieve wellness."
"We stamp out disease in our community."

The following mission statements are more likely appropriate for hospitals and clinics. These statements likely reflect reality, but also give a broader sense of responsibility for "health," and not just procedure-based care. The examples listed below are more focused than the previous examples:

"We provide health services to the population of our county."
"We provide our community with medical and health-related services."
"We provide health-related services for the poor."

There is one more important consideration about the mission of organizations in the not-for-profit world: ethics. When an organization is defining a mission, ethical questions often become an issue. In other businesses, the mission may very well be to dominate a product or technology category and attempt to be the sole source of information, knowledge, or a production methodology. In health care, we are obligated to share new information and spread medical knowledge to others so that all can benefit from new technologies or processes. For example, photodynamic therapy is now available for cancer of the esophagus. It involves injecting a photo sensitive drug that accumulates cancer cells. Then, a laser light is used to trigger a reaction to kill the cancer cells.[12] The results are promising. An entrepreneur could build a multimillion-dollar, worldwide business by monopolizing the technology. But in the not-for profit world, such a business mission would be in conflict with the more conventional and typical not-for-profit healthcare mission that seeks to disseminate and provide wide access to new, lifesaving clinical approaches to everyone, including the competition. In clinical practice, there is debate about treating many different conditions. Prostate surgery is an example. Physicians all practice surgical intervention, radiation, and watchful waiting. As physicians search for the best practice or protocol, the profession demands that they share and publish their results rather than guard their practice secrets so that everyone, regardless of clinical affiliation, can use the best practice.

DEFINING THE VISION

The leadership's decision-making conversation around the vision of the organization is possibly the single most important discussion the board will have, and might be the most difficult. Why? The mission is a statement about what the firm does today, but the vision statement is about where the firm is going in the future. The vision is a future state 5 to 10 or more years out. It is a dream, and therefore might likely represent unchartered territory for the organization. A vision is a vivid image for all stakeholders in the organization to rally around. Typically, the vision is clearly stated in simple terms that the average employee, consumer, or constituent can understand. Furthermore, the vision is specific, comprehensive, and reasonably detailed. Finally, the vision is powerful, compelling, often emotional, and a call to action.

The Kennedy statement is an excellent illustration of a clear and compelling vision: "Achieving the goal, before this decade is out, of landing a man on the moon and returning him safely to earth." In contrast, the Allina Health System (at the time a series of hospitals and Medica Health Plan) vision in 1997 was to be the recognized innovator in improving community health. Clear? Yes. Goal-oriented? Yes. But at that time, Allina spent less than one-half of 1% of its funds on improving community health. Nevertheless, the organization believed deeply that the key to a rational healthcare system in the United States was community-based efforts "upstream" from the health and medical services Allina provided. It was difficult to see how Allina was going to accomplish its vision—just as people said it would be impossible to accomplish Kennedy's vision of putting a man on the moon. Kennedy committed funds for his vision, and Allina did not. Allina's vision failed and the delivery system split apart from the insurance system.

TOOLS TO WORK THROUGH THE VISION CONVERSATION

Given the complexity of healthcare systems and organizations, and the variety of interests of various constituencies, how does an organization work through the process?

Strategy Conversation Tool #1: Checking for Congruence

This is a simple technique to see to what extent the leadership currently has a shared vision and an understanding of the current vision. Using a conference room setting, give each member of the board or leadership team (likely 5–15 people) a 3×5 index card. Without discussion or reminder of the vision the organization might currently have, ask board members to write on the index card what they believe the current vision is—not what it should be, but what it actually is currently. When everyone has finished writing on the card, ask one person to read his/her card and to then tape the card on a wall or white board. Then ask another person to read his/her card, and if the card is significantly different from the first, place that card on the same wall, but maybe 3 feet away from the first card. At this point, do not have discussion around who is right or wrong, or any judgments around good or bad ideas. Instead, the group is simply working to get all the thoughts on the table. Continue the process around the room, allowing each person to read his/her card and then place the card on the board next to other like cards, or if significantly different, in a new area.

When the process is completed, the group should be able to make several observations. First, the group will be able to identify the extent to which the leadership can articulate a vision at all. Second, the group will be able to see the extent to which there is currently congruence around a vision, regardless of whether or not it is the published version. Third, the group will be able to visualize the variety of thoughts around different visions or different directions that leadership at the table believes the organization is moving in. Remember, the exercise is to have each person articulate the current vision of the organization—that is, to say the direction that the person believes the organization is now moving. Upon completion of the exercise, if the index cards were found to be clustered around several different concepts, it would indicate that the clinic leadership does not currently have a common vision or direction for the organization.

Criteria for a Strong Vision

Good vision statements share some common features. First, a good vision statement represents a dream and future direction. As one practical Midwestern healthcare executive would say to his team, "Do we dream of going to Seattle or flying to London?" Second, the statement is usually 5 to 10 or more years out. Third, as much as possible, the vision should have some detail, like a picture that would help people see what the future would look like. Fourth, the vision should clearly reflect how the organization's passion, belief, or core value adds to the community. Regarding this point, if the passion is quality, then the obvious question will be: How are we intending to live the passion of quality? How will patients be able to discern the passion? If the vision is about quality, then will the hospital, for example, only accept board-certified doctors to the medical staff, or will the medical staff give surgical privileges to doctors with demonstrated certifications and satisfactory outcome performance? And, finally, some suggest the vision statement should be measurable as a reflection of quality—for example, "100% of the doctors will be board certified," or, "we will be in the top 5% of the state in terms of clinical outcomes."[13] One test of an organization's seriousness around its vision statement is whether the organization is willing to live the words, even if it means letting go of some physicians on the staff, or rejecting a pet project of a long-standing board member because it no longer fits with the vision.

Using the Data to Guide Discussion

An environmental assessment and actual data about the reality of the organization's situation should now be brought forward as the formal discussions begin on setting or reestablishing the vision. Questions like what the economic health of the community is, what the clinic's market share is, whether the community is leaving town for services that we offer, whether it is likely that people will be able to evaluate our care versus others', and whether our business will continue to be profitable are all examples of data that should be reviewed and discussed. The board might look at literally hundreds of different data points or facts, but at the same time it is useful to distill the facts down to what the management and board believe are the dozen or so key data points that will be most relevant in the future. Usually the key facts will include, at a minimum:

1. Market share trends
2. Community growth trends
3. Historical financial performance
4. Customer opinions
5. Broad changes in the general environment

Once the team has looked at the data and distilled the facts, it is time to begin the vision-setting conversation.

Strategy Conversation Tool #2: The Nominal Group Process

After discussing the data, the next task is to begin to frame what the medical clinic or hospital system might look like well into the future. The goal is to be as specific as possible. With several community and medical leaders at the table, it is sometimes difficult to have a balanced conversation. One person might dominate with her thoughts, while the best ideas are kept silent by the most insightful person because he is uncomfortable speaking in a larger group. Professor Delbecq and Andrew Van de Ven from the University of Wisconsin studied these issues and pioneered a method of conversation called the Nominal Group Process.[14] It is designed to:

1. Deal with complex conversations
2. Get many ideas on the table quickly
3. Force participation from everyone and balance the conversation without bias

The general overview of this process is presented here.

To begin the vision process, assemble the group around a table for a conversation with a planned time of about 2 hours. Each person will need a blank sheet of paper and pencil. It is assumed that the members are familiar with the organization's data, but if that is not the case, some time should be used at the outset of the meeting to review the core facts that the organization has agreed on. The leader for the session will remind the group that there are no right or wrong answers and that the purpose of the meeting is to generate thoughts and ideas. It is not a goal to create a final vision during this session. In fact, the vision conversation may continue for many months as the organization looks at options and moves toward a final view. This meeting is about understanding options and getting an early read on possible directions that the organization could take.

The leader begins the meeting by indicating that there are no right or wrong answers and that everyone's view is important and will be required. Then the leader frames the conversation topic around which everyone will concentrate for the next 2 hours. Usually the vision topic for this meeting is as follows: "As you look into the future 10 years from now, list on your paper the elements that you think could describe what the organization should look like or be known for."

Each person is then asked to write on his/her own page brief phrases about what he/she thinks the business will look like in the future. The group is given 10–15 minutes to complete this individual work without discussion, and it would be normal for each participant to have 10–20 items on his/her individual list. When the individual work is completed, the task is to get all of the ideas in front of everyone.

The leader will start at one side of the room and ask the first person to mention one of his/her ideas. That idea is then transcribed by the leader onto a board or flip chart with a corresponding number and with enough space for 30–100 different thoughts. After the first item has been placed on the chart paper, the person sitting next to the first person is asked to mention one of his/her ideas, and that is placed on the chart paper and numbered as item 2. The process continues to the next person and the next until every person around the table has given his/her first thought. If there are 15 people at the table, there will be 15 thoughts on the chart paper. At this point, two observations are important. First, there is no discussion or comment on any of the ideas. All ideas are considered equally. Second, everyone participates; in fact, participation in this process is forced. It is an orderly process going around the table allowing and, indeed, forcing everyone to offer a thought.

After everyone has offered his/her first thought, the leader starts the process again and continues to add to the list using the same method that was used in the first round. After the second round, the leader will start over again for a third round. At some point, a participant will have no new ideas that are not already on the flip charts. The leader will indicate that that person has exhausted his/her list and the leader will move on to the next person and will keep moving around the table in an orderly fashion until all thoughts have been exhausted. Once that has happened, all of the ideas on the flip chart will represent all of the ideas in the room. Some thoughts will make sense, while others may not. But all ideas are considered, and all thoughts are displayed on the chart or board. Examples of thoughts from the group might look like the following:

1. We will be the biggest hospital in the town of Sidney.
2. We have 95 doctors on staff.
3. One hospital, 5 clinics.
4. We will have a clinic in Lodi.
5. We will have top quality.
6. A new obstetrics wing.
7. Earn $1 million a year.
8. Known for wellness.

This would continue on for 85 more items, for example.

The next step is to turn the attention of the group to the flip chart and to clarify the list. The leader will move down every item on the list and ask the group if the item is clear. Does the group understand, for example, what item 1 means, then item 2, and so on? Next, the group will look for duplication of items. For example, if item 12 looks like item 54 and the person who put item 54 on the list agrees, then item 54 is crossed off the list. During this process, the group is in conversation to understand the meaning of each item, but the items are not debated as good or bad, right or wrong. What is likely to happen is that the group can become aware of all the different options and can begin to broaden its perspective. This clarifying conversation might take 30 to 45 minutes to complete.

Once the list has been clarified, it is time for a preference vote. It should be noted that up until now, there has been no grandstanding for a particular view, and there is no allowance to give a particular person or point of view a chance to grandstand or influence the group. The underlying assumption of the nominal group process is that all of the participants have a value at the table, and the idea at this point is to get a balanced and unbiased perspective. Each person is now given five dot stickers, and all participants are asked to go up to the flip-chart paper and place one dot by each of their top five choices that they could see as part of a vision for the organization. Everyone votes at the same time. Once the voting is finished, the list of 30–100 items will likely narrow to 5–10 items that get the most votes, and the participants will immediately begin to get a visual sense of direction. The leader will write those 5–10 concepts on a new flip-chart page, and the group can now begin to have a more focused conversation. From this point on, the focusing and fine-tuning process can require many months of study, conversation, and debate, with the ultimate goal of establishing a draft vision.

Strategy Conversation Tool #3: Dots and Votes

Once the Strategy Tool #2 Nominal Group Process is completed, the organization has a better sense of possible alternative strategies. The alternatives might be very divergent, and therefore there might be many passionate conversations. But the idea is to use tools to keep the conversation balanced, allowing for alternative views without domination by one group member or another and recognizing that the goal is congruence. At the conclusion of the nominal group session, the result was a list of 5–10 possible directions or ideas. More can be added, but at a minimum at this point in the process there should be some sense of a range of thinking.

At the next conversation(s), which may be weeks or months away, the idea is to present the conclusion from the nominal group discussion. Show the list of 5–10 possible items. Devote a 5- to 10-minute conversation to each item. Check to see if something is missing or if there is new information. Then give everyone 3 sticker dots. Have each person go up to the chart and place a dot (votes) next to the items each member is most passionate about. Using this process continues to allow all participants to have an equal opportunity to express their views. Once that process is completed, check again for congruence, narrowing and further understanding. Is the team moving in the same direction? If not, seek more discussion, review the data, seek clarity of opinion, and be prepared to vote again at this or a future session. Recognize that what we are trying to accomplish, using these techniques, is to seek a leadership view and ultimate direction for the company that is generally supported by the leadership constituencies.

Strategy Conversation Tool #4: Define and Refine

As the organization moves closer to a vision concept, it is time to draft a vision and distribute the proposed draft to each participant. Review the draft together and make sure everyone understands the concepts and the words. Then, ask each participant to work alone and to cross out any words on the proposed vision he/she does not like and circle the words on the vision that are particularly powerful. Collect the individual pieces of paper and on a large flip-chart page tally the results. Usually the group will be able to see areas of conflict and areas of agreement. Again, using this method, the team should be moving toward a common understanding and clarification of direction.

Strategy Conversation Tool #5: A Model Vision Statement Outline Format

As the vision is coming into focus, the following model is a tool designed to help organizations move as far as possible in the vision-setting process. Achieving this level of precision might be difficult for many organizations based on factors such as community, competitors, and internal issues. For example, board members might feel uncomfortable making available this level of detail to the general public. However, in the case of a privately owned clinic, this model can work very well as a way for all of the partners in the group to understand what the direction is.

The fill-in-the-blanks–style vision contained in **Exhibit 5.1** provides for all of the essential elements of a good, robust vision. This model communicates who we are, what we will look like in the future, what our specific competency is, and what we will be known for. It might not be possible for an organization to fill in all of the elements listed in Exhibit 5.1, but the exhibit provides a model of best practice in vision thinking.

Strategy Conversation Tool #6: Reality Check

Once the participants have created a proposed new vision, it can be tested by asking the leadership team to discuss two questions. First, ask the group what activities could be carried out under the umbrella of the vision statement. If the list is long, the focus might be too broad, or if the list is small, the focus could be too narrow. The second question is: "What strategies or ideas would we not explore because of what our vision says?" A good vision will give the organization guidance around what it could be doing in the future and what it would not pursue. The vision statement that has been crafted should readily provide guidance in both directions.

EXHIBIT 5.1

Model Vision Statement Platform Example*

Vision Statement for _____ [*organization name*]

By_____ [*year*] the _____ [*name of organization*] will concentrate on_____ [*type of care, i.e., hospital, medical, group practice,
health*]. We will have _____ [*number of facilities*] including _____
[*special services*]. We will have _____ [*mix of providers*]. Within
the marketplace we will provide excellent care, but in addition we will be
known for our capability in _____ [*special skill, competitive advantage*]. Our total revenue will be _____ with a margin of _____ %,
and we will see an annual growth rate of _____ %.

*This example is a template for a medical clinic group.

WHAT SHOULD A GOOD VISION STATEMENT LOOK LIKE?

The goal is to create a picture of what the enterprise will look like at some
point in the future. As in photography, an out-of-focus picture is not good,
while a clear, sharp picture is great.

The following are examples of vision statements that are not usually
helpful.

Example: We will be an area leader in quality health care.
Problem: This is a common and generic vision statement. The statement is broad and provides little passion or direction. Further, there is
no hint of who the organization is or what it really does. Is this a health
plan, hospital, or family practice clinic? Is it any wonder organizations
often dread the process of visioning if this loose and generic statement
is the result?

Example: We will provide the highest possible quality of care at the
lowest possible cost.
Problem: The statement might be conflicted. As worded, some might
say that the vision directs the organization to offer PET scans while
others believe that the statement tells them to have nurse-run clinics
in the local grocery store. Does cost mean cost, or does it mean lowest

possible charge to the consumer? Does the Ritz-Carlton Hotel chain ever suggest that it can be the lowest possible cost?

Example: We will be a world-class healthcare system.

Problem: This is an actual vision statement from a rural hospital with one family practice medical doctor and weekend emergency room call coverage. The hospital is located in a mining, timber, and agriculture area. While this could be part of a vision statement for a research, university, or large teaching center, it is not realistic for this community and therefore provides no honest strategic guidance or meaning to the organization's leadership. A better strategy statement might be, "Do our best and refer the rest."

The following vision statements are better.

Example: Andrew Hospital will continue to be a not-for-profit provider committed to meeting the medical needs of our community. We will provide patient care, and we will expand our efforts in cardiac medical research and medical education for primary care doctors and nurses. We will be known as the best provider of medical quality in our community by the year 2020, as indicated by the clinical outcome measure standards utilized by the Centers for Medicare and Medicaid in terms of being in the top 5% in the state.

Comment: With this statement, the leadership knows that the hospital will be involved in research and education around a specific focus. It is also clear that the organization understands that it sees itself as a medical care organization, and it is not focused on healthy community issues or public health concerns. This is not to say that this statement is right or wrong, but we can say that the statement belongs to and gives the Andrew Hospital direction.

Example: To be the healthcare provider of choice in our service area by leading in quality, access, and service.

Comment: Rochester, Minnesota is a community of 85,000 people, and the town is known as the home of the Mayo Clinic. The clinic's influence is everywhere, dominating the skyline, the employment base, the hotels, housing, and the airport. Unlike the Cleveland Clinic, or Johns Hopkins Medicine in Baltimore, Maryland, or MD Anderson Cancer Center in Houston, Texas, Rochester sits in a rural area with bluffs and farm fields less than 15 minutes from the vast complex of the Mayo Clinic's medical facilities. In the middle of this community, so obviously dominated by the Mayo Clinic, is the Olmsted Medical

Center. The not-for-profit Olmsted Medical Center is an interesting organization with a hospital of more than 60 beds, 60 physicians, and a dozen fully staffed area clinics, including quick-stop facilities. The organization continues to thrive. Its vision statement is realistic and forward thinking: The Olmsted Medical Center wants to be the hospital of choice for the locals, and it intends to lead in quality, access, and service. It is not focused on price, not on the wider region, not wellness, not tertiary care. It intends to be the local leader in quality, access, and service. The vision is future oriented, and a bit of a stretch given that it is surrounded by the Mayo Clinic, and yet realistic in terms of what its strength can be.

CRITICAL SUCCESS FACTORS

Once a vision has been agreed upon, the entity can begin to figure out how to achieve it. What are those key actions that will determine if the vision can be achieved? These are called *critical success factors*. Critical success factors are those three to four elements that, as a result of the vision decision, become an absolute critical focus of the organization. What exactly must the organization concentrate on over the life of the vision if it is to succeed? If the organization has decided to focus on quality, then it stands to reason that a critical success factor for the vision is an immersion in quality learning, quality processes, data analysis, and investment in information systems and decision support. Once again, focus is key, and usually firms will work on three to four clear critical success factors. For example, FedEx has a critical success factor revolving around improving the speed of delivery of a package, Google focuses on search engine expansion, and Walmart focuses on cutting cost. The tendency in health care is to have a host of critical success factors that often overwhelm managers and make it difficult to truly understand what is absolutely critical if the organization is to achieve the vision. The best strategy is to have superior execution around a small list of factors.

Focused organizations will typically have three or four critical success factors. If they start to have seven or more, it is much more likely that the strategic plan will not be accomplished under the weight of too many initiatives. At the same time, each critical success factor will have several measurable goals designed to support the critical success factor to which it relates. Therefore, the organization will end up with a clear mission that identifies its actual focus today, a vision of the future, and ideally three to four critical success factors that, if accomplished, will make the vision a success—and, in turn, each critical success factor is supported by a group of precise, measurable goals. **Figure 5.8** shows how the major elements of the strategic plan fit together.

FIGURE 5.8

How the Building Blocks Fit

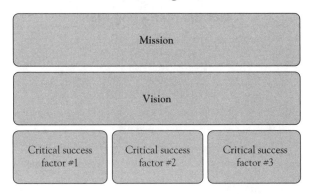

WHAT NEXT? WHO DOES WHAT?

At this point in the process, the team should now be clearly focused and understanding of its mission, vision, and the key critical success factors that are required to execute the vision—which are, in reality just a handful of elements. At this point in the strategic management of the organization, on a day-to-day basis the process begins to move on two tracks. The first track is the strategic one. On this track, senior management will have goals and tactics around the vision to help move the organization, over time, to accomplish the vision of the organization. At the same time, each business entity or product line will have its own business plan along with its goals and tactics to accomplish its targets. As stated earlier, the business plan targets should be compatible with strategic plan and vision goals so that even though multiple people are working on multiple strategies, the strategic and business plans are, in fact, working in concert with one another.

Once the strategy is in place with its own goals and tactics, we can begin to consider the marketing and business plan. Strategic plans and their goals are about the long-term direction of the organization. The marketing plan and business plan are about the daily activities of the organization. The marketing plan takes its cues from the strategic plan, as diagramed in **Figure 5.9**.

When completed, the strategic plan will have goals and specific tactics designed to guide the organization to achieve its long-term vision. The strategic plan is also useful to the marketing plan to provide direction so that the marketing plan is not in conflict with the long-term goals of the clinic.

FIGURE 5.9

The Relationship Between the Strategic Plan
and the Marketing Plan

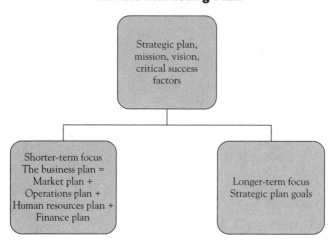

SUMMARY

The strategic process outlined in this chapter contains the basic elements required in any strategic plan. Different consultants might have different slides and models and might use different terms, but the outcome remains the same. High-performing organizations have a solid understanding of their mission, a clear sense of direction through their vision, and a handful of critical factors that the organizations know are required if they hope to reach their vision. From the critical success factors, strategic planning goals are established. At the same time, the strategic plan provides guidance to the marketing plan that is oriented toward the short run. Ultimately, the marketing plan and complete business plan will also have their own set of precise and more short-term goals and targets.

Is strategic planning really all that important? Bain and Company, a highly respected business consulting firm, has been tracking the ebb and flow of the use of business tools since 1993. It has tracked the importance of tools like change management, the balanced scorecard, and core competencies, as well as 23 other tools. While some tools come and go, strategic planning and mission/vision work has remained at the top of the list of important tools from 1993 to today as reported in a survey of executives.[15] Only in 2008 and 2010 did benchmarking eclipse strategic planning, and that was because of the severe recession that caused executives to focus more on cost-management issues. In successful boardrooms, strategic planning is a focal point that is taken very seriously. As health care is forced to confront new models of delivery and cooperation, such as accountable care organizations (ACOs), strategic planning takes on an increasingly important role.

This process is not complete—it never is. The vision will be used to help monitor results on a regular basis. Every 12 to 18 months, it is normal to double-check the vision to see if, in light of new data and environmental changes, it is necessary to take another look and refresh our thinking.

General Strategic Planning Checklist

1. Is the mission broad enough and does it provide enough flexibility so that changes can be made as required? At the same time, is the mission specific and clear?
2. Have all important constituencies had an opportunity to provide input for or comment on the mission?
3. Has the organization worked through possible alternative operating plans to see how the mission might be applied? Specifically, does the mission provide guidance as to which types of plans are acceptable?
4. Does the mission statement answer the question: What business are we in?
5. Do the constituencies understand the vision (the dream) of the organization?
6. Is the vision set well into the future?
7. Is the vision exciting?
8. Is the vision difficult to achieve, yet possible to achieve?
9. Is the vision compelling and worthwhile?
10. Is the vision statement a useful guidepost?
11. Do the goals specify measurable outcomes and time frames?
12. Do the goals reflect the important operating needs of the company?
13. Are the critical success factors clear and precise?
14. Does the entire leadership team understand, with precision, the strategy of the organization?

QUESTIONS FOR DISCUSSION

1. What are current examples of myopic thinking in health care?
2. Can a multi-specialty hospital or clinic have a focused competitive advantage?
3. Why do healthcare strategic plans often seem overwhelming in scope and expectation? What can be done to manage the scope of the plan?
4. Many strategic plans lack financial underpinning. Why?

NOTES

1. John F. Kennedy, Speech to the American people, May 25, 1961.
2. Bryson, J. M. (2004). *Strategic planning for public and nonprofit organizations* (3rd ed.). New York: John Wiley & Sons.
3. Allison, M., & Kaye, J. (2005). *Strategic planning for nonprofit organizations* (2nd ed.). New York, NY: John Wiley & Sons.
4. Campbell, A., & Yeung, S. (1991). Brief case: Mission, vision, and intent. *Long Range Planning, 24*(4), 145–147.
5. Ginter, P. M. Swayne, L. M., & Duncan, W. J. (1998). *Strategic management of health care organizations* (3rd ed.). Malden, MA: Blackwell Business.
6. Bart, C. K., & Tabone, J. C. (1999, Summer). Mission statement content and hospital performance in the Canadian not-for profit health care sector. *Health Care Management Review, 24*(3), 18–29.
7. Levitt, T. (1960, July–August). Marketing myopia. *Harvard Business Review*, 45–56.
8. One company two cultures. (1966, January 22). *Business Week*, 88.
9. Porter, M. (1987, May–June). From competitive advantage to corporate strategy. *Harvard Business Review*, 43–59; Robert, M. (2006). *The new strategic thinking, pure and simple.* New York: McGraw-Hill.
10. Raynor, M. (2007). *The strategy paradox.* New York: Doubleday.
11. Kim, W. C., & Mauborgne, R. (2005). *Blue Ocean strategy: How to create uncontested market space and make competition irrelevant.* Cambridge, MA: Harvard Business School Press.
12. A ray of hope for cancer patients. (1996, June 10). *Business Week*, 104.
13. Kaplan, R. S., Norton D. P., & Barrows, Jr., E. A. (2008). *The executive premium: Linking strategy to operations for competitive advantage.* Cambridge, MA: Harvard Business School Press
14. Delbecq, A. L., & Van de Ven, A. H. (1971, July/August). A group process model for problem identification and program planning. *Journal of Applied Behavioral Science, 7*(4), 466–492. Delbecq, A. L., Van de Ven, A. H., & Gustafson, D. H. (1975). *Group techniques for program planners.* Glenview, IL: Scott Foresman and Company; p. 11.
15. Rigby, D. K. (2010, December 13). *Management tools 2011: An executive's guide.* Boston, MA: Bain and Company.

FURTHER READING

Morrison, I. (2000). *Health care in the new millennium.* San Francisco: Jossey-Bass.

CHAPTER 6

STEP 3: THE STRATEGY/ACTION MATCH

WHAT YOU WILL LEARN

- Environmental and organizational data relate directly to strategy options.
- Different strategies fit varying market conditions.

PERSPECTIVES ON STRATEGY

Once Steps 1 and 2 have been completed, it is time to build your strategy. Many managers move immediately to this step (diagrammed in **Figure 6.1**), overlooking the importance of Steps 1 and 2 entirely. Typically, they call the marketing staff with the following question: "I would like to involve you in a strategy to help our orthopedics program; could you help us put together a brochure that we can send out to doctors about the program?" Many managers think that this is marketing. It is not. Furthermore, this type of question implies not only that Steps 1 and 2 were not followed, but also that strategy was not discussed either. A tactic (the brochure) was discussed, not strategy.

This chapter presents the concept of strategy from a marketing point of view. Strategy tradeoffs, the progression from strategy to tactics, and the marketing tools used to achieve strategic objectives are examined.

Management experts have advanced several strategies and models to help businesses conceptualize problems related to mission, growth, and competition. Consider the following examples of such strategies.

FIGURE 6.1

Step 3: Strategy/Action Match and Setting Marketing Objectives

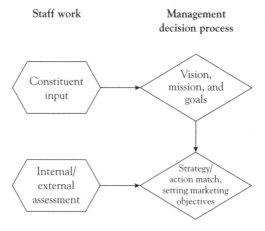

Cost versus Differentiation Strategy

Noted strategist Michael Porter believes strategic advantage can take only two forms—either a cost advantage (not to be confused with discount pricing) or a differentiation advantage. A cost advantage is a delivery system that is more efficient than the current standard or some other means of providing opportunities for significant profit margins in comparison with competitors.[1] An alternative strategic option is to search for a differentiation or a unique selling proposition. The key to a sound differentiation strategy is creating a unique advantage that can be sustained over time. Differentiation for a healthcare organization can be obtained through such features as convenience, unconditional service guarantees, better hours, more nursing care, quick follow-up, better technology, better information, an on-site hotel for families, automatic callbacks to patients, more equipment, or board-certified staff.

Meeting Customer Needs

Ohmae emphasized that strategy is not beating the competition, but meeting the needs of customers.[2] Ohmae noted that although organizations must always be mindful of the competition, they cannot waste time just trying to match their competitors. The real battle is searching for new ways to solve customer problems. For example, Yamaha studied what people did with their pianos. It found that most people did nothing! It takes many years of practice to learn to play the piano, and many consumers are not willing to invest the time and effort. Therefore, Yamaha developed a sophisticated and sensitive concert-style player-piano disk that can be retrofitted to the 40 million pianos that the company had already sold. It made it possible for people to have concert-style sound and get use from their pianos; Yamaha solved a big problem.

What can referral doctors do for their referral sources? A family practitioner who sends a patient to a specialist becomes a customer of that specialist even though, for the most part, the specialist's practice is an extension of the family practice. The specialist can affect the reputation of and the respect that patients have for the family doctor. Furthermore, the family doctor wants not only to maintain the respect of the patient, but also to be viewed as part of the team. In order to maintain a good relationship with his or her customer, the family practitioner, the specialist must (1) do a good job technically, and (2) position the family doctor as the ultimate team coordinator in the eyes of the patient. One small way of accomplishing these tasks, for example, is for a surgeon to send a package of follow-up materials to the family practitioner so that he or she can give them to the patient at the next visit or send it on to the patient. This practice keeps the family doctor feeling involved in the case, positions the family doctor nicely with the patient, and definitely helps solidify the relationship between the practitioner and the specialist. The specialist has created a unique service that exemplifies market-centered strategy: continuously thinking about customers (in this case, the family practitioner) and their needs.

BCG Matrix

The Boston Consulting Group (BCG) designed a matrix that allows managers to examine an entire hospital or company portfolio of services in order to determine which products and services can and should be continued, as well as those that may be eliminated or modified. This model is based on market share and potential growth in the market.

Figure 6.2 shows the BCG matrix, the four alternative quadrants within which to plot products or services. The horizontal axis represents a product's current market share relative to other products with which it is competing. For example, if an organization had a chemical-dependency program with a 15% market share, but two other competitors had much higher market shares, the organization would plot its market share in the right-hand side of the matrix. The vertical axis of the matrix represents the program's growth and the likelihood of continued growth in the future.

FIGURE 6.2

The BCG Matrix

Market share

		High	Low
Growth	*High*	★ Star	? Problem child
	Low	$ Cash cow	— Dog

Source: Reproduced from Henderson, B. (1979). *Henderson on corporate strategy.* Cambridge, MA: ABT Books.

If the organization expects the growth of the chemical-dependency program to be low, it plots the growth potential along the lower portion of the vertical line. Plotting these two items, low market share and low growth potential, places the program in the lower right-hand quadrant, which BCG calls the "dog" quadrant. Products or services in the dog quadrant are going to have a difficult time surviving and, therefore, become likely candidates for elimination or sale.

Programs with a low market share but a high growth potential are called "problem children." The potential growth of an ambulatory-surgery service may be fantastic, even though it may not be achieving the anticipated market share. This kind of service could turn into either a "dog" or a "star."

The upper left-hand quadrant is the "star" quadrant. Products that fall into this category have a high growth potential and a high market share. Stars can be products or services, such as an imaging center. They need to be protected and cultivated to achieve maximum potential. Cash generated by stars should be reinvested in them.

In the lower left-hand quadrant are the "cash cows," which have a high market share but a low growth potential. Usually, this kind of product or service is the mainstay of the corporation, has a long history, but is no longer growing. Such a product is likely to be profitable, but is not considered a "star." Surgery often falls into this category. These services should be maintained, but excess revenue from them should be shifted to develop the "problem children."

The use of this matrix makes it possible to identify and eliminate poor performance areas and to generate business opportunities with high potential in growing markets. The model depends heavily on the notions of relative market share and growth. Although directly relevant in manufacturing firms, these concepts are often less pertinent in service businesses. Growth in market share in manufacturing often means greater efficiency, lower unit cost, and greater profit. In service businesses, where personnel are directly involved in each sale (or interaction), efficiency may or may not occur with growth. And, to a large degree, the classification of services (and products) into any quadrant in the matrix may lead to oversimplification that may well need to be guarded against. For example, placing a service into the cash cow quadrant suggests that one should no longer devote resources into that area. However, it is important to monitor the external environment, which may well lead to a shift in opportunity to spur new revenue streams. Similarly, a dog may not contribute directly to the bottom line, but the cross-subsidization value in a healthcare organization cannot be dismissed.[3]

While there may be limitations to the BCG matrix, the overall conclusion of this planning tool is that it has been useful in initiating corporate planning and strategic change. It is useful as a diagnostic aid more so than a prescriptive guide.[4]

General Electric Model

An alternative to the BCG matrix is the General Electric (GE) model, with which management can evaluate industry attractiveness and business strengths (**Exhibit 6.1**). The GE model makes more explicit comparisons between external opportunities (industry attractiveness) and internal capabilities (business strengths). This approach attempts to overcome the inherent weakness of the BCG matrix in ignoring industry attractiveness factors such as industry competition and profitability, along with the effect of outside forces.[5] Factors relating to industry attractiveness include industry growth, vulnerability to new competitors, profitability, and competitive intensity. Business strengths relate to the following questions: Does this organization have capability and experience in this business? Can the business be integrated into the company's current businesses? Does it make the company more productive? Is it of value to the firm? The goal of this model is to find those businesses and services that show the greatest promise for the organization.

The GE model suggests a host of strategic options according to the position of a service on the basis of the two dimensions: industry attractiveness and business strength. The three cells in the upper left part of the matrix (high attractiveness, strong strength; high attractiveness, average strength; medium attractiveness, strong strength) are positive on both the industry attractiveness and business strength dimensions. As a result, the strategies suggested in these three cells are aggressive. A second set of more

EXHIBIT 6.1

Strategic Options Based on the General Electric Model

		Business Strength		
		Strong	**Average**	**Weak**
Market Attractiveness	**High**	Premium—invest for growth: • Provide maximum investment • Diversify worldwide • Consolidate position • Accept moderate near-term profits • Seek to dominate	Selective—invest for growth: • Invest heavily in selected segments • Share ceiling • Seek attractive new segments to apply strengths	Project refocus—selectively invest for earnings: • Defend strengths • Refocus on attractive segments • Evaluate industry revitalization • Monitor for harvest or divestment timing • Consider acquisition
	Medium	Challenge—invest for growth: • Build selectively on strengths • Define implications of leadership challenge • Avoid vulnerability—fill weaknesses	Prime—selectively invest for earnings: • Segment market • Make contingency plans for vulnerability	Restructure—harvest or divest: • Provide no unessential commitment • Position for divestment or • Shift to more attractive segment
	Low	Opportunistic—selectively invest for earnings: • Ride market and maintain overall position • Seek niches, specialization • Seek opportunity to increase strength (e.g., through acquisition) • Invest at maintenance levels	Opportunistic—preserve for harvest: • Act to preserve or boost cash flow • Seal opportunistic sale or • Seek opportunistic rationalization to increase strengths • Prune product lines • Minimize investment	Harvest or divest: • Exit from market or prune product line • Determine timing to maximize present value • Concentrate on competitor's cash generators

Source: Reprinted from Rausch, B. A. (1982). *Strategic market planning.* American Marketing Association; p. 88.

selective options are those represented on the diagonal from the lower left to the upper right positions. These strategic options involve more selective seeking of niches or segments within the market. The final three cells in the lower right (low attractiveness, average strength; low attractiveness, weak strength; medium attractiveness, weak strength) all suggest a gradual withdrawal from the business line and a reduction of investments. The factors in the nine-cell GE matrix are weighted by management.

Both the BCG matrix and the GE model are useful in making decisions about new business and investment opportunities, but they do not offer hospitals and other healthcare services that are already committed by mission to a service or location ways to solve problems in order to improve.

MAC Model

The Management Analysis Center (MAC)—a Cambridge, Massachusetts–based management consulting firm, since acquired by Capgemini—developed a model that helps a business identify a strategy within the context of its current situation. Called the retail-positioning map, this model concentrates less on new business and more on existing business (**Figure 6.3**). It involves two dimensions: value-added service mix and breadth of product line. Value added refers to features such as hours of service, location,

FIGURE 6.3

Retail Positioning Map

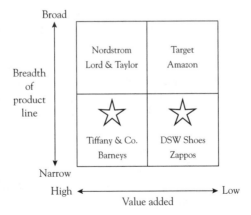

Source: Adapted from Gregor, W. T., & Friars, M. (1983). *Money merchandising.* The MAC Group; p. 00.

credit policy, prestige, schedule system, and telephone follow-up; these factors tend to differentiate one service from another. Breadth of product line describes the number of products and services available. Nordstrom and Lord & Taylor department stores, for example, both have wide product lines with an extensive value-added dimension in the areas of credit options, credit policies, store locations, prestige, and personal service. Target and Amazon might be considered two retailers with broad product lines, but fewer "extras"—thus positioned in the low value-added quadrant. Tiffany & Co. and Barneys are narrow in their product line, but specialize in several value-added features. DSW Shoes and the online retailer Zappos both offer a narrow product line and are low in value-added features.

Although all organizations try to build a loyal base of customers, they do so in different ways. Each method creates a differential advantage for a specific customer group. Sony, for example, decided to compete in a new home gaming market, so it created the PlayStation. Healthcare organizations can also compete differently, often by changing the game rules and creating new products and services to meet market demand. Instead of having a traditional emergency room, a hospital may develop a different, value-added service in order to set itself apart from the competition. A physician housecall service may allow a clinic to compete on an access dimension (i.e., by being more available to the patient). Such a service exists in the triangle area of North Carolina—the group is called Doctors Making Housecalls (http://doctorsmakinghousecalls.com)—and consists of 23 board-certified clinicians who make home visits to be convenient to the patient.

The MAC model suggests that an organization may, by mission, choose to be in the hospital business, but it can select how and within which areas of that business to compete. Most hospitals in a community may rush to be a Bloomingdale's of health care, offering much value-added service in all specialties. When all the competition is instituting this strategy, however, several alternative and profitable options might be available (**Figure 6.4**). Alternatives to the Nordstrom strategy (e.g., the Mayo Clinic) include a high value-added dimension and a narrow product line (e.g., Hospital for Special Surgery in New York City), a low value-added dimension and a narrow product line (e.g., an internist in solo practice), or a low value-added dimension and a broad product line (e.g., an acute care community hospital). Because a hospital or clinic has an opportunity to select market segments that it would like to attract, it can design a package of value-added services and a range of products to appeal to targeted markets. This is often called *field positioning*.

Field positioning is the basis on which a service competes. The elements are selecting the target market segments and the services to be included

FIGURE 6.4

Healthcare Positioning Map

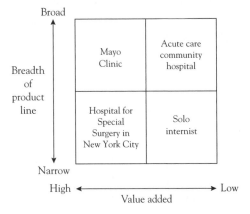

Source: Adapted from Gregor, W. T., & Friars, M. (1983). *Money merchandising.* The MAC Group; p. 00.

in the value-added package. Field positioning involves a variety of strategic decisions, such as how broad or narrow the service line should be, in which market segment or segments to compete, which services to add to the package to make it attractive to a segment, and where to act against the competition. For example, a geriatric hospital has a narrow focus on a specific market segment with a specific specialty; this is a service offered to a single target. In contrast, a medical group organized to make house calls, such as Housecall Doctors Medical Group, which serves the Orange County, Riverside, Los Angeles, and San Bernardino Counties of California (http://housecalldoctorsmedicalgroup.com), has a broad focus; caring for home-bound people, the group offers a broad package of medical care with value-added services that also include several tests such as electrocardiogram, x-ray, echocardiogram, and respiratory analysis. The idea is not to play the field, but to select which markets to capture and where and how to compete by selecting a value-added package and a product line.

DEVELOPING THE STRATEGY/ACTION MATCH

All the models presented thus far are helpful in developing strategic thinking regarding opportunities and problems. One of the difficulties with the models, however, is that they address either what business to be in or what to do within a given business, but not both. The connection between choosing the right business area and deciding what to do within that area is important. Yet, hospital and clinic leadership often had not adequately developed this match—until now. A model that helps determine what business to be in and what to do in each business is needed. This process is called the *strategy/action match*.

Analysis of Lifecycle

The focus of the strategy/action match is on the concept of a product and a marketplace lifecycle. Few concepts in marketing have received such attention. A comprehensive discussion of product lifecycle has been presented by Gardner.[6] Hofer stated that "the most fundamental variable in determining an appropriate strategy is the stage of the product life cycle."[7] Day described the lifecycle as a versatile framework for choosing appropriate strategy alternatives and an aid in directing management attention to the underlying dynamics of a competitive market.[8]

The concept of product lifecycle is based on four key foundational premises:

1. All products (and services) have a limited, defined life.
2. Products pass through four distinct phases, each one presenting different strategy issues and challenges.
3. Profits rise and fall at different stages of the lifecycle.
4. Each stage presents different opportunities and competitive issues for the provider or producer.[9]

Additional research on the nature of the product lifecycle has also found that:

5. At the beginning of the industry, the number of entrants may rise over time, or may peak at the start of the industry and then decline over time.
6. Eventually, the rate of change of the market shares of the largest firms declines and the leadership of the industry declines.[10]

Lifecycle can serve as the normative model by which healthcare managers focus on their internal strategies relative to the external competitive market.

The notion that products, services, and even entire markets all have a lifecycle is the basis for the analysis of lifecycles. **Figure 6.5** shows the typical curve with its four stages of activity. The horizontal line represents time, which could be a matter of months or many years. The vertical line represents growth. Growth may be calculated by sales, revenue, or

FIGURE 6.5

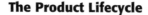

The Product Lifecycle

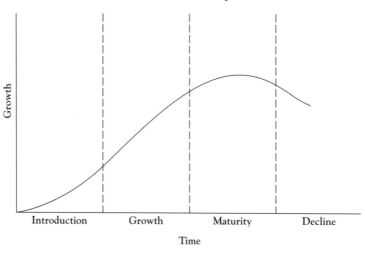

patient days. The first stage in a lifecycle is the *introduction* of a product or service. At this point, sales and revenue are slow. By and large, the market is unaware of the product offering, and primary demand must be developed. When the first urgent-care service opens in a community, for example, the curve rises slowly until people become aware of the facility and how it can be used. In the second stage, *growth*, demand begins to increase, and the size of the total market expands. Often, a competitor enters the market, so that people become more aware of the existence of urgent-care facilities. Having both competitors promote their services creates a synergistic effect on the market. Selective demand develops between the competitors. It has been found that the growth phase is where the number of products or firms entering the market is increasing and there is a rapid increase in supply and demand.[11] In the third stage, *maturity*, demand reaches a plateau. A slight increase occurs as the last potential buyers in the market finally use the urgent-care facility, and loyal buyers continue to return at their average utilization level. Maturity can occur for several reasons other than saturation, however. Demographics, for example, may play a role; in many northern tier communities, pediatrics is in the mature stage as the population ages. In the fourth stage, *decline*, the service begins to lose appeal, and sales drift downward. A new healthcare alternative may have become available.

Figure 6.6 shows the product lifecycle of inpatient care in acute-care hospitals in the United States from 1970 to 2007. The curve shows the rate of hospital discharges from short-stay hospitals per 1,000 population.

FIGURE 6.6

Discharge Rates in Nonfederal Short-Stay Hospitals 1970–2007

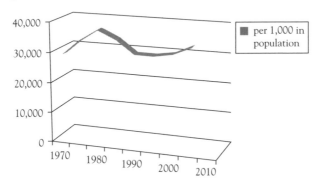

Source: Data from Kozak, L. J., Hall, M. J., & Owings, M. F. (2002, November). National hospital discharge survey: 2000 annual summary with detailed diagnosis and procedure data. Department of Health and Human Services. *Vital and Health Statistics, 13*(153), 7; Hall, M. J., DeFrances, C. J., Williams, S. N., Golosinskiy, A., & Schwartzman, A. (2010, October 26). National hospital discharge survey: 2007 summary Department of Health and Human Services. *National Health Statistics Reports, 29*, 7.

This discharge rate removes the effect of changes in price and changes in the size of overall market. The curve shows a classic product lifecycle for inpatient care through the mid-2000 decade. However, now as the population is aging, inpatient care has begun to rise again and may see a renewed lifecycle, although how long and significant it will be remains to be seen, as other factors can impact its volume, such as technology to provide more intensive care on an outpatient basis as well as to be able to monitor patients more easily in their own homes.

Some products, such as Pet Rocks, parlor games, and first-generation computed tomography (CT) scanners, went through the lifecycle quickly as other products, services, or technologies replaced them. Others, such as passenger trains, tuberculosis hospitals, polio treatment, and some respiratory therapy, went through at a much slower pace. Still others seem to run through the lifecycle only to recover; Arm & Hammer baking soda, for example, recovered through the invention of new uses (e.g., as a powder for brushing teeth, as a refrigerator freshener, and as a carpet deodorizer). Mental health matured on an inpatient basis, but saw new growth in the form of outpatient mental health programs. Similarly, DVD technology replaced VCRs, and now as cable streams movies on demand as well as with the increasing technology of Internet-based access by companies such as Netflix, the product lifecycle of DVDs may be significantly shortened.

FIGURE 6.7

Intuitive Surgical's Product Lifecycle

da Vinci surgical robot unit sales

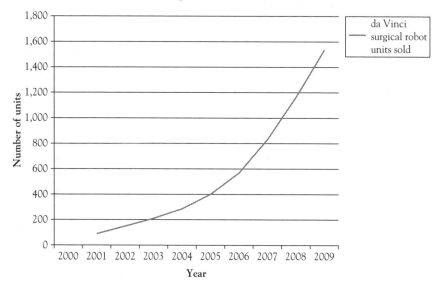

Source: Data from Intuitive Surgical announces $12.1 million first quarter revenue; 12 da Vinci Systems sold; quarter solid highlighted by FDA thorascopic clearance. *Intuitive Surgical: Press Release*. Retrieved June 3, 2010, from: http://investor.intuitivesurgical.com/phoenix.zhtml?c=122359&p=irol-newsArticle&ID=169636&highlight=12.1%20million; da Vinci™ Surgical System. *Robotic Surgery*. Retrieved June 3, 2010, from: http://biomed. brown.edu/Courses/BI108/BI108_2005_Groups/04/davinci.html; Bregel, E. (2010, March 8). Robotic medical arms race. *Timesfreepress.com*. Retrieved June 3, 2010, from: http://www.timesfreepress.com/news/2010/mar/08/robotic-medical-arms-race/.

The concept of the product lifecycle is useful in that it helps managers anticipate what is likely to happen in the future, including when competitors may enter the arena, and it provides insights into pricing changes. In addition, the analysis of lifecycles underscores the fact that as new products and services are developed, other products and services mature or decline; **Figure 6.7** shows the product lifecycle of Intuitive Surgical's da Vinci robot, which is still in the growth stage of the lifecycle. There are competitors at this stage, including Integrated Surgical Systems, which manufactures ROBODOC, and Renishaw, which has developed neuromate, an image-guided surgical robot.

Externalities can affect the lifecycle of any product or service, as shown in **Figure 6.8**, which depicts the lifecycle of imaging technologies from 1993 through 2009. The growth of unit sales of CT and magnetic resonance imaging (MRI) scanners was dramatic for a 10-year period from 1993 through 2003 (the introduction and growth phase of the lifecycles). Many factors were cited for this growth: the training of new young physicians, the high-technology culture of medicine, fear of malpractice, and patient demands for imaging technology. However, another important factor was the financial incentive for physicians to refer patients for imaging on equipment they acquired or in which they had a direct financial ownership interest, termed "self-referral."[12] While the federal government passed the Stark II law in 1991 preventing certain fraud and abuse aspects, it continued to allow for "in-office ancillary service exceptions," such as imaging.

To respond to this provision, manufacturers developed a second version of CT and MRI machines that were less expensive than the $1 million investments historically required for imaging devices. This exception allowed physicians to purchase such technology, and the lifecycle curve took off, as shown in Figure 6.8. To slow the cost that was rapidly occurring, the federal government passed the Deficit Reduction Act in 2005, as shown in the Figure 6.8. It required lower payments for the technical component of imaging exams (for MRIs this was a 20–40% reduction in fees; for CT exams it was smaller—in the range of 25%—but still a major cut). The full effect of the cuts took place in 2007, as shown in Figure 6.8, and Medicare's

FIGURE 6.8

The Effect of Externalities on the Product Lifecycle: The Case of Scanning Technologies

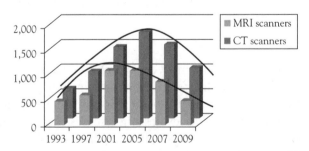

Source: Adapted from Hillman, B. J., & Goldsmith, J. (2010). Imaging: The self-referral boom and the ongoing search for policies to contain it. *Health Affairs, 29*(12), 2231–2236.

imaging spending declined 12.7%. Sales of CT machines fell 27% from 2006 to 2008; MRI unit sales have declined 36% from 2002 to 2008.

The concept of a marketplace lifecycle is useful for entire product categories. For example, the tuberculosis-hospital industry has completed its lifecycle. The entire hospital industry of many large cities may be in the maturing phase as ambulatory and urgent-care facilities and the patient-centered medical home model establish new lifecycles at the introductory stage. Like the product lifecycle, the marketplace or industry lifecycle has four stages. In the *introduction* stage, the service is first offered in the market area. The appearance of a competitor, as well as a rapid increase in patient volume, signals the second stage, *growth*. Providers also begin to allocate additional resources to the service at this stage. For most services, revenue begins to level off at some point, typically signaling the onset of the *maturity* phase. Some providers of the service may then begin to drop the offering. An ongoing decrease in revenue signals the onset of the fourth stage, *decline*. Externally, competitors may have left the market as new services or technological advances replace the existing service.

In many cases, it is difficult for a specific product or service to perform much differently from the entire market in which it is competing. For example, on the average, domestic car manufacturers, real estate companies, and medical supply houses tend either to do well or to perform badly as an industry sector. Hospital use throughout the industry is often up or down. Within these general ups and downs, some specific companies do better than others, or at least do not suffer sales variations as much as their competitors do. The marketplace lifecycle referred to in this text is assumed to be within the company's competitive area. If the company offers a national product, then the marketplace lifecycle is within the nation as a whole. If the company offers a community service, then the cycle relates to the community within which the company competes. Assume five clinics exist in a given suburb and that they offer the same service to the community. Also assume that business is down an average of 10% in all five clinics. Unless a new service is developed or a new market segment is found, it is unreasonable to assume one clinic can outperform another.

When studying the marketplace or industry lifecycle, it is important to compare a service to a similar service of new competitors. The marketplace lifecycle of an urgent-care service is different from that of a family practice. The emerging lifecycle of patient-centered medical homes may look dramatically different from what was experienced by health maintenance organizations (HMOs) of 20 years ago in many metropolitan communities. Within each of these broad categories, each service is likely to have its own lifecycle, as indicated in **Figure 6.9**.

FIGURE 6.9

Possible Alternative Lifecycles

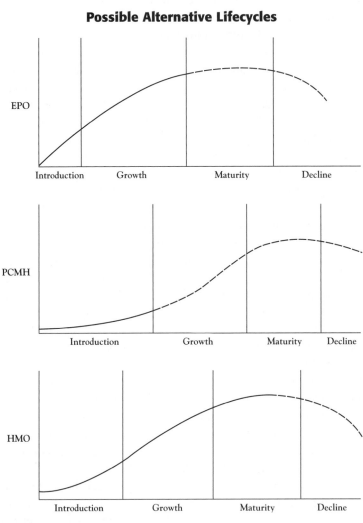

Studies have shown several variations in the marketplace lifecycle. Examination of the charts in Figure 6.9 reveals a noticeable difference in the introduction stage of each lifecycle, for example. For the employer-provider organization (EPO), the introduction stage is relatively short. An organization entering this market must prepare for the entry of new competitors within a short time. A key goal may be to have as many sites as possible to block new competitors. The patient-centered medical home (PCMH) model marketplace curve is different, with an extended introduction stage. The organization entering this market must recognize that extensive promotion is necessary and that families (buyers) may require time to become aware of the benefits of this alternative program, to understand how the clinical team will coordinate their care, and to understand how they will interact with their healthcare system and be able to track their health progress and records with an electronic health record (EHR). Each service has a different shape for its curve. Although there is no exact method for forecasting these shapes, managers must be sensitive to the possibility of variations. The key issue for managers is the importance of assessing strategy relative to a changing environment and in light of future trends.[13]

An Organization's Lifecycle versus the Marketplace Lifecycle

The strategy/action match is designed (1) to match an organization's lifecycle with the marketplace lifecycle, and (2) to determine what marketing planning strategies are appropriate based on this match. The organization's lifecycle represents the product or service, while the marketplace lifecycle represents the total market. In order to do the strategy/action match, it is necessary to examine both of these, not separate, but intertwined lifecycles. The resulting strategy matrix is essentially an overlapping of the organization's lifecycle and the marketplace lifecycle. Too often, managers view their own service's lifecycle in isolation, without considering the marketplace lifecycle. For example, a hospital introduced a pediatric service 10 years ago; over the past 7 years, this service has grown at a small but increasing rate. At first, it may appear that the hospital should increase the resources allocated to the pediatric service. Examination of the marketplace lifecycle in relation to the service lifecycle suggests a different strategy, however. During the past 2 years, two hospitals in the same metropolitan area eliminated their pediatric services. Furthermore, the demographic profile of the community shows a rapidly aging population. In view of these two factors, the organization should probably harvest (ultimately reduce or eliminate) this service and explore new opportunities.

Figure 6.10 shows the logic used in this strategy/action match. When the organization's lifecycle curve and the marketplace lifecycle curve are examined in combination, a strategic match is made. From this match, it is possible to begin to make strategy and action decisions. The two curves can develop in several different ways in respect to each other. Each combination results in different strategy and action decisions.

An organization can be in a different phase of the lifecycle than the marketplace. For example, as **Figure 6.11** shows, the Hunter Clinic is in the

FIGURE 6.10

The Logic of the Strategy/Action Match

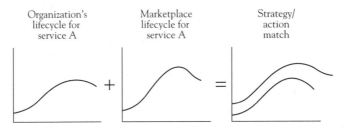

Organization's
lifecycle for
service A

Marketplace
lifecycle for
service A

Strategy/
action
match

FIGURE 6.11

The Hunter Clinic and the Marketplace Lifecycle for Mammography

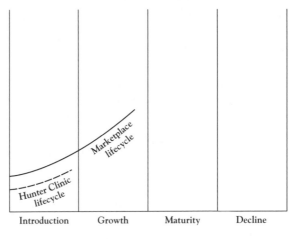

Introduction   Growth   Maturity   Decline

——— Current position in lifecycle
– – – Future possible lifecycle

introduction stage of its lifecycle for a walk-in mammography program. Two competing facilities in town have been offering the same service for 6 months, and public acceptance of this service is growing rapidly. In the marketplace lifecycle, the mammography service is in the growth stage. The importance of recognizing where the organization is relative to the marketplace has been empirically documented. It has been found that the probability of survival of a firm in a business differs significantly across

FIGURE 6.12

Matrix for the Strategy/Action Match

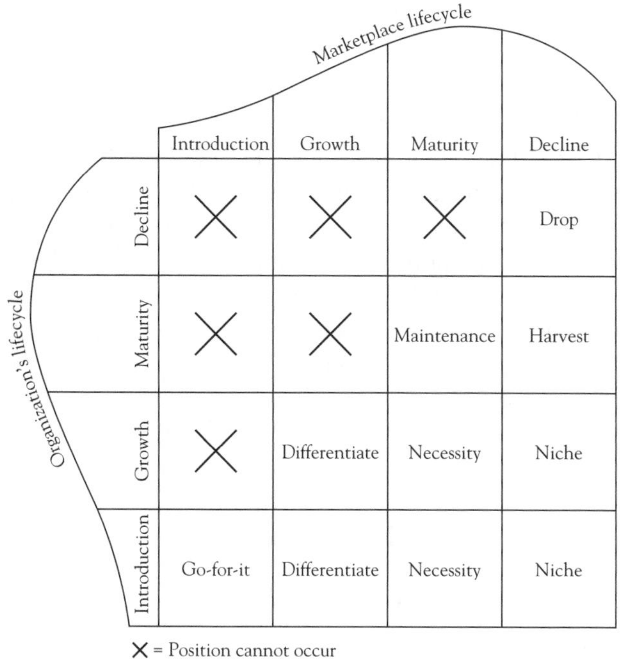

X = Position cannot occur

the stages of the lifecycle. There is a consistent decline in survival rates with increase in competitive intensity. Early entrants in a market (assuming a well-defined marketing strategy) enjoy a higher probability of survival.[14]

Once an organization's position and the marketplace's position in their respective lifecycles have been plotted, strategy alternatives can be formulated from the resulting matrix (**Figure 6.12**). Data generated through the internal/external assessment are essential for this process. Even though all the data may not be available, the matrix can still provide direction for management. An examination of Figure 6.12 indicates that the Hunter Clinic must select a differentiation strategy—the box on the matrix where the organization's introductory position in the lifecycle and the marketplace's growth position meet. As a later entrant to the market, the Hunter Clinic's offering must be different from existing programs, or consumers will view the clinic's program as just another alternative. There will be little incentive for current buyers to switch or for new buyers to see the Hunter Clinic's program as a more valuable offering.

STRATEGY OPTIONS

Much of the remainder of this chapter discusses alternative strategies and how to select an appropriate strategy on the basis of an organization's and its marketplace lifecycles.

Go-for-It Strategy

When a service is first being introduced and the overall market demand is just beginning, an organization may adopt a *go-for-it strategy* (**Figure 6.13**). During this period, there are few (or no) competitors, and there are two rather dramatic options—boom or bust. The market may never develop beyond this stage, or it may become strong, in which case the new service may perform in a dramatic fashion. Studies have shown that early entrants in a marketplace often enjoy a significantly greater market share than later entrants.[15]

If an organization is in a position that indicates a go-for-it strategy, the key is to obtain strong marketplace recognition. Because this recognition

FIGURE 6.13

Go-for-It Strategy

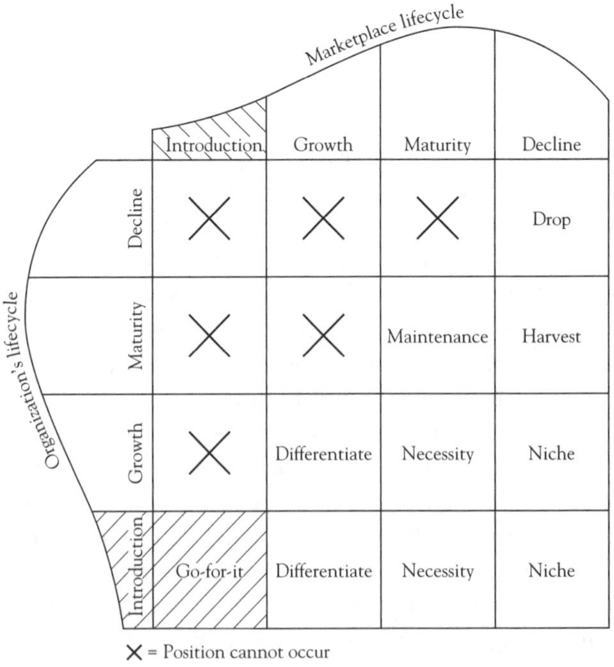

X = Position cannot occur

is often linked to quality in healthcare settings, healthcare organizations must maintain tight quality control at the go-for-it stage. Each element of the marketing mix is used to maintain a competitive position at the go-for-it stage. Negative early consumer experiences will kill future gains.

Product/Service

In the go-for-it strategy, the goals of the product/service element of the marketing mix are (1) to obtain leadership by being one of the earliest organizations (if not the first) to introduce the service, (2) to carefully control quality, and (3) to limit product or service variations and reserve the introduction of options for a later time. This approach is a useful technique for four reasons:

1. It allows the organization to concentrate its resources on one option and to develop consistent quality. A critical review of the results of the organization's internal assessment is important before entering the go-for-it stage.
2. It allows the organization to obtain recognition in the marketplace for a specific service.
3. It allows the organization to save new ideas or service modifications until it needs to be more competitive.
4. It keeps future ideas confidential until it is necessary to introduce them for competitive advantage.

Price

Organizations in the go-for-it position often use a high-price strategy because of a lack of competition and the need to recover the high setup costs of the program. A high price also has other advantages. For example, it provides image value to the product or service, which may be particularly important in health care. In addition, it is often difficult to calculate the actual cost of providing the service (i.e., the cost per unit of delivery). Without an accurate account of the cost of delivery, a high price provides some room for error or experience without incurring significant costs to the organization.

Finally, a high initial entry price can be a control on demand. Market demand determines the appropriate staffing levels of a program, but estimates of demand are not always reliable. When an organization is not certain of demand, it can use a high relative price to ensure that demand remains within its capacity. Many organizations create ill will in the marketplace by offering a desired service when they do not have the capacity to meet the demand. A 4-, 6-, or 8-week wait to see a physician often results in consumer dissatisfaction and negative word of mouth.

Although these advantages appear to justify setting a high price, the quickest way to encourage competitors to enter the market is to set a high relative price. Other groups come to believe that they can offer the same service at a lower price and still achieve a reasonable return on their investment.

This effect on potential competitors is a major justification for setting a low price. This strategy has the additional benefit of reducing the risk of the buyers and, thus, encouraging them to try the new service. The major risk associated with this strategy is that demand will exceed capacity.

Promotion

When a new service is introduced in a market, consumers often know little about it. It is important, therefore, to develop a high advertising and public relations profile. For example, people who visit a new walk-in clinic at a shopping mall may receive free emergency kits. Promotional goals include educating the consumer about product benefits and gaining widespread marketplace awareness of the existence of the service. In the long run, the goal is to position products and services that provide unique benefits to customers, such as convenience, speed of service, better technology, or more attractive price. It is important that benefits be in line with the market's needs.

A major promotional goal is to establish a "brand" name in order to achieve marketplace dominance and to develop an early competitive advantage as the supplier of this service. Public-information advertising, feature articles in various publications, and television news reports are all valuable ways for services in the go-for-it category to achieve marketplace recognition and dominance. Increasingly, in this Web 2.0 era, posting videos to YouTube or using other social media platforms like Twitter to engage and inform the potential market will play a key role in the information stage of a service.

Price/Promotion Options

At the go-for-it stage, there are typically four alternatives with regard to pricing and promotional strategies, as shown in **Figure 6.14**. Determinations of high and low are made relative to the competition or to substitutable service or product offerings.

The option in quadrant A is a high-price, high-promotion, or a premium, approach. It is useful when buyers are price insensitive (because third-party coverage for the service is high), yet largely unaware of the service (because it is being offered in a way that is unique in the market).

FIGURE 6.14

Price/Promotion Tradeoff

Price

	High	Low
High	A Premium	B Penetration
Low	C Selective	D Mandate

Promotion

Geriatric medicine as a separate department is a new, unknown service in many communities, for example, and consumers must be educated as to the unique perspective of such a department. The advantage of a premium approach is somewhat intuitive. A relatively high promotion budget, if effective, should stimulate demand. Coupling this type of promotion with a high initial price (and a sufficient profit margin) could result in significant early-stage profit or revenue to cover development costs. The risk, however, is that competitors will enter the market and try to establish a cost-differential advantage.

Options in quadrant B involve significant promotional expenditures and a low price. They can lead to the highest level of market share, but profits may be low. This approach has a competitive advantage in that the low price will delay others from entering the market for fear that the profit margins will not support the new offerings. There are, however, some disadvantages for the organization following this penetration strategy. One potential problem is that once consumers learn of the service, there is a heavy demand for it. While this is the goal of any new offering to some extent, consumers can become dissatisfied rapidly if staffing levels do not support the demand. Individuals who cannot get an appointment with the geriatric staff for several weeks or months may hesitate to respond to any future service offering from the same health facility.

Historically, there always has been some concern associated with a low price, because an organization does not truly know the cost per unit of delivery, especially given the complexity of healthcare services. Setting an initial low price does not allow the organization much room for error. Yet, increasingly in this era of value in healthcare delivery, the low-price position may not be as much of an issue as it has been considered in the past. Unless real economies of scale can be achieved with an increase in patient volume, organizations should use this low-price, high-promotion strategy with great caution.

In quadrant C, a new service is offered at a high initial price with little promotional support. This strategy is effective when consumers are already aware of the service and want it, and when the market is also relatively price insensitive. In this situation, the organization can offer a program such as industrial medicine with a selective, low-cost promotional budget.

A low-price, low-promotion strategy, as shown in quadrant D, is unusual. The only time that an organization generally offers a new service under these conditions is when a regulatory agency mandates it or the service is necessary to round out the product offering to the market. For example, a hospital may offer on-site physicals for employees as a component of its industrial-medicine program without promoting this service. The low price of this service is presented to make the package attractive to potential buyers of the total program. The on-site physicals are not in themselves a profitable venture for the hospital.

Distribution

Distribution involves alternative ways of providing the service to customers. At the go-for-it stage, an organization should control distribution tightly. The most accepted model is to allow only those over whom the organization has total control to distribute the product. In this way, quality and performance problems can be completely resolved, and the product will be provided as intended. Increasingly in healthcare today, many health systems have moved to integrating their own physicians. For example, Aurora Health Care in Milwaukee now employs almost 1,500 primary care physicians and specialists within the healthcare system, as well as having its own hospitals; Premier Health Partners, which serves southeastern Ohio, has a similar structure, although it does not have as many physicians within its network of doctors. A complex distribution network, such as franchises or outreach clinics, that is developed too early (i.e., before all problems have been resolved) is difficult to manage. Once all systems are running smoothly, the organization should move as quickly as possible to establish a distribution system that provides the greatest possible market penetration.

Differentiation Strategy

Two points of the strategy/action match—the introduction–growth and the growth–growth stages—call for the differentiation strategy. In both situations, the major need of the organization is for differentiation from its competitors, and an organization's concern is to establish a differential competitive advantage. An advantage of entering after the market is in the growth stage is that the later entrant can see how the market has responded to the early entrants.[16] In considering a basis for differentiation, analyses of competitors' strengths and weaknesses are valuable. Differentiation can be developed around the competitive profile.

In situation 1 (**Figure 6.15**), an organization is introducing a service even though offerings of a similar nature are already in the marketplace. In Dallas, for example, a clinic has opened an "urgicenter" as a low-cost alternative to the hospital emergency room and as an extended-hours source of care. This facility has been open for 1 year. The market has been growing, and another organization is about to open a similar clinic. What strategies should the new entrant implement?

FIGURE 6.15

Differentiation Strategy: Situation 1

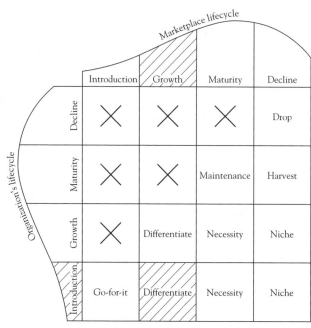

X = Position cannot occur

When an organization is in the introduction stage but the marketplace is in the growth stage, product differentiation is essential. The organization that enters the marketplace at this stage has lost some flexibility in its marketing strategy, as others have already entered the market. The earlier entrants have set the minimum level of product quality for the offering as perceived by the buyer. To some degree, the same constraint can be placed on price. An organization that enters the market when it is at the growth stage and offers the service at a higher than market price can succeed only if consumers perceive that a real value has been added.

The entering organization must meet the promotional expenditures established by the competition. In the fall of 1989, 3 months before its new automobile, the Lexus, was generally available, Toyota started to advertise the car extensively. This late entrant into the luxury-car market had to establish high brand-name recognition to separate itself quickly from the existing players in the market. Toyota was willing to invest millions in advertising long before the first car was even on a showroom floor. Similarly, a healthcare facility should be proactive, rather than reactive, in promoting new service offerings. The later a facility enters the market relative to the competition, the more difficult and expensive it becomes to establish a differential advantage.

In situation 2 (**Figure 6.16**), both the organization and the marketplace are in the growth stage. One hospital introduces a sports medicine program, and soon afterward two other hospitals enter the market with similar services. People in the community are now aware of such services, and demand is growing for all three programs. What is the original hospital's next move? As in situation 1, the differentiation strategy is important. All elements of the marketing mix should be directed toward differentiating the organization from its competitors.

Product

In attempting to differentiate its product, an organization may create a more segmented service offering. The hospital may segment the sports medicine program according to the age of the potential user, for example. A program may be developed for teens and preteens; links may be established with park sports leagues, high school coaches, or parents. Creating a program version for a specific age group provides a more dominant image within that segment and differentiates it from competitors' general programs. These segments should be selected according to their size, needs, and the organization's ability to meet those needs.

FIGURE 6.16

Differentiation Strategy: Situation 2

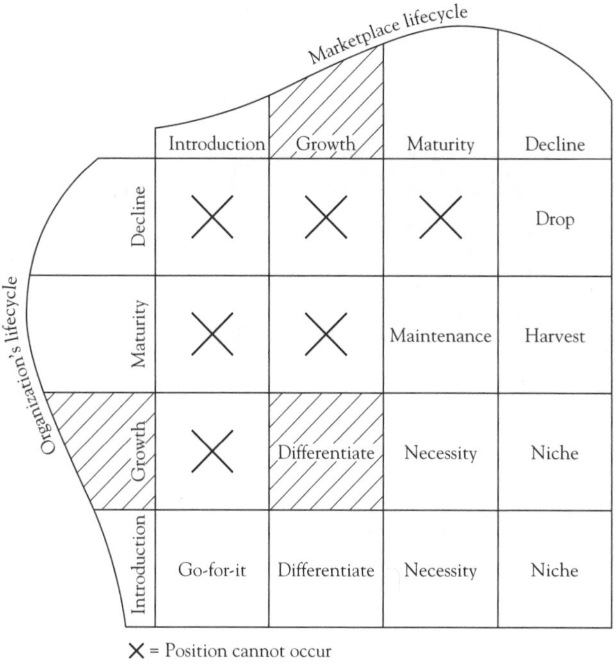

X = Position cannot occur

Price

Matched with program (i.e., product) variations, price can be a successful differentiation tactic. The organization can create different versions of the same clinical service. In a sports medicine package, for example, fees for medical service can include rehabilitation at a number of community health clubs. In obstetrics, where expectant mothers often may not have insurance, cost may be a real concern. St. Luke's Hospital in Sioux City, Iowa offered obstetrical cash discounts at a level shown in **Figure 6.17** at the end of 2011 and into 2012 to help address the economic concerns of uninsured patients. Price variations can broaden the appeal of the service offering beyond the original market.

Promotion

Promotion plays an important role in differentiation. In the go-for-it stage, advertising is necessary to create awareness. In the differentiation stage, the emphasis of advertising copy must shift to offering trials of the service. The

FIGURE 6.17

Package Pricing

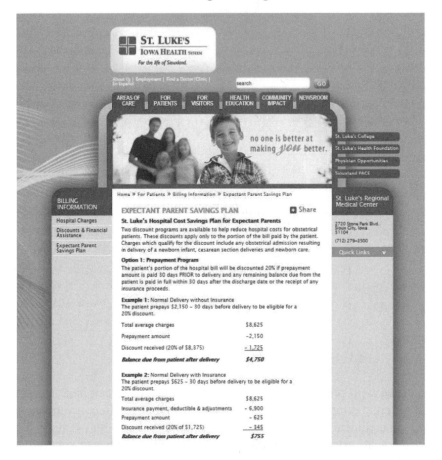

Source: St. Luke's Iowa Health System. *Expectant parent savings plan.*
Retrieved October 4, 2011, from: http://www.stlukes.org/body.cfm?id=91

need, in this phase, is to create a preference among buyers, often called selective demand. This approach must be coordinated with changes in the other elements of the marketing mix. Now is the time to focus on extended hours, lower prices, more specialized services, and a more comprehensive program, all designed to differentiate an organization from its competitors. Promotional programs are less important in this strategy than in the go-for-it strategy. Consumers are already aware of the offering. The organization must now concentrate on advantages in order to encourage the market to use its service rather than a competitor's offering.

The role of the sales force often becomes more important at this stage. The key goal for the sales staff is to control the channels of distribution for patients. If a company is going to use just one alcohol-/chemical-dependency program, the objective of the sales force is an exclusive contract with that company. Likewise, a sales effort may be necessary whenever the buyer has more than one offering from which to choose.

Distribution

The most common way for healthcare services to achieve differentiation is through distribution. In order to distinguish its offering from that of its competitors, an organization should consider the hours/days of availability, number of locations, accessibility/convenience, and manner in which the service is delivered. Many organizations' approach to differentiation is to provide more intensive distribution (multiple locations and longer hours). The best form of differentiation may be to have a number of sites with one brand name throughout the community.

Necessity Strategy

When the marketplace is mature and the service is in the introduction or growth stage, the organization may adopt a necessity strategy (**Figure 6.18**). Such a strategy is carried out in the belief that it is necessary to offer the service in order to compete effectively, even when the service is not expected to gain a large share of the existing market. The only limitation on capturing market share is the prior existence of competitors.

In Engertown, a fictitious example, several clinics have family practitioners to meet patients' primary care needs. Five years ago, the Peterson Clinic, which had offered specialty care services for 20 years, decided to add primary care to ensure that it would have a referral base. Three family practitioners were brought into the group. Although the Peterson Clinic was a late entrant into this service in Engertown, a community with a stable population, the demand for family practitioners within the clinic is still growing. Although difficult, it is possible to make gains in such a situation. One approach is for the late entrant to position itself against the leading competitor by differentiating its service. An alternative option is to select a market segment that may have special needs and develop the service to meet those needs. This alternative helps to develop reputation, cost control, and recognized community capability.

Each element of the marketing mix is important for a successful necessity strategy.

FIGURE 6.18

Necessity Strategy

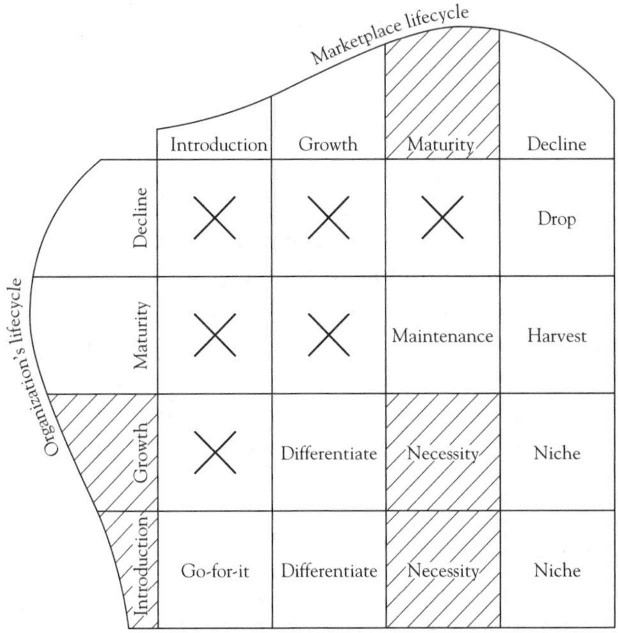

X = Position cannot occur

Product

Because the organization is entering the market late with its own offering, the market already has expectations of the service. Any necessity offering must be at least equal to those of relevant competitors. The potential for profit may be greater if the late entrant tailors its service to a specific market segment. In one community, for example, several gynecologists had established practices when a new obstetrics-gynecology service opened. The new service included a supervised childcare area staffed by college students who were majoring in child development. Because of this service, a woman could take her child with her to the doctor, and while she had her examination, the child could participate in supervised play activities. This benefit for the market of single-parent households created a differential advantage that helped shift market share from existing providers.

Price

To a great extent, an organization does not control price under a necessity strategy. Usually, buyers are aware of the already available price options because the existing competitive entrants have established the viable price ranges. The organization must recognize the existing price structure. When Sprenger Hospital decided that it should offer health courses, two ranges of prices for weight-control programs already existed in the community. Some groups charged high prices with medical, psychological, and nutritional services included; others provided only lecture programs, but at a low price. Because Sprenger Hospital was a late entrant in this market, it decided to offer a middle-price program. The marketplace was mature, and thus aware of the alternatives. Consumers probably viewed this late offering as either an "expensive," low-end program or a "cheap," premium program.

Promotion

In the necessity strategy, promotion is difficult. The program may have been introduced at a late stage simply to keep physicians at the hospital or patients at the clinic. Promotion should be on a mass basis to inform the market that the organization does provide the service. If the organization decides to focus on a market segment, a personal sales effort may be helpful to explain the unique service benefits and encourage trial use. A key goal is to persuade consumers to switch to the late entrant.

Distribution

The role of distribution is small in the necessity strategy. The need is to match the competition. If the organization can appeal to a market segment based on how, where, or when the service is delivered, then that market segment will be the focus of a competitive advantage.

Maintenance Strategy

When the organization's lifecycle and the marketplace lifecycle are both in the mature stage, the maintenance strategy is in order (**Figure 6.19**). For example, in Knoxville, six hospitals provide pediatric service. The last hospital to add such a service did so in 1968. Despite occasional shifts in relative patient days, most of the hospitals view this service as stable, but heading toward decline. If a hospital has maintained a steady census in pediatrics, the question is what it should do with this service in the next 5 years.

Occasionally, organizations using a maintenance strategy attempt to increase their market share or revenue, but the incremental cost of each patient day may not equal the marginal revenue. It is probably not cost efficient for an organization to go to the expense of encouraging physicians to shift patients at this stage. In following the maintenance strategy, the organization assumes that the level of maturity is satisfactory.

FIGURE 6.19

Maintenance Strategy

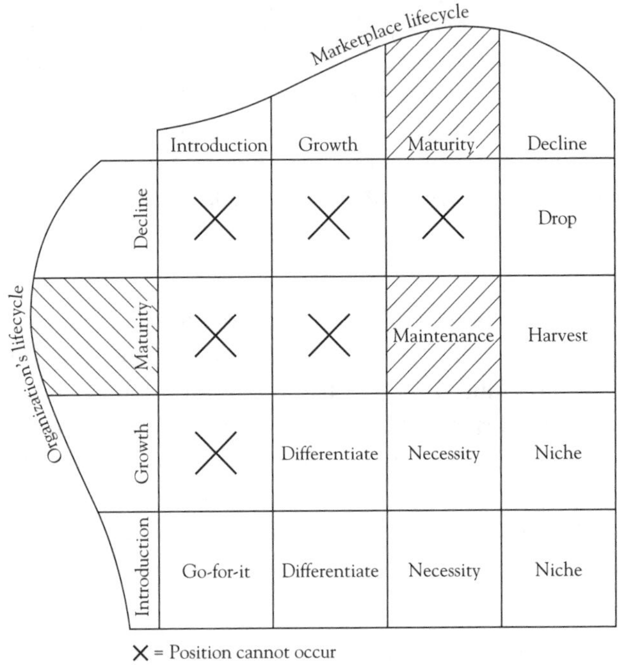

X = Position cannot occur

Typically, one healthcare provider dominates the market for the mature service. This leader can follow one of two basic strategies:

1. Segment and fortify. The leader has the power to segment the market by focusing on the more profitable groups and can attempt to fortify its market share within these segments.
2. Innovate. A key advantage to being the leader is often the large revenue base that comes with that position. To maintain it, the leader should strive to develop new offerings.

The remaining organizations must reexamine the factors in the marketing mix in order to survive in mature markets. Healthcare providers who are not the leaders must ask themselves the following questions:

1. Is there a segment of the market that is not being served?
2. Can the product/service be improved?
3. Can the product/service be distributed more efficiently, or can accessibility be significantly increased?
4. Can the product/service be offered at a lower price?
5. Can a superior advertising campaign be mounted?

The maintenance strategy requires action. Increased sales and market share can come only from a competitor. A fight for share and a search for new alternatives are the courses for growth.

Product

With the maintenance strategy, the organization must reexamine the service periodically if the organization is to stay alive. The leader in a mature business may notice a loss of business as competitors begin to attract small market niches in the target market. By reexamining the service, managers can explore opportunities to gain back prior users or to reposition the service against that of competitors.

Price

In a maintenance strategy, price is the focus only as a defensive position. An organization may reduce the price of its service to keep loyal consumers away from competitors or newly developed service alternatives. However, a price war should not be started.

Promotion

A key element of the maintenance strategy is promotion. The goal is to keep current users satisfied. Healthcare organizations must make ongoing efforts to ensure that patients return to them and that physicians continue to refer patients to their services. Post-use follow-up through letters, telephone calls, or the sales force is necessary to monitor the continuing satisfaction of the clientele. Such activities as newsletters and tie-in educational seminars also become important in keeping the loyalty of existing users.

Distribution

As part of the maintenance strategy, distribution continues at its present level. Hours and locations are changed only by necessity; if a competitor offers night hours, for example, a clinic may do likewise. Because no new buyers are entering the market in the mature stage, retention of existing users becomes the goal.

Niche Strategy

Occasionally, an organization finds that the demand for a service that it offers is increasing, although overall market demand may be decreasing. Growth may occur in a declining market for two reasons. First, competitors may have left the market because the reduced demand does not support their cost curve or target return. Second, even in this stage, there may be market segments that are still attractive or need the offering.

In this instance, the organization must consider a niche strategy to target or exploit these growth segments (**Figure 6.20**). There are obvious problems with this strategy, however. Foremost is the fact that market demand is in the decline stage. If the niche strategy is to be profitable, too many competitors cannot be vying for the same segments. Second, it is critical to estimate the size of these niches with some degree of accuracy because, again, total market demand is on the downward slope. Finally, the internal efficiency of operations is essential as an avenue to any future increase in profitability because market demand will not be increasing.

As noted in Figure 6.20, an organization can adopt the niche at either the point of introduction or during the stage of growth, but the marketplace must be in decline. This is an unusual, but not unlikely, situation. One healthcare facility may see that many large competitors are abandoning a particular service. Operating from a lower cost-overhead position, this organization may believe that if it captures a sufficient market share,

FIGURE 6.20

Niche Strategy

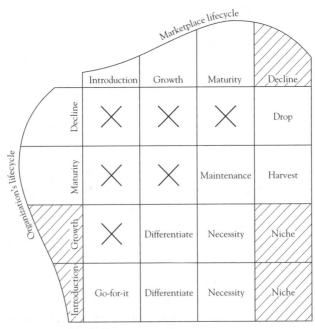

X = Position cannot occur

it can make a profit because of the total size of the available market (even while in decline). It is more common, however, for an organization to find that one of its services (such as pediatrics) is growing while the market demand is declining. In this instance, an aggressive niche strategy, such as increasing the number of pediatric beds, may allow this facility to be seen as the source of pediatric care. In fact, such an aggressive posture may force the last few marginal competitors from the market.[17]

Harvest Strategy

One of the most difficult decisions that a healthcare manager faces is whether to harvest (phase out) a service that is no longer productive. Although there may be political and public relations pressure against the harvest strategy, it is still an important option to consider in one case: when the organization is in the maturity stage and the marketplace is in decline (**Figure 6.21**). If managed properly, the harvest strategy can be employed to maximize the organization's effectiveness.[18]

FIGURE 6.21

Harvest Strategy

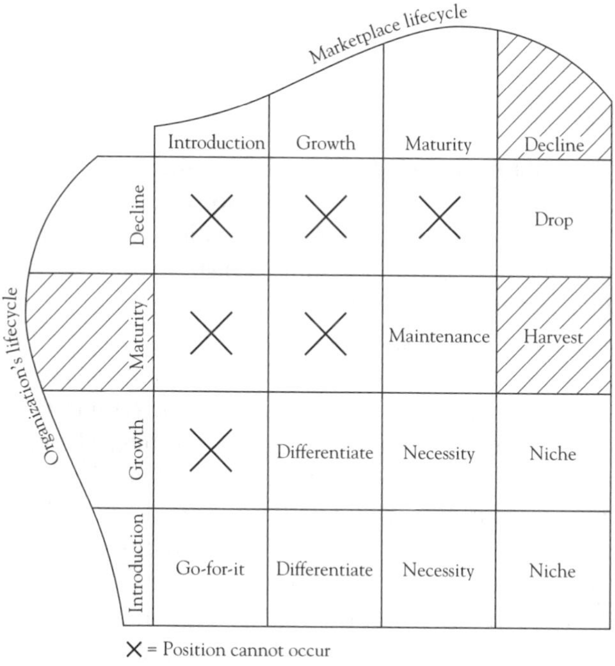

Organization's lifecycle \ Marketplace lifecycle	Introduction	Growth	Maturity	Decline
Decline	X	X	X	Drop
Maturity	X	X	Maintenance	Harvest
Growth	X	Differentiate	Necessity	Niche
Introduction	Go-for-it	Differentiate	Necessity	Niche

X = Position cannot occur

FIGURE 6.22

Drop Strategy

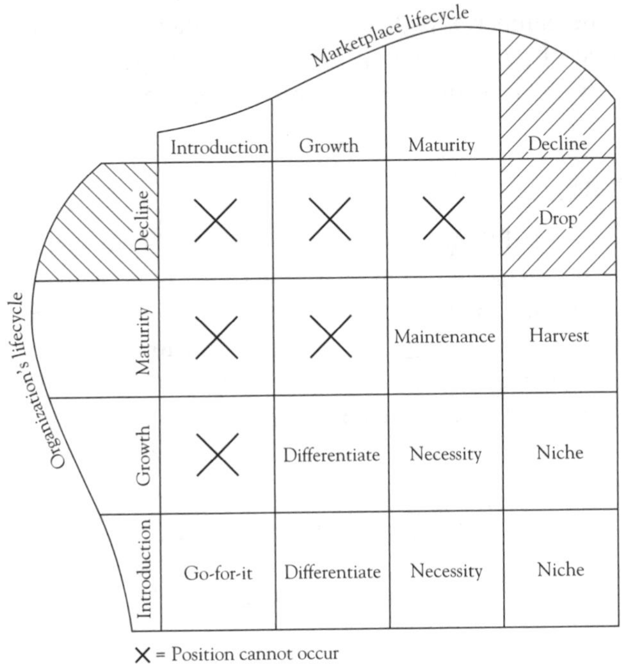

X = Position cannot occur

Drop Strategy

Clearly, if both the marketplace lifecycle and the organization's lifecycle are in the decline stage, it is appropriate to drop the service, sell it, or merge with another entity (**Figure 6.22**). It is important to recognize also that declining services tend to consume a disproportionate share of management time and of financial resources.[19] Any business must recognize the seriousness and risk of a drop strategy. Before dropping any service, management must assess the internal and external impacts of the decision. From an internal perspective, it is necessary to determine the importance of the service to the organization's mission, the interrelationships of the service and other business lines, and its contribution to these other lines. A service may be in decline along with the market, but still may generate dollars (such as through the laboratory and radiology services) that are not reflected in an analysis of this particular service. An analysis of such contributions may reveal a justification for continuing the service under review. In a healthcare setting, such a service is also often essential for the operation of other business lines. If, in fact, there is no other profitable or less expensive way to offer this service within the facility, the drop decision must be moderated.

An external, or customer-focused, analysis is also necessary prior to any drop decision. An organization must determine who is still using the service. If the remaining buyers account for a significant percentage of revenue through their use of other services in the facility, the good-will value of maintaining this service may be sufficient to moderate the drop decision. Again, however, because of the fiscal drain at this stage, a healthcare facility should explore creative options to provide the service with less financial risk. For example, some other provider or entity may contract to provide or run the service, or buyers may be persuaded to use a substitutable offering.

Too often, when there is justification for dropping a particular service, there is a familiar refrain—the service should be maintained as a loss leader. A loss leader is a pricing device designed to generate an activity that may not be profitable, but that may lead to other profitable services. For example, a $2 cholesterol check may be a loss leader that helps generate new physician activity. An external analysis may support such a contention, but, in addition, an internal analysis must show that the loss does lead to revenue gains in other areas.

SETTING MARKETING OBJECTIVES

After completion of the strategy/action match, the organization can set its marketing objectives. These objectives are specific targets that are consistent with the mission of the organization and the strategy/action match. They also form the basis for tactical actions. The following are examples of marketing objectives:

1. Establish gross hospital revenues of $15 million in 20__.
2. Serve 110,000 (patient days/inpatient) in 20__.
3. Expand market share in Anytown from 18% of inpatient hospital days to 22% by 20__.
4. Establish a gross margin across all product lines of 35% by 20__.
5. Establish a reputation among physicians and consumers as the premier heart-surgery program in Nevada by 20__.
6. Average 28 patients per physician per practice day at an average billing of $30 per patient by 20__.
7. Harvest the service by the 4th quarter of 20__.
8. Become the market leader (in market share) by 20__.

Note that objectives should specify the time by which they are to be achieved.

Marketing objectives must be as precise as possible. In general, they should be:

1. Measurable in dollars, time, and units
2. Realistic
3. Challenging
4. Clear, concise, and understandable
5. Consistent with one another

Marketing objectives should cover the following areas:

1. Profitability
2. Cash flow
3. Units sold
4. Market share
5. Image
6. Quality
7. Price
8. Service

Some objectives include a measurable outcome, such as units sold, market share, net income, or profit. Other objectives, such as image enhancement, can be measured through market research.

Usually, a marketing plan for a specific product or service contains three to five specific marketing objectives and can be summarized briefly. The success of the marketing plan is measured by how well marketing objectives are achieved.

SUMMARY

Building a strategy is developing a plan to meet the needs of customers. In this chapter, three alternative industry frameworks were presented that have been used previously in industry: the Boston Consulting Group (BCG) matrix, the General Electric (GE) Industry model, and the Management Analysis Center (MAC) model.

From a strategic perspective, each model has its own respective strengths and weaknesses. On a model-by-model basis, however, each provides some incremental insight to consider as you further refine your own perspective in formulating your organization's strategy. The BCG matrix is useful as a diagnostic tool in considering the overall balance of services in an organization's portfolio. Are there enough new opportunities being developed? Are too many of the organizations' services classified as "cash cows," generating significant cash but, in fact, rather mature in the lifecycle? Is there a proper distribution of services throughout the matrix? These are the questions that are often generated with the use of the BCG matrix.

The GE model considers two dimensions of industry attractiveness and business strength. More complex than the BCG matrix in its consideration of competition and profitability within its framework, the GE model moves strategists within an organization to more directly consider multiple factors explicitly as they examine new business opportunities.

The MAC model considers the positioning of a business venture in terms of the breadth of the service offering and the value added of the business. It is the four quadrants of this model that suggest alternative positions an organization might consider as a function of its value-added service mix or the breadth of what it provides to the customer that forms its ultimate strategic position.

All of these models help shape strategy, yet this chapter suggests a fourth alternative structure (strategy/action match) shaped around the lifecycle of the service and the industry. The complexity and reality of the lifecycle leads to an array of strategic alternatives determined by two factors: first, where you as an organization are in terms of your (the organization's) lifecycle (i.e., is this a new service rollout?); and second, where the industry is. Are you beginning a service as the industry is also beginning this same service? Or, are you rolling out this service later than the industry (which has significant strategic implications, according to this model)? Thus, there is a match of strategy and opportunities based on this lifecycle framework. It is this fourth model that reflects the reality of developing a strategy based not only on competition, but also in terms of where your position is in the timing of your service as you enter the market and where the total market is in terms of its maturity.

The concept of the product lifecycle is well accepted. The four Ps of marketing (product, price, place, and promotion) contribute to the strategies in each cell of the strategy/action match as the organization decides whether it is a go-for-it, necessity, maintenance, or drop strategy.

The strategy/action match provides the organization with direction for its marketing actions. This approach follows a basic marketing approach. The match requires an external examination of the marketplace, as well as an internal assessment of the organization's position. Successful identification of position on each lifecycle is based on audits of the marketplace, the competition, and the organization. Throughout this process, data generated through staff work are required to determine positions on the lifecycle. These positions, while not exact, must be reasonably accurate. Incorrect position placement can lead to strategies inconsistent with market demand.

Once the strategy/action match has been completed and appropriate marketing objectives have been established, it is necessary to develop the specific tactical actions that can be taken to meet the objectives.

QUESTIONS FOR DISCUSSION

1. What are the strategic options available to any business? Provide an example of each option for a free-standing, urgent-care center that has been opened within a retail shopping mall.
2. What are the factors that can move a product or service from one stage to another through the product lifecycle? Which of these factors can be controlled by the organization as a function of the effectiveness of its strategic plan? Does the effectiveness of control vary according to whether it is in health care versus a high-technology industry such as computers, or versus manufacturing?
3. A health system is the first in a major metropolitan area to offer a comprehensive senior memory disorders clinic. Staffed with neurologists and other specialists, the clinic is integrated within this health system's expanded geriatric health program, which is also the first major program in the area. Describe this health system's available strategic options.
4. Explain when in the strategy/action match the "differentiation" strategy is to be implemented. Provide examples for an outpatient service if there is more than one possibility for the differentiation strategy.
5. In the mature stage, a maintenance strategy is often the norm. Describe the different strategic options available between the leader and those that are not in the dominant position in the market.
6. Niche and harvest strategies are two possibilities for any healthcare organizations using the strategy/action match. Under what conditions would these approaches be relevant? Provide examples where each approach might prove beneficial.

NOTES

1. Porter, M. (1980). *Competitive strategy*. New York: Free Press.
2. Ohmae, K. (1988, November–December). Getting back to strategy. *Harvard Business Review*, 149.
3. Seeger, J. A. (1984). Reversing the images of BCG's growth/share matrix. *Strategic Management Journal, 5*(1), 93–97.

4. Morrison, A., & Wensley, R. (1991, April). Boxed up or boxed in? A short history of the Boston consulting group share/growth matrix. *Journal of Marketing Management, 7*(2), 105–129.

5. Kopf, J. M., Kreuze, J. G., & Beam, H. H. (1993, July). Using a strategic planning matrix to improve a firm's competitive position. *Journal of Accountancy, 175*(7), 97–101.

6. Gardner, D. M. (1987). Product life cycle: A critical look at the literature. In Michael Houston (Ed.), *Review of marketing 1987* (pp. 162–194). Chicago: American Marketing Association.

7. Hofer, C. W. (1975, December). Toward a contingency theory of business strategy. *Academy of Management Journal, 18,* 798.

8. Day, G. (1981, Fall). The product life cycle: Analysis and application issues. *Journal of Marketing, 45,* 60–67.

9. Kotler, P. (2000). *Marketing management.* Upper Saddle River, NJ: Prentice Hall; pp. 303–304.

10. Klepper, S. (1996, June). Entry, exit, growth, and innovation over the product life cycle. *The American Economic Review, 86*(3), 562–583.

11. Agarwal, R., & Gort, M. (1996, August). The evolution of markets and entry, exit, and survival of firms. *Review of Economics & Statistics,* 489–498.

12. Hillman, B. J., & Goldsmith, J. (2010). Imaging: The self-referral boom and the ongoing search for effective policies to contain it. *Health Affairs, 29*(12), 2231–2236.

13. Lamont, B. T., Martin, D., & Hoffman, J. J. (1993). Porter's generic strategies, discontinuous environments, and performance: A longitudinal study of changing strategies in the hospital industry. *Health Services Research, 28*(5), 623–640.

14. Agarwal, R. (1997). Survival of firms over the product life cycle. *Southern Economic Journal, 63*(3), 571–584.

15. Robinson, W. T., & Fornell, C. (1985, August). Sources of market pioneer advantages in consumer goods industries. *Journal of Marketing Research,* 305–317.

16. Smith, K. G., Grimm, C. M., & Gannon, M. J. (1992). *Dynamics of competitive strategy.* Thousand Oaks, CA: Sage.

17. Van Doren, D. C., & Spielman, A. P. (1989, March). Hospital marketing: Strategy reassessment in a declining market. *Journal of Health Care Marketing, 9,* 15–24.

18. Feldman, L. P., & Page, A. L. (1985, Spring). Harvesting: The misunderstood market exit strategy. *Journal of Business Strategy,* 79–85.

19. Hise, R. T., Parasuraman, A., & Viswanathan, R. (1984, Spring). Product elimination: The neglected management responsibility. *Journal of Business Strategy,* 56–63.

CHAPTER 7

STEP 4: DETERMINING MARKETING ACTIONS

WHAT YOU WILL LEARN

- A variety of tactics exist to achieve marketing goals.
- Advertising is one tactical area, but it is by no means the only option.

DEVISING TACTICS

Step 4 in the process of developing a competitive marketing plan involves translating marketing objectives into specific actions (tactics). Marketing actions are determined on the basis of research into market wants and needs (**Figure 7.1**). Coordination between the strategy/action match and action plans is important. Choosing a strategy from among options presented in Step 3 involves completing a comprehensive analysis of the environment, the market, the competition, and the organization's internal capabilities and marketing system, and then making the strategy/action match. From the match, we move logically to tactics.

The major tactics that managers can employ in launching a marketing effort are commonly referred to as the four Ps of marketing: product, price, place (distribution), and promotion. Every detail can have an impact on the customer, either positive or negative. The little alligator on a sports shirt, a 30-minute guarantee for pizza delivery, a callback from a nurse, and a handwritten note to a referral physician are all examples of marketing tactics that can have an impact. The depth and breadth of marketing decisions are enormous, as are the opportunities to make mistakes. Service, design, packaging, promotion, location, and pricing are all interwoven to make for hundreds of possible combinations for any given service.

FIGURE 7.1

Step 4: Determining Marketing Actions

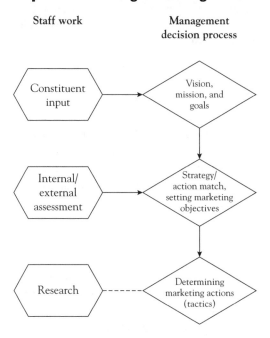

Staff work   Management decision process

Constituent input

Vision, mission, and goals

Internal/ external assessment

Strategy/ action match, setting marketing objectives

Research

Determining marketing actions (tactics)

Frequently, healthcare marketing managers put together marketing actions that are tactically weak. For example, they do not always try to meet an objective of increasing business, profitability, or the number of patients by devising a tactic that will be successful in a competitive environment. An organization may think that it can just steal market share from a competitor and fail to consider the possibility that the competitor may retaliate with protective countermeasures or with intense, successful marketing actions of its own.

Therefore, it is important to establish sound actions to accomplish specific marketing objectives. Action can be divided into two components: (1) the general marketing action, such as the introduction of a price-competitive product, and (2) implementation of the tactical details. The development of general marketing actions is the creative part of the marketing planning process. Implementation is often more tedious. Nevertheless, both parts of the process are critical to the success of marketing plans. Once appropriate actions and tasks have been specified, the potential impact of these plans should be studied.

At this point, marketing must act as a catalyst to help integrate the marketing plan into the overall business plan. Marketing staff should provide input to other members of the organization, such as those in finance and operations, in order to determine the effectiveness and "fit" of the proposed course of action within the organization's overall plans and culture.

All marketing plans need to address (1) product/service, (2) pricing, (3) distribution, and (4) communications/promotion. These elements are discussed within this chapter.

PRODUCT/SERVICE

To a great extent, the product or service is the central part of the marketing mix. It is around the service that the other elements of the marketing plan flow. In regard to products and services, the manager or management group must evaluate their core quality, determine a service level, select among possible new offerings, modify existing services, choose a branding strategy, and select a name.

Evaluating Core Quality

There is increasing concern about the value and effectiveness of healthcare services, the core element of the marketing mix. This concern revolves around making sure that the need for a service exists and that the service is provided with technical competency. Several systems are being developed to address these concerns and to make additional information available to buyers of care. In today's healthcare climate, which might be termed an *era of transparency*, consumers can check on a hospital's website to determine how the hospital performs on certain core measures according to the standards of the Joint Commission, or an individual can look to a state agency such as in Pennsylvania where the healthcare cost containment council publishes outcomes by physician for orthopedic surgical procedures (www.phc4.org/hipknee). And now there are ever-increasing amounts of independent rating agencies such as HealthGrades (www.healthgrades.com) and even Angie's List (www.angieslist.com/health) for consumers to make their evaluations. These systems are not unlike *Consumer Reports* product evaluations.

Figure 7.2 shows the state of Pennsylvania's outcome data for mortality and readmission rates for particular cardiac surgery procedures. Consumers in the state of Pennsylvania can also access information on orthopedic surgery in terms of deep joint infection and readmission compared to whether it may be above the average, below the average, or the same as others across physicians. The challenge with information presented like this, of course, is the complicated nature of what might occur in any surgical procedure. Yet, in examining the chart presented in Figure 7.2,

FIGURE 7.2

Pennsylvania Health Care Cost Containment Council Data Quality

Cardiac Surgery in Pennsylvania 2008–2009 Combined

Symbol Legend
● Significantly higher than the expected rate.
◉ Not significantly different than the expected rate.
○ Significantly lower than the expected rate.
NR Not Reported (too few cases).

Surgeon	Number of Cases			Mortality		Readmissions		Post-surgical length of stay
	2008	2009	Total	In-hospital	30-Day	7-Day	30-Day	
Doctor A								
CABG without valve	44	49	93	◉	◉	◉	◉	7.5
Valve without CABG	6	9	15	NR	NR	NR	NR	NR
Valve with CABG	10	4	14	NR	NR	NR	NR	NR
Total valve	16	13	29	NR	NR	NR	NR	NR
Doctor B								
CABG without valve	55	37	92	◉	◉	◉	◉	5.5
Valve without CABG	21	28	49	◉	NR	NR	NR	7.2
Valve with CABG	15	11	26	NR	NR	NR	NR	NR
Total valve	36	39	75	◉	NR	NR	NR	8.0
Doctor C								
CABG without valve	63	65	128	◉	◉	◉	◉	5.5
Valve without CABG	11	12	23	NR	NR	NR	NR	NR
Valve with CABG	16	10	26	NR	NR	NR	NR	NR
Total valve	27	22	49	◉	◉	◉	◉	7.5
Doctor D								
CABG without valve	48	65	113	◉	◉	◉	◉	5.7
Valve without CABG	13	12	25	NR	NR	NR	NR	NR
Valve with CABG	12	19	31	◉	◉	◉	◉	9.0
Total valve	25	31	56	◉	◉	◉	◉	8.1

Source: PHC4: Pennsylvania Health Care Cost Containment Council. (2012). *Cardiac surgery in Pennsylvania 2008–2009 combined.* Retrieved March 4, 2012, from: http://www.phc4.org/cabg/?year=0809

most readers would quickly judge it to be very similar to a *Consumer Reports* type of format.

What are the marketing ramifications of these data? How would a physician be viewed by the market (or possibly market his/her practice) if the circle next to his/her name were a solid black circle? Fortunately, in the names listed in this depiction, no such physician had that set of experiences; however, searching through the databases, names would be revealed with these marks. Dealing with such negative information in the market is a challenge when the actual clinical product quality comes into question. Should Doctor A advertise her outcomes if the circles are all open, indicating "significantly lower than the expected rate" in terms of infections? Should Doctor A be allowed to set higher fees than others do because her outcomes are better? Knowing Doctor B's poor performance, would a marketing consultant recommend heavy advertising expenditures and discount pricing in order to mask the performance problems? Undoubtedly, physicians with strong performance records will, in the future, compete on clinical quality as well as on other product aspects. However, those with poor performance records cannot be protected by using marketing strategies such as advertising and pricing, and under pay-for-performance reimbursement systems, these physicians will increasingly suffer economically. In order to survive, Doctor G will first need to be clinically competent. Overall, these systems are bad news for poor clinicians, who may have been able to hide behind general quality discussions, and good news for customers, who deserve better information than has been available until now.

In a similar vein, individual medical groups are also moving increasingly to marketing themselves in terms of their own quality metrics. For example, Minnesota Gastroenterology, a large single-specialty group in Minneapolis–St. Paul, has long published quality metrics on the practice's website for viewing by referral doctors and patients (www.mngastro.com/about-us/quality-amp-outcomes).

Determining Service Level

The notion of service has become a popular management focus. Organizations have been advised to provide the customer with extra attention and support. The new preacher in a suburban church demonstrated this approach. The church was huge and at times had been viewed as cold and not always friendly. The new preacher had a keen understanding of this problem. One vivid way in which he showed his understanding was in the parking lot. For years, the clergy had assigned themselves parking spots right next to the front door of the church. After all, they needed to get in and out of the office quickly and back and forth from one function to another. Having a different viewpoint, the new preacher took down the signs next to the front door and replaced them with signs that read "Visitor." On Sundays, he parked at the far end of the lot, leaving ample parking room for visitors near the door. This was not a big marketing action, but it was a display of the attitude that the customers come first. The change provides this church with an extra feature, warmth and caring, that can lead to the perception of a better "product." In almost half of clinics and hospitals, the customers (who are typically ill and often cannot walk well) are forced to park away from the front door. The parking lot can be one indicator of the way in which an organization will handle customer-service issues. Increasingly, there is recognition of this factor in health care, to the point that there is a totally specialized niche company called HealthCare Parking Systems of America, which specializes in providing valet parking services to hospitals, medical clinics, and medical office buildings (www.healthcareparking.com).

The key to good service is striving to have a product exceed the expectations of the customer. This approach also recognizes the important belief that it is the customer that defines quality. Obviously, in health care, defining quality health is not in terms of the clinical quality, but rather the service-delivery quality. Research has found that consumers use five broad dimensions to assess a service's quality:

- *Reliability.* Was the promised service delivered accurately and dependably?
- *Responsiveness.* Was the provider organization (or the representatives of that organization) willing to help and provide prompt service?
- *Assurance.* Were the employees knowledgeable and courteous, and able to instill trust and confidence?
- *Empathy.* How much caring and attention was provided to patients or customers?
- *Tangibles.* What was the appearance of the physical facilities, personnel, and the supporting communication material?

These criteria are listed in order of importance.[1]

In a study conducted within one large multispecialty group, the Fallon Clinic, the importance of the services delivered was found to be critical by 77% of the patients who described themselves as loyal. Loyalty to the Fallon Clinic and satisfaction of the patients was highly correlated to the attributes of reliability and assurance factors.[2]

Focusing on these components will increase satisfaction and ideally loyalty, an objective that is much more difficult to attain. For example, in one hospital physicians enjoy having their patients on a particular nursing unit. The patients receive good care. In addition, however, the head nurse views the physicians not only as team members, but also as customers who could just as well take their patients to another hospital. This nurse tries to shape the nursing unit (the product) to satisfy the physicians. In another example, some automobile dealerships call their customers 48 hours after a car has been serviced to make sure everything is satisfactory. At others, salespeople send plants to the owners of new cars, thanking them for the purchase. This type of customer service is a surprise to customers. When they need service again or are looking for new cars, these automobile dealerships will be on their lists. As a final example, a hospital radiologist decided to make a sales call on a group of internists at their office. This radiologist had been reading films for the internists for more than 15 years, but always at the hospital, and the internists had had to come to the radiology department to see the radiologist. The radiologist called in the morning to see whether he could meet with the internists during a take-out lunch that he would bring. At the meeting, the radiologist simply asked the internists how they viewed the radiology service and what, if anything, could be done to improve it. At first, the internists were skeptical, then amazed, and finally pleased that the radiologist would make such an effort. Three weeks later, the internists offered the radiologist a chance to buy into the new mammography program that they had been planning independent of the radiologist's involvement.

Service or product enhancements are everywhere—from the mint on the pillow at the hotel, to pick-up and delivery from the office for car repair, to weekend and night hours at the clinic. In fact, what differentiates one hospital from the next, one physician from another, or one consultant from another is not just the underlying skill that the professional brings to the table. The skill, in fact, has become somewhat homogenized as hundreds of universities turn out thousands of technically well-trained professionals. Today, it is necessary to have not only outstanding technical skills, but also the ability to provide the extra service that goes beyond the current standard.

Service enhancements include dozens of little items that can help patients distinguish among outstanding technicians: clean waiting rooms, responsive callbacks, respect for the time constraints of others, assistance with filling out insurance forms, nurses who call back after a day to make sure everything is all right, a birthday card, a newsletter every 4 months, or a free bus pass. All these activities define the product or service offering and help determine how competitive it will be.

Understanding that the service delivery extends beyond the technical or a clinical offering of the organization has been a key component of the strategy of the Mayo Clinic.[3] The Mayo Clinic manages both visual and experiential clues by having staff wear business attire to make it seem less clinical and making the physical space appear as unstressful as possible.

Selecting Among New Offerings

Given product and service lifecycles, managers must recognize that declining demand for a service may occur because of factors beyond their control. These factors could be demographic changes in the market, new technological impacts, or changes in reimbursements. For example, healthcare reform and the impending possible shift to population-based care may result in less of a focus on inpatient care revenue and more of a focus on consideration of managing dollars toward a patient's health to go where they are appropriately utilized. Therefore, a successful organization must always consider new service offerings. **Figure 7.3** is a checklist that allows managers to give each possible new service a score on several variables as an aid in the ranking of alternatives. The criteria provided on the checklist are not intended to be definitive. Rather, each organization should add or delete criteria to fit its situation. An organization's checklist should provide a total picture of this critical decision area.

Identifying product or service opportunities often requires creativity on the part of key management personnel. In considering new program opportunities, the five questions presented here may be helpful:

1. Can this service substitute for another service? For example, substitute a laser center for a surgi-center.
2. Is it possible to combine this product or service with another to enhance the service line? For example, bundle physical examinations, laboratory services, and physical therapy into one new service called sports medicine.
3. Is it possible to adapt existing products or services into new products or services? General Electric has followed this strategy very successfully in India. It launched a portable electrocardiogram (ECG) machine that weighs less than 1 kilogram and runs on a battery, ideal for the hot and dusty conditions of rural India. It allows ECGs at approximately 20 cents, compared with $50 using the typical machine. By modifying existing technology, General Electric can greater penetrate India's $3 billion medical device market.[4]
4. Is it possible to modify current products to become more competitive? Since 1992, the amount of cosmetic surgery has grown six-fold, yet the real price of such procedures has declined by one-third.[5] The major reason for this decline in price has been that existing products have been modified through innovation, and thus growth has continued as costs have decreased.[6]
5. Is it possible to magnify the product's role? For example, this is being attempted in medical services such as laboratories by companies such as Any Lab Test Now (http://anylabfranchise.com/), which is a franchising approach to setting up a free-standing lab; some retail clinics are franchised operations; and there are temporary, per diem healthcare personnel agencies such as the franchises offered by Interim Healthcare based in Houston, Texas (www.interimhealthcare .com/news/articles/040130_tacoma_houston.aspx).

Modifying Existing Services

Often, as a market matures or as more competitors enter the market, it is necessary to modify the existing service or product. Program modifications may be accomplished in two ways: feature addition (i.e., adding features

FIGURE 7.3

Checklist for Evaluating New Services

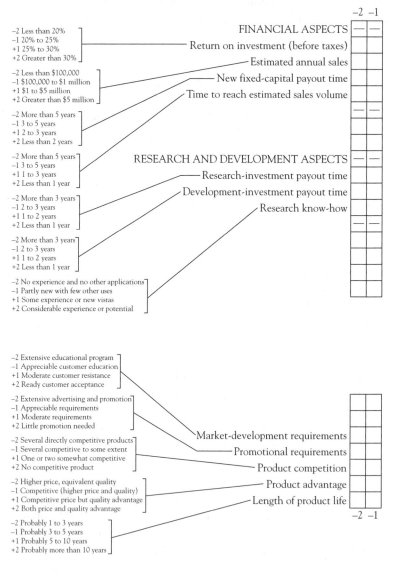

to the existing offering) and quality shifting (i.e., making a change in quality). The MedPath Group, for example, offers international destinations in Costa Rica, India, the Philippines, and Thailand for procedures that include orthopedics, cardiac care, cosmetic surgery, dental, weight-loss surgery, and liver and kidney transplants. In addition to the cost advantages at their Joint Commission–accredited facilities, they include features such as stays at luxury hotels (www.medpathgroup.com/destination.php). As

FIGURE 7.3
(continued)

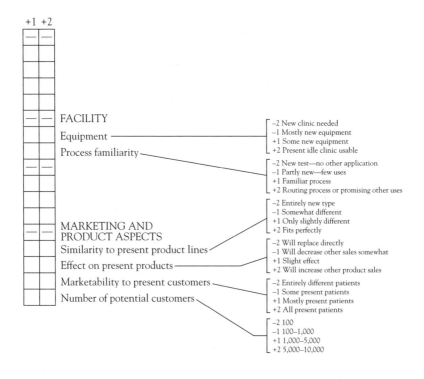

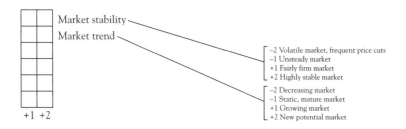

competition becomes more intense, the clinic may improve the quality of the program to seek differentiation.

For our purposes, quality has two dimensions: technical (clinical) and perceptual, or service related. Both are important, but service quality is sometimes lost in an industry dominated by clinicians. Discussions of clinical quality tend to focus on the relationship between cost and quality. In other words, at what point does spending an extra dollar for care add little or no quality or even detract from quality through the provision of unnecessary surgery or unnecessary medications? **Figure 7.4** explores this

FIGURE 7.4

Relationship Between Cost and Quality

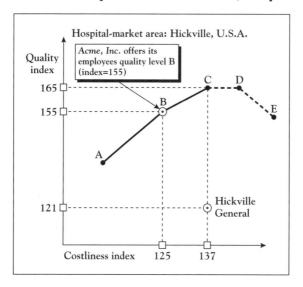

Source: Reprinted from *Hospitals* (1988, December 5) with permission from Health Forum, Inc.

ethical dilemma. In this example, there is a relationship between higher quality and higher costs to a point, but the relationship ultimately evens out and then declines (point E). This relationship gives rise to countless questions, such as how much clinical quality should Medicare allow for and whether an employer should pay only for baseline quality care and require employees to pay for any care beyond this point.

Although providing a minimal level of safe-care is important, several different levels of clinical quality may be acceptable, based on the service offering and the expectations of the patient. For example, a patient who has a deep cut on a finger may be satisfied to have an internist place two or three stitches for $60. A patient with a highly visible cut on the face that requires two or three stitches may want a different level of quality, however, such as plastic surgery at $200.

The best technical quality without outstanding service, in a competitive market, will result in a loss of customers over time. In one study, consumers ranked "up-to-date facilities" as a critical factor in deciding which hospital they preferred.[7] A physician's outstanding clinical skills may be negated as a competitive factor if he or she practices in facilities that appear shoddy to the patient.

Quality involves a host of items that, when bundled together, create an impression that meets, exceeds, or does not meet the customer's expectations. It is a reasonable goal to exceed customer expectations. Organizations are increasingly providing guarantees to try to enhance the service side. Many companies, such as L.L. Bean, have built their strong reputations on unconditional service guarantees.[8] Hospitals have experimented with guarantees for hot food and prompt answers to call buttons in an attempt to provide breakthrough service and to keep service quality on the agenda.

Choosing a Branding Strategy

"Branding" as a part of marketing has not received the appropriate degree of importance among healthcare decision makers. In health care, several industry activities underscore the importance of brand name consideration. The increasing consolidation among healthcare institutions often results in organization name changes. Setting up physician practices, establishing ambulatory surgical centers, or offering health insurance products to the market all pose questions about branding. Traditional industries have long recognized the concept of *brand equity*, which is the total accumulated value or worth of a brand. Brand equity has five components:

1. Brand loyalty is the commitment buyers have to a particular brand. Brand loyalty is useful in reducing marketing costs and creating barriers to entry from others, as customers say, "I would go only to the Smith Group for my medical care."
2. Name awareness indicates how well known the brand is in the marketplace. The Mayo Clinic has exceptionally high awareness compared to other healthcare provider organizations. In a 2003 national study, the primary decisions makers in households were asked if they had no income constraints and could go anywhere for health care should they be suffering a major medical condition such as cancer, a heart condition, or the like, where would they go (unaided); 19% said "Mayo." Additionally, 8% said the Mayo Clinic when asked what "other institutions" they would consider in a follow-up question. This result was three times greater than any other organization cited.[9]
3. Perceived quality is the value a consumer perceives a brand has. This perception has definitely led to a trend in recent years as major tertiary and academic centers in the United States such as the Mayo Clinic, Johns Hopkins University, Harvard University, and others have moved to international affiliations in India, the Middle East, and elsewhere. Patients associate the strong reputations of these institutions with a quality of clinical service.[10]

4. Brand associations link a consumer's memory to a brand. For example, McDonald's is linked by Ronald the clown, Prudential is linked by the rock, Travelers Insurance by the umbrella. Unlike traditional businesses, few organizations in health care have worked to develop this component of brand equity. In September 2010, BioSpace Med changed its name to EOS Imaging. This attempt at rebranding was to capitalize on the strong brand-name recognition of its flagship low-dose imaging device. The EOS ultra-low-dose orthopedic imaging system has strong brand-name recognition in Europe. In March 2010, the company won Federal Drug Administration (FDA) approval for a pediatric version of the device and hopes to significantly push the marketing of the product in the United States with strong brand association.[11]

5. Brand assets are proprietary resources, such as the service mark of a brand.

Brand equity is increasingly being eroded within health care as organizations merge or consolidate. For example, when hospitals merge, often neither organization wants to be seen as having been taken over by the other. As a result, the organizations frequently create a new brand name. In San Jose, California, Good Samaritan Hospital, a large, well-respected tertiary hospital in the area began to merge with other community hospitals. The new entity was given the name Health Dimensions, which meant little to consumers. After promoting the name for more than a year and changing corporate stationary, signs, and the like, the organization realized it had lost value in the marketplace when focus groups revealed that in spite of its efforts, a large majority of consumers in its service still did not relate to Health Dimensions, but most knew Good Samaritan as a good hospital. Now, Health Dimensions is gone, replaced by the Good Samaritan Health System.

That a brand is important to a product or company is unquestioned. As organizations develop multiple sites or products, the protection of that equity is critical; it can be accomplished by using one or more of the five components listed earlier.

Will Americans allow their health care to be influenced by a brand name? The power of brand was demonstrated in the Massachusetts market in a study in 2007 comparing the prices negotiated from insurers and the quality across many procedures between the largest academic institutions and competing community institutions. Although it was determined that in many instances the quality was equal, and in some cases the demonstrated outcomes were better, the negotiated prices by the larger, better known branded institutions were far better. As was noted in this study, the clout was often based on "a powerful brand name and elite reputation."[12]

The possibility of national brands looms large. In a sense, it is the American way. Large, brand-name systems have the power to negotiate for more business, capital, and market control. Furthermore, as the Fortune 500 companies, along with major insurance companies such as Blue Cross Blue Shield, begin to shop for healthcare providers, dealing with national brands is efficient and effective. Most astute observers seem to understand this concept. The Voluntary Hospitals of America (VHA), the Cleveland Clinic, the Hospital Corporation of America (HCA), and new national health maintenance organization (HMO) systems are all maneuvering to be part of this national level of competition.

Blanket Branding

An organization that brings out every new product offering under one name uses blanket branding. Many companies have adopted this approach— Toro, Scott, Caterpillar, Medtronic, and HCA. The advantages are obvious. The use of the organization name reduces the cost of introducing a new service. If the organization has a good reputation, the consumer will be receptive to the new products. The Johnston Clinic, for example, is a highly respected multispecialty group in its city. Consumers will probably consider a clinic under the Johnston name in a suburban area as an extension of this well-known group.

Blanket branding has risks, however. A new offering that is not up to the high standards of the organization may hurt the entire group. Therefore, the riskier the offering and the less time spent in research and development, the less attractive this approach should be.

Marketers are increasingly applying the name of a product or brand beyond its original use. This approach has been referred to as *brand extension*. The underlying logic is that a strong brand name can substantially reduce the risk of introducing a new brand. Kaiser Permanente, for example, has moved beyond its traditional closed-panel HMO by offering a Kaiser preferred provider organization (PPO) in several states. Creating the wrong extension, however, can lead to damaging brand associations or cannibalizing the image of the existing brand. A brand extension works when consumers perceive a relationship between the original brand and product class and the one to which it is being extended. Thus, a consumer might be able to relate the Mayo newsletter to the Mayo Clinic, but making such an association might be more difficult should Mayo decide to extend its name to a line of salt-free food products. Mayo recognizes the value of its name, and in 1985, established the for-profit Mayo Clinic Health Solutions Service Divisions (www.mayoclinichealthsolutions.com). The range of products includes online applications, print publications, telephonic programs, and health benefit administration. Encompassing them are tools to empower individuals to address a spectrum of their health needs across the health continuum.

Multibrand Strategy

An alternative to blanket branding is the multibrand approach. For example, if the Johnston Clinic is merging with a group of family practitioners in the suburbs, and not only are there concerns about some of the physicians within this new group, but many people in the community also view the clinic as a high-priced group, the Johnston Clinic may decide to name the new group the Suburbia Family Practice Clinic. The multibrand strategy minimizes risk to the parent organization. Even though the Johnston Clinic will have to spend additional money introducing this new group to the community, the high-price image of the Johnston Clinic will not be carried over to this new brand name.

Reseller Strategy

Another branding approach used in traditional business is selling a product or service under someone else's name. Many small manufacturers have used this approach for many years in dealing with Sears. The manufacturer provides Sears with the product, and Sears markets it under its own name or the Craftsman tool brand. This approach takes advantage of the existing market presence of the reseller. The application of this strategy in health care has been limited, but has increased potential with the onset of integrated delivery systems. Organizations may be able to offer turnkey rehabilitative-medicine services to multiple systems, but provide the service under the name of each particular integrated delivery system. For some solo specialty medical groups, this branding strategy might provide a viable direction for the future.

Mixed Branding

In mixed branding, an organization markets a product under its own name and also that of a reseller. Michelin, for example, markets its tires at Sears and also manufactures tires to be sold under the Sears name. So too in health care, some large-territory laboratories are providing pathology services on their own and are also providing these services under contract to small community hospitals with no identification with the laboratory name.

Co-branding

In co-branding, one organization markets its name in conjunction with another entity. Taco Bell and Pizza Hut are co-branding at many outlets. This strategy is also appearing in health care. MD Anderson Cancer Center is promoted as offering cancer care at Orlando Regional Medical Center in Florida. As the Mayo Clinic has moved to acquire medical groups in Iowa and Wisconsin, it too has used a co-branding strategy by promoting the name of the existing groups with the Mayo logo listed beneath. The logic of co-branding is clear. It allows the power of both brand names to be used in the market. What is less clear is the risk. Tying an organization's name to another entity where it might have limited control over how the service is delivered could lead to some negative consequences.

Selecting a Program Name

Major corporations spend many dollars to select the right name, yet the importance of this aspect has escaped many healthcare organizations. The guidelines for name selection are simple. The name should be:

1. *Meaningful.* A program's name should be relevant to the market for which it is developed. For example, "regional oncology program" means little to the community at large. The nonmedical person does not talk about oncology, but rather about cancer. The name selected should help identify the company and position it clearly in consumers' minds. Ticketron (a computerized ticketing company later acquired by Ticketmaster) suggests both the service and the electronic means by which the product can be purchased and processed. Humana (a health insurance company) suggests warm, personalized care.
2. *Concise.* Most good product names are short and crisp.
3. *Memorable.* Brand names should be easy to spell and pronounce. Otolaryngologists overcome this problem by listing themselves in the yellow pages under "ear, nose, and throat." Many rheumatologists provide alternative listings under "arthritis."
4. *Legal.* Any service or product name should be free of legal problems. Brand names and service marks can be registered. Infringement of a name is always a concern if two organizations use identification marks that are similar. This issue came to the forefront when Columbia University filed a lawsuit claiming that Columbia/HCA was infringing on its name. The for-profit hospital chain had used that name for 9 years prior to the filing of the lawsuit by the university, and the court ruled in favor of the chain, finding no infringement.

5. *Distinctive.* A good brand name should clearly identify the service and the supplier and distinguish the product from its competitors. In health care, the number of hospitals with the word "Community," or, for those with religious affiliations, "Saint," in the name makes distinctiveness a difficult criterion to meet. An alternative approach is exemplified by the walk-in urgent care facilities in Fort Wayne, Indiana called Redi Med, which clearly conveys the benefits offered by the organization.

6. *Flexible.* An important concern today—because of the nature of health care—is that a name not be too restrictive. Geographical references might limit an organization as it acquires facilities in other communities or states. This is not a concern for "U.S. Healthcare," until it contemplates expansion overseas. A name should be selected with consideration of the long-term strategic direction of the organization. Ohio Health in Columbus, Ohio is addressing the issue of flexibility. This company owns two of the better known hospitals in the community, Riverside Methodist and Grant. Few consumers in Columbus identify with the parent company Ohio Health. Although the company owns and manages medical facilities in 46 of the 88 Ohio counties, it keeps the Ohio Health name apart from each hospital's and health center's own unique identity.

Two additional criteria that have been suggested in the pharmaceutical industry are:

7. *Credible.* It is vital to ensure that a brand be credible across all target markets.

8. *Sustainable.* Where might the brand ultimately go? A brand should be "future-proofed" for long-term opportunity.[13]

DISTRIBUTION

The element of the marketing mix that refers to the manner in which service is delivered or offered to the customer or patient is called distribution. In traditional industries, the channel of distribution refers to the way the product moves from the manufacturer to the wholesaler to the retailer to the consumer. Although this is the common path, there are channel variations. In health care, we can define the channel of distribution as the path a patient takes as he or she moves to the appropriate level of care (**Figure 7.5**).

Often the question of what value the middle levels of the channel provide arises. In traditional industries like consumer food products, this question pertains to the wholesaler, while in health care, one might raise

FIGURE 7.5

Some Distribution Alternatives in Health Care

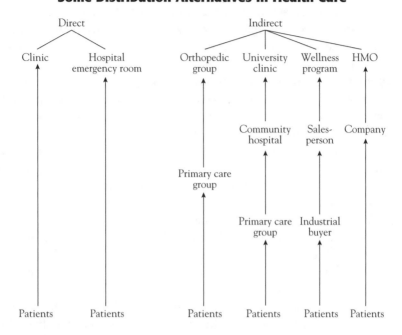

the question about the managed-care organization. In health care, the benefits provided at these levels include:

- *Access.* Some organizations provide value by bringing providers closer to the customer through the establishment of satellite clinics.
- *Consolidation.* Some organizations provide value by bringing together a large number of patients or subscribers.
- *Economy.* Some organizations provide value by making it easier to purchase the service through their pricing of premiums or the purchase terms provided.
- *Grading.* Some organizations provide value by indicating the quality of the services available. Increasingly, health insurers, with the various plans they offer (be they high-deductible offerings or other forms of coverage), are now tiering physicians and hospitals, other parties in the channel, based on two criteria: cost and quality. In essence, this tiering of these other entities within the channel could be viewed as a form of "grading," a function commonly performed by a channel member. For example, the highly rated Harvard Pilgrim Independence health plan, a not-for-profit insurance company, bases co-pays on the tiering of specialists in the

benefit guide information for state employees covered in Massachusetts. These co-pays range from $20.00 (Excellent) up to $45.00 (Standard). This tiering, or "grading" strategy by Harvard Pilgrim Health Plan is not atypical by healthcare insurance companies in today's marketplace.

- *Time savings.* Some organizations provide value by being available when the consumer wants to access the service. This value is provided by after-hours clinics and by visiting-nurse organizations.
- *Information.* An important value provided by some middlemen is that of information. Retailers, for example, often train their salespeople to be knowledgeable in the product. Some medical organizations have developed detailed health education programs for consumers. In many states, the governments have, to a degree, also entered the channel to provide information. Minnesota Board of Medical Practice is a very transparent website (www.state.mn.us/portal/mn/jsp/home.do?agency=BMP) in terms of information, and is moving to become increasingly more so—a person can examine any disciplinary actions taken against a physician, and physician profiles are available. In Vermont, a consumer can search by physician and examine the training level of a physician, whether there have been any disciplinary actions filed, research publications, malpractice claims, education and training levels, or hospital and staff privilege (www.healthvermont.gov/hc/med_board/bmp.aspx). One might argue that, to some degree, the Board of Registration has entered the channel of distribution between the patient and the doctor.

Healthcare organizations need to recognize the benefits that can be added at intermediate levels and determine with regard to their own strategy which benefits they want to deliver and which they will let others enter the channel to provide. A principle in marketing with regard to channels that is relevant for healthcare organizations today is the Law of Functional Shifting. This law states that the middle levels of the channel can always be eliminated, but the function can never be. Understanding this law is important as the healthcare marketplace moves to population-based health and the acceptance of risk by provider systems responsible for the care of patients. Presently, managed-care organizations are responsible for consolidating patients or subscribers; with this base, the managed-care organizations then turn to contract with providers. In future years, the integrated delivery systems might decide to eliminate the managed-care organizations, since it is the physicians or the health system (a hospital and its own employed physicians, along with some community doctors) that will be responsible for a population of patients in their region. It is this accountable care entity, however, that will also need a data support structure beyond the existing electronic medical record, such as that which exists in the information technology (IT) departments of today's managed-care entities.

For accountable care organizations (ACOs) in the coming years, a critical strategic question will then present itself: Do these new ACOs perform this function (information management of patient populations), or shift it elsewhere in the channel? This is a strategic question. Does the shifting occur through contracting? Strategic alliances? How is it performed?

Distribution alternatives common to the healthcare setting can be characterized as direct or indirect. The channel is direct when the service provider deals directly with the user; for example, a primary care clinic that serves its immediate neighborhood directly or a retail medical clinic. The channel is indirect when the service provider needs the assistance of an intermediary; for example, an orthopedic group that depends on referrals from primary care physicians serves patients in an indirect channel. A hospital that provides services with the assistance of the medical staff is another indirect channel. A hospital-based sales force may be involved in either a direct or indirect channel; they may sell the service to patients, the direct users, or to corporations, who are not the direct users. Using either direct or indirect channels involves making several kinds of decisions.

Decision Areas

When *direct distribution channels* are used, management decisions focus on the following aspects:

1. *Location.* Access is possibly the most critical element for direct channels. Where should the facility be located? The convenience of the practicing physicians has often determined a healthcare facility's location. As competition for patients increases, however, the preferences of the patients rather than those of the professional staff may determine the site of the facility. Nowhere has the change been greater than in the expansion of retail clinics in health care. The first retail clinic, QuickMedx, now Minute Clinic, pioneered the concept when it opened in a Minneapolis-based Cub Food store in 2000.[14] Rand estimated that by 2010 the number had grown to 1,200 clinics operating in 33 states.[15] The importance of the location as valued by the consumer, less so the provider, is best demonstrated in **Figure 7.6** with data from the Commonwealth Fund's report on retail clinics. These clinics' locations were more convenient than that of other sources of care, and thus consumers decided to go to them for treatment.
2. *Hours.* When should the service be available? Hours and days must meet the market's needs. If a group's patient base consists of families in which both husband and wife work, for example, evening hours may be desirable. However, with advances in technology, the concept of time (and thus hours) is changing dramatically.

FIGURE 7.6

Primary Reasons Consumers Cite for Using Retail Clinics

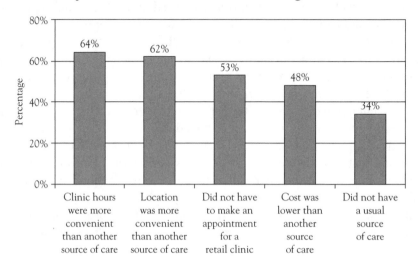

Note: Categories are not meant to be mutually exclusive; respondents were able to select multiple categories.

Source: Tu, H. T., & Cohen, G. R. (2008, December). Checking up on retail-based health clinics: Is the boom ending? (Issue Brief), The Commonwealth Fund. Retrieved June 20, 2011, from: http://www.commonwealthfund.org/Publications/Issue-Briefs/2008/Dec/Checking-Up-on-Retail-Based-Health-Clinics--Is-the-Boom-Ending.aspx

> For example, Zipnosis, a web-based service (www.zipnosis.com) offered in conjunction with Park Nicollet in Minneapolis–St. Paul, uses smart-decision tools to provide online diagnoses for a limited number of conditions and sends the necessary prescriptions to the pharmacy. Time, then, is what is convenient to the patient.
>
> 3. *Mode.* How will the service be provided? Should the physician at the primary care group provide all inoculations, or can a nurse provide this service? The mode by which a service is delivered can be altered for a competitive advantage in price (as this example may provide) or in another dimension, such as convenience or perceived quality.

Each of the preceding decision areas pertains to indirect channels as well as to direct channels. In *indirect channel settings*, however, additional strategy concerns focus on push/pull alternatives. In an indirect channel, such as a tertiary-care hospital, patients can be admitted in two ways. The common method is for the family physician to refer patients to the hospital. An alternative way is for the patients themselves to select the facility. Any indirect channel has two strategies to attract users: a push strategy or a pull strategy.

Clinics and hospitals dependent on referrals traditionally use the *push strategy*. This approach centers on efforts to build loyalty among the members of the channel, usually physicians. In no area of health care is this strategy more prevalent than that of pharmaceutical companies to physicians. A recent estimate has pharmaceutical companies spending slightly more than $38 billion dollars in samples, detailing, and meetings geared toward physicians on pharmaceutical marketing efforts.[16] Ideally, successful implementation of a push strategy leads to the development of loyalty in intermediate channel members, who will then write a script for a particular drug; or, if it is a hospital trying to develop a push strategy with physicians, they will refer patients to the institution over a competitor.

As an alternative to depending on the other channel members for referrals, some organizations try to develop a preference for their facility among the ultimate users, thus using a *pull strategy*. In many cities, for example, physicians may have privileges at several hospitals. Hospital X and Hospital Y both have modern obstetrical units, and they both try to meet physicians' needs in a similar manner. As an additional strategy, however, Hospital X attempts to pull patients into the hospital (around the physician) by promoting its obstetrical service to consumers in the community, primarily through newspaper advertising. The objective of this approach is to have the patient request Hospital X when in the physician's office. If a pull strategy is to be successful, the organization's quality of care, as well as its capabilities, must meet those of its competitors.

The pull strategy is being used increasingly in health care within the pharmaceutical sector. Historically, the channel for pharmaceutical companies was clear. The manufacturers dealt with the physician, who ultimately wrote the prescription for the patient. In order to affect this channel, manufacturers relied on the push strategy by calling on physicians' offices, providing them with little promotional giveaways like pens and prescription pads, and by sponsoring seminars at attractive locations on medical topics. With increasing government concern over some of these practices, pharmaceutical manufacturers have turned to a pull strategy, promoting drugs and their ultimate benefits directly to patients in the belief that they will request the drugs from their physicians. And, research has demonstrated that patient requests have a significant effect on physician prescribing behavior.[17]

Figure 7.7 shows a graph of the promotional spending by marketing type that has occurred in the pharmaceutical area from 1989 to 2007. As shown in this chart, the direct-to-consumer pull strategy began to wane as 2006 approached, when the government raised greater concern over this method and its public health implications.

FIGURE 7.7

Annual Spending on Direct-to-Consumer Advertising and Promotion to Health Professionals, 1996–2005

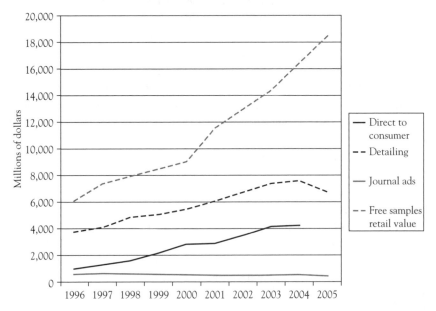

Source: Data from Donohue, J. M., Cevasco, M., & Rosenthal, M. B. (2007, August 16). *New England Journal of Medicine, 357,* 673–681.

As recently as 2011, Congress has considered banning or putting severe restrictions on direct-to-consumer advertising for pharmaceuticals, thus eliminating this pull strategy. There is a concern, however, that this may lead to countervailing increases of push tactics to physicians.[18]

A pull strategy has also been a major focus of academic medical centers. Because managed-care organizations now contract with providers and often avoid certain tertiary centers for cost or contractual reasons, these entities often try to appeal directly to patients in managed care to request access to a particular medical facility as part of their healthcare plan.

Controlling the Channel

Health care today is characterized increasingly as a market in which some intermediaries have gained significant leverage in contracting. Managed-care companies and some insurance firms are responsible for large amounts of patient volume. For example, by 2008, the American Medical Association had reported that 94% of 314 geographic areas in the United States (mainly metropolitan statistical areas) were found to be highly concentrated in terms of health insurance firms.[19] Similarly, in some communities, large provider systems are also attempting to gain leverage by having a significant percentage of the delivery system within their control. As the healthcare market moves to a situation in which bulk buyers (insurance companies) deal with bulk sellers (hospitals), marketing strategy will have to focus on controlling the channel flow for patients. Sometimes providers will control the channel, and sometimes customers will control it. In effect, control of the channel will require power over the other intermediaries. For example, in markets where there is concentration of insurance power, it has been found that physicians have lower earnings and employment growth, while there is resultant higher earnings for nurses and employment growth for nurses. This suggests that insurance companies may be using their power to substitute one clinical provider for another.[20] One member of the channel can use four common sources of power alone or in conjunction with others to control the other players.

One kind of power is punitive, or coercive, power. Increasingly, large corporations are using punitive power by wielding influence to gain discounts. A company may, for example, threaten to switch providers if it does not receive favorable contractual terms. The threat of coercion has come to the forefront between hospitals and physicians under the term *economic credentialing*, in which a physician is judged as a viable member of the staff as a function of the amount or degree of business that the individual brings to the institution. In a relatively recent case in Little Rock, Arkansas, a physician felt the coercive power of Baptist Health, where she practiced as a gynecologist; her husband, also a doctor, practiced at another institution. Baptist Health was also the exclusive provider for Blue Cross Blue Shield. The gynecologist had done all her procedures at Baptist Health and her office was on the campus of the health system. But, when her husband decided to join a group of doctors who wanted to open their own surgi-center, the board of the health system wrote a "conflict of interest policy" that described indirect financial interest. The gynecologist could not do any procedures at the surgi-center given the nature of the practice, but the hospital said she would have her privileges revoked, essentially ending her practice. This approach was the ultimate use of coercive power. She sued and won.[21]

A second kind of power derives from the expertise of the hospital or healthcare organization—the more expert the medical provider, the more effective power it has in controlling the channel. In order to heighten expert power, it is important to promote the specialized technological aspects or medical expertise of the healthcare organization. *U.S. News & World Report* publishes each year a list of the "best" medical facilities. Some organizations have used these rankings in advertisements to heighten their expert power.

A third kind of power comes from rewarding an intermediary for cooperation. This approach was the strategy pursued by Fox Chase Cancer Center in the establishment of its extensive Fox Chase Network Affiliates Program in Southeastern Pennsylvania and Southeastern New Jersey. A competitive market in which there are four teaching hospitals and more than 82 other hospitals in the region, four medical schools, and four major medical systems, Fox Chase needed to develop a strategy to fulfill its research mission. It worked with community hospitals and doctors in the region to support other cancer programs, although within the institution there was concern this would be developing increasing competition. Fox Chase wanted to develop referrals for its adult solid tumor program. As **Figure 7.8** shows, the network has proven to be not only viable, but highly effective using this cooperation strategy.[22]

Finally, identification is a source of power valuable in controlling the channel in health care. Intermediaries within the channel may find it

FIGURE 7.8

Fox Chase Network Affiliates

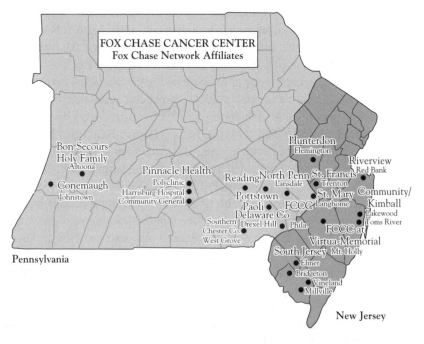

Source: Higman, S. A., McKay, F. J., Engstrom, P. F., O'Grady, M. A., & Young, R. C. (2000, August). Fox Chase Network: Fox Chase Cancer Center's Community Hospital Affiliation Program. *The Oncologist,* 5(4), 329–335.

advantageous to be associated with an organization that has a good name or image. Many large medical organizations offer physicians in the community the opportunity to be an "affiliate," for example. Physicians see this affiliate status as a market advantage because of the prestige associated with the larger group, and they often increase their referrals to the larger organization.

The Changing Nature of Channels

No aspect of the healthcare marketing system may be undergoing greater change today than channels. Two significant trends are affecting this shift: integration and technology.

Figure 7.5 presents some alternative channels of distribution within health care. However, these channels are being revised by *forward and backward integration*. In traditional businesses, forward integration occurs when a manufacturer begins to move closer in the channel of distribution to the consumer. As a result, the company would open retail stores, as was done by the Singer Sewing Company when it opened Singer Sewing Centers, or by Levi Strauss when it opened its national chain of Levi stores. This same trend has been occurring in health care today. A large number of major tertiary and academic medical centers have, since around 1997 or so through the present, established their own network of primary care physicians, surgi-centers, and community hospitals, similar to Johns Hopkins Medicine in the Maryland–DC metro area shown in **Figure 7.9**. An alternative to forward integration is backward integration, in which a member of the channel moves closer to the production end. Holiday Inn, for example, began to manufacture its own furniture for its franchises. In health care, Kaiser Permanente is a health maintenance plan in the state of California that employs doctors and also owns and operates its own hospitals.

The most far-reaching change in health care, however, with regard to distribution channels, may be the result of advances in technology. The entire concept of place might have to be redefined because of the changes occurring in this aspect of the environment. Increasingly, the channel of distribution for care delivery is now a direct, web-based solution, such as American Well's Online Care suite of solutions, where consumers can consult a provider via video chat. Technology has also affected the channel aspect of referrals and medical consults. Partners, the physician group affiliated with Mass General Hospital in Boston, does online second opinions in areas that range from cancer to neurosurgery, to pulmonology, to nephrology. Specialists' opinions cost $575, while a radiologist review is $200 and a pathology consult is $300. The cost of the online visit is

FIGURE 7.9

Forward Integration:

A Map of Johns Hopkins Medicine in the Greater

Maryland–DC Metro Area

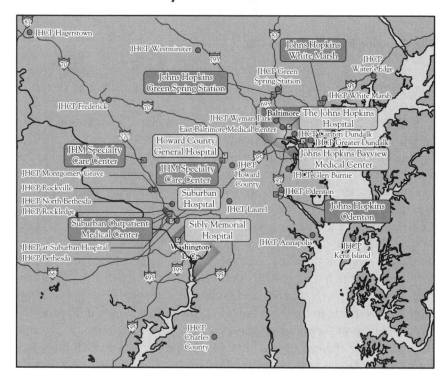

Source: Courtesy of Johns Hopkins Medicine. Retrieved November 10, 2011, from: http://www.hopkinsmedicine.org/patient_care/_images/locations714.jpg

only $36 compared with $135 for an on-site visit for the same services. In fact, many marketing people now view the Internet as a possible way to "deconstruct" the traditional channel of distribution. A medical group in Boston provides consults over the Internet for a fee. Other such programs will no doubt appear with increasing Internet access and use.

PRICING

Some managers still believe that pricing strategies do not apply to healthcare providers. Indeed, such strategies may have been less important under the traditional cost-based reimbursement system. However, with the appearance in recent years of high-deductible health plans and health savings accounts coupled with increasing transparency of price information, consumers are becoming more sensitive to the prices they are paying for health care. It has been suggested that there are five particular situations when effective price shopping may take place in health care:

- The services are not complex.
- The need for the service is not urgent.
- A diagnosis has already been made.
- Bundled prices are the norm for the service.
- The insurance benefit structure provides incentives to choose lower cost providers.[23]

In fact, a growing number of reports show that patients are negotiating the cost of medical services or receiving a discount for cash.[24] Intermediaries have also entered the market, such as HealthCare Advocates, Inc. (www. healthcareadvocates.com/services.html), which provides a fee-negotiation service for its members. The commonality across these changes is that price is a strategic issue for healthcare providers.

Price, then, appears to be gaining strength as a critical market factor of value to the end customer, the patient, as it has always been to the employer in terms of decision in the healthcare environment. As a cost-control measure, most employers are adding significant copayments (30%) for physician visits and hospital stays. Additionally, insurance companies are moving increasingly to tiering providers and hospitals on the basis of quality and efficiency (cost) and communicating these data to consumers to use in their ultimate decisions. In 2006, WellPoint launched a hospital cost-comparison tool for its 300,000 members in Dayton, Ohio to allow subscribers to compare the prices of 40 medical procedures at various hospitals in the region. Other insurers such as UnitedHealthcare, Aetna, and Cigna also offered similar comparison tools.[25] As reimbursement plans change, it becomes increasingly appropriate to consider various pricing options.

Pricing strategies differ according to an organization's goals and its direction. In general, costs determine the floor for pricing, and consumers set the ceiling. In addition, a hospital's or clinic's objectives affect pricing. The following are several objectives that would result in various pricing actions:

- Build traffic or market share.
- Obtain short-run or long-run profits.
- Obtain growth.
- Stabilize the market.
- Speed the exit of marginal competitors.
- Discourage competitive entry.

- Enhance image.
- Develop product leadership.
- Use price as an artificial indication of quality.

Other factors that determine the price of a product or service include competition and the willingness of third-party payers to reimburse the provider.

Several different pricing strategies are available. Their appropriateness for a particular organization depends on various factors. Hospitals and healthcare professionals are often somewhat limited in their use of pricing strategies. As experimentation with nontraditional areas of health care increases, alternative pricing approaches may become necessary. The following are examples of alternative pricing approaches:

1. Offering package prices for husband-and-wife physical exams.
2. Providing patients with a discount for cash payment. This is done by St. Joseph Medical Heritage Medical Group with offices in Southern California. Discounts are 30% for physician office visits, x-rays, urgent care, ECG testing, and other services. Depending on the laboratory test, discounts can range from 30% to 60%.
3. Offering a prepayment discount for an obstetrical program. This pricing strategy is employed by St. Luke's of Iowa Health System, which provides a 20% discount for patients who prepay 30 days before delivery for both normal and cesarean deliveries.[26]
4. Providing industrial rates for companies that bring their accident victims to your hospital.
5. Offering family credit-card programs. These programs are offered by companies such as CarePayment, which is a credit-card system that contracts with hospitals and then allows patients to spread out hospital charges over 36 months, interest free. The card is offered under the hospital's brand name. CarePayment gives the hospital 85 cents on the dollar.[27]
6. Providing discounts (based on diagnosis-related group [DRG] code) to group buyers such as an industrial plan.

Skim Pricing

The buyers who are most interested in a service are less price sensitive than those who are not interested, and they will find it acceptable to pay a higher price. Skim pricing—which involves setting a high price—allows the organization to recover the costs of project development. Generally, the higher the technology required, the higher the potential for skim pricing. This strategy has been used by academic institutions that are financially successful and in which higher quality, higher perceived value, better reputation, and/or other organizational differentiation factors have allowed their hospitals to charge incrementally higher prices for the same services as their competitors and thus skim the market.[28] Moreover, a premium price can be used to develop a status position for the service in the consumer's mind. Expensive cars, condominiums, some nursing homes, and consultants sometimes use this strategy. A cosmetic surgery program may have a high price to provide status and to increase perceived quality. Buyers are likely to gravitate to the more expensive program because they perceive it to be better. The disadvantage of skim pricing is that it often encourages competitors to enter the market. A new competitor may seek to establish a differential advantage based on a better price.

Penetration Pricing

Some organizations may price a service below the prevailing level in order to penetrate the market or increase market share. This situation occurred in Vancouver, British Columbia as more providers entered into the increasingly competitive Lasik surgery space. In 1997, the cost of doing this procedure for Canadian patients was $4,800; the following year, a new provider entering the market had to do so with a penetration pricing strategy that had dropped to $2,995 in order to achieve any level of differentiation. By 1999, the price of new entrants had dropped Lasik surgery to $1,498. In 2011, Lasik MD charged $490, and currently the group offers patients a "lowest price guarantee," stating it will match the lowest price within the last 6 months, provided the competitor is in the same city.[29] Clearly, penetration pricing requires a good understanding of the organization's cost structure.

Elasticity Pricing

In order to take advantage of known or perceived price elasticity or inelasticity at a given point in time, an organization may adopt elasticity pricing. For example, a parking space at a city hospital may be rented for $8 during the day shift and $1 during the evening hours. This pricing strategy is based on demand elasticity.

Cost-Plus Pricing and Variable Pricing

Hospitals and clinics most often use cost-plus pricing, and reimbursement is generally made on this basis. This strategy can cause perception problems with consumers, however. For example, because markups on items such as aspirin and chest x-rays are highly visible to consumers, a hospital may be wise to use variable pricing, which calls for shifting prices based on demand, customer expectations, and costs.

Price Bundling

Increasingly in health care, as services are packaged together (e.g., industrial programs), price bundling is becoming more common. With this strategy, an organization prices individual services together so that the bundled price is lower than the total of the individual prices. Consumers are inclined to purchase such a package because of the discount. As the marketplace has moved toward managed care, bundled prices are appearing under the term *global pricing*, which is a single fee for diagnosis and intervention. This approach to pricing has appeared with greater frequency for cardiac and musculoskeletal procedures. In 2011, CaroMont Health and Blue Cross Blue Shield agreed to a bundled price (payment) for knee replacements. Patients who qualify receive a single bill for presurgery, surgery, and most follow-up care. Typically, patients would receive separate billings for each of the services that would involve the physician, anesthesiologist, radiologist, pathologist, physical therapist, and the lab that may do the presurgical testing.[30] Under healthcare reform, the issue will be less about price bundling and more concerned with bundled payment. In this scenario, the government will provide a lump-sum payment to ACOs (whatever composition they may consist of) to provide for the quality care of a population in an efficient way. Defining what will be in that bundle of payment is still to a large degree not yet fully clear or agreed upon.

In an industrial healthcare program, for example, employee physicals may be priced at $125. An on-the-job analysis to detect problem areas for the Occupational Safety and Health Administration or workers' compensation claims may be priced at $350 per half-day session with a follow-up report. In addition, 1-day educational workshops to reduce on-the-job injuries may be provided for a fee of $400 per session, with a maximum of 25 employees per session. The individual prices of these three services total $875. If they are offered separately, some corporations may be tempted to buy one or two of them, but not all three. However, if costs are well below the prices charged, the provider might bundle the prices and offer this industrial healthcare program at $650, a real savings to the customer. If, in fact, costs are significantly below each individual component's market price, the bundled price can lead to higher total revenue for the firm.[31] **Table 7.1** offers ideas for selecting a pricing strategy given various objectives, product or service lifecycles, and market conditions. It is apparent that, depending on the objective of the organization,

TABLE 7.1 PRICING STRATEGY

Objective	Strategy	When Tactic Is Employed	How to Implement	Pros	Cons
Short-term profit gain	Price-skimming strategy	• No similar competing product/service • Significantly improved new product • Large market potential • High barriers to entry • Inelastic demand • Use price as spigot to control demand • Recoup research and development	• Charge short-term premium price • Reduce price as competitors enter in later lifecycle stages	• Help with any organizational capacity constraints • Recover development costs • Image value for product or service (in health care may be of value)	• May limit market • Encourage competitive entry who will undercut price
Encourage others to produce and promote the product (service) to stimulate primary demand	Price at market	• Several providers with similar services (products) • Market is growing • Lifecycle of service is long • Cost structure is reasonably well known	• Start with price to charge and work back to cost	• Existing market already aware of service • Market price recognized by customers	• Limited flexibility to price • Limited flexibility for error • Internal pressure on cost curves • Focus on differentiation of service elsewhere than price

(continued)

TABLE 7.1   *(CONTINUED)*

Objective	Strategy	When Tactic Is Employed	How to Implement	Pros	Cons
Stimulate market growth and become entrenched for long term	Penetration pricing	• Long product lifecycle • Large market • Low barriers to entry • High price sensitivity/demand is highly price elastic • There is an economy of scale point that must be reached in terms of volume throughput internally	• Price low relative to substitutable services (products)	• Discourages competitive entry • Encourages trial	• Must know cost curves • Must be able to handle demand relative to capacity
Keep competitors out of market or eliminate existing competitors	Preemptive pricing	• Common in consumer products	• Set prices as close as possible to cost of production • If prices drop with volume, begin prices at level where drop occurs	• Discourages entry of competitors who do not have the economic scale of production	• Must know efficiency of production • Small errors lead to large losses • Must attract and ensure volume

Source: Adapted from Chase, C., & Barasch, K. (1988). *Marketing problem solver.* Radnor, PA: Chilton; pp. 190–191.

pricing can be used as a tool to affect not only the financial performance of the company, but also the perceived quality and value of the service.

Positioning Value of Price

Just as a healthcare organization must consider alternative pricing strategies, so too it must consider the positioning value of price in strategy. At issue for any organization is whether the price will be an active or passive part of the focus of the organization and whether the price will be higher or lower relative to the competition.

Figure 7.10 shows the four possibilities for the positioning role of price. Quadrant A is the high-active position: The organization's price is higher than its competitors' prices, but there is no attempt to downplay this factor. Rather, the high price is seen as a cue for quality. Curtis Mathes,

FIGURE 7.10

Price Positioning

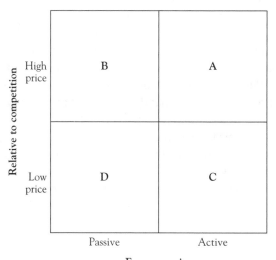

Focus on price

Source: Reprinted with permission from *The Journal of Medical Practice Management,* *3*(2), 120–124, Copyright 2011, Greenbranch Publishing, http://www.greenbranch.com. Get a free sample issue of *The Journal of Medical Practice Management*: email info@greenbranch.com or call 800-933-3711.

for example, promoted its television sets for years as "the most expensive television sets money can buy." Clairol's slogan was, "The most expensive hair coloring, but I'm worth it." This position is viable when there are no objective criteria by which to judge the product or service, or there is a large physical, social, or financial risk in the purchase. In fact, without outcome measures for medical services, setting clinic prices historically was not a determinant for consumer choice. In the earlier days where dollar-covered health insurance first appeared and there were no quality measures on outcomes, price might have been a cue for quality.

In the high-passive position, quadrant B, the price may be high relative to the competition, but the organization shifts the focus to other attributes for the potential buyer to consider. Maytag focuses on reliability, while a hospital might highlight a clinical center of excellence. There is no open discussion of price; it is passive. For example, the marketing strategy may be to highlight comprehensive service, or, as is the case for many urgent-care centers, the focus may be on immediate service.

Quadrant C is the low-active position, which follows an aggressive pricing strategy that is heavily promoted. Advertising visibly displays the low, fair pricing. This has been the orientation of the discounter, like Walmart and, to some extent, Sears. This strategy requires a good sense of costs because aggressive pricing often requires a decreased margin and therefore leaves less room for error. Walmart has followed this approach with the $4 prescription program for a 30-day supply and $10 for a 90-day supply on a wide range of common drugs. The retailer visibly promotes this in the store and on its website. Kaiser has long been viewed as a low-price healthcare plan.

In quadrant D, the low-passive quadrant, the organization sets its price lower than that of the competition, but does not publicize it. This quadrant is almost nonsensical in a competitive market, but this positioning sometimes occurs with services that are required (because they are complementary to others that are provided) or that are mandated by the government, such as the free services which a hospital must provide to those in need in return for any government reimbursement that the hospital receives.

Sensitivity of Price

In establishing its pricing policies, an organization must determine whether its business is volume sensitive or margin sensitive. This determination can be made by examining the ratio of fixed costs and the ratio of variable costs to total costs:

high fixed costs : total costs = volume-sensitive business

high variable costs : total costs = margin-sensitive business

The implications of these ratios are important in the organization's position with regard to price. If a business line is volume sensitive, the goal should be to cover fixed costs; any additional business is a significant addition to earnings. Airlines typically provide significant reductions in ticket prices for those who purchase their tickets weeks in advance. In this way, the airlines can begin to feel confident that their fixed costs are covered. The higher profits come from those who wait until the last minute to purchase a ticket. Many theaters follow a similar strategy, but the timing of the discount is reversed. Individuals who want to see a particular performance on a particular evening usually pay full price for their tickets (unless they purchase multiple tickets). Yet, 10 minutes before the performance or, in some cases, on the day of the performance, consumers can obtain tickets at a discount. Individuals who are willing to take a chance that a particular play will not be sold out or who do not care what play they see on Broadway can receive a discount on their tickets. Theater managers believe that an empty seat contributes nothing to overhead, whereas even the discounted seat will contribute at some level.

There is an analogy in the healthcare industry. Many services have a high ratio of fixed costs to total costs. Therefore, it may appear that healthcare organizations should discount aggressively to cover fixed costs and should recognize that, once overhead allocation is covered, any additional revenue is a significant enhancement to earnings. Often, however, each level of new business is given some overhead allocation, which prevents the discount from being considered acceptable to potential buyers. Allocating a predetermined amount of fixed costs to a service does, however, permit a more aggressive approach to prices in contract-bargaining sessions.

In margin-sensitive organizations (i.e., those with variable costs that are high relative to total costs), a small increase in price can lead to a significant gain in earnings. As hospitals and clinics become more competitive, managed-care organizations, PPOs, and other entities that contract for care will continue to be margin sensitive. Different segments of the market will respond differently to price changes, however. Many buyers may still be attracted to the higher priced healthcare option in the belief that high prices mean better service, better physicians, and better care. As a result, managers who consider raising or lowering prices must be sensitive to market reactions.

Figure 7.11 examines the potential relationship of margin to several alternative services and differing degrees of physician and patient (segment) involvement. Because healthcare institutions will begin to experiment more with pricing options beyond cost basis, the marketing staff will begin to play a more important role, working with finance in the development of pricing strategies.

FIGURE 7.11

Hypothetical Continuum of Healthcare Services

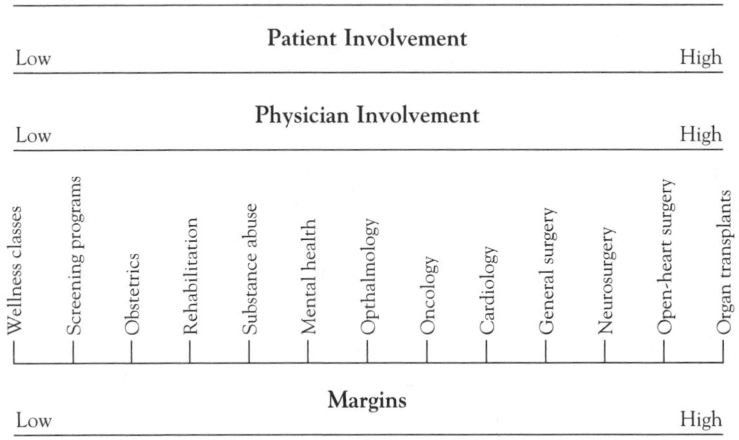

Patient Involvement
Low   High

Physician Involvement
Low   High

Wellness classes | Screening programs | Obstetrics | Rehabilitation | Substance abuse | Mental health | Opthalmology | Oncology | Cardiology | General surgery | Neurosurgery | Open-heart surgery | Organ transplants

Margins
Low   High

Source: Health Care Forum Journal, 32(5). (1989, Sept./Oct.).

PROMOTION

The most visible aspect of marketing is promotion. It has been the cause of some concern among healthcare professionals, who sometimes perceive it as hucksterism and manipulation. For example, the *Journal of the American Medical Association* many years ago ran Camel cigarette ads that quoted a physician as saying, "Not one single case of throat irritation due to smoking Camels." Although promotion can indeed be misused, it can also be a valuable tool in resolving marketing problems. Promotion consists of four elements: advertising, public relations, direct marketing, and personal selling.

How Promotion Works

Figure 7.12 illustrates a model of consumer purchases that explains how promotion works. The model flows from left to right. By the very nature of each stage, fewer and fewer buyers are "eligible" to purchase the service because of diminishing awareness of or interest in it. Therefore, the lower the pool of eligible or aware customers on the left, the lower the pool of potential customers down the line. As a result, the goal is to increase "soft" promotion, such as awareness, in order to influence stages down the line. The strength of the first item, awareness, affects the strength of all the remaining items until the point at which the service is utilized.

FIGURE 7.12

Model of Consumer Purchases

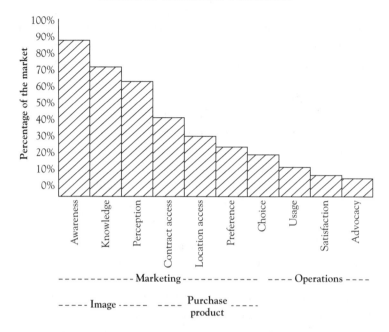

The model of consumer purchases consists of 10 elements:

1. *Awareness.* Customers do not necessarily have an opinion about the service; they simply know it exists.
2. *Knowledge.* Potential customers not only are aware that a service exists, but also can explain something about it. In short, they have some understanding of the service.
3. *Perception.* Potential customers have some beliefs about the service. For example, not only does Community Hospital provide cancer services, but it also provides good cancer services. In this stage, consumers begin to make evaluative judgments.
4. *Contract access.* This stage is unique to health care. A patient may think that Johns Hopkins provides the best care in the United States for Parkinson's disease patients, for example. If the potential patient's healthcare plan precludes care at that first choice, the patient moves to other choices. Therefore, where the patient would like to go or where the physician would like to send the patient may be different from where the patient can go or be referred to.
5. *Location.* Increasingly, location is one of the most important variables in decision making about health care. Years ago, when physicians

were scarce and consumers more passive, location was clearly secondary. Now, with a greater number of choices and the increasing availability of healthcare providers, consumers can be more fickle.

6. *Preference.* At this point, the purchaser of care narrows the field to one, two, or maybe three choices. All of the choices have met the earlier criteria, and the consumer is reaching a decision point.

7. *Choice.* Finally, after becoming aware of seven places to receive care, studying four places, and visiting two places, the consumer makes a decision.

8. *Usage.* The process is not over yet. If the service meets the consumer's expectations, the consumer is likely to buy again. Honda promotes the number of its repeat customers.

9. *Satisfaction.* Consumer satisfaction is the ultimate goal.

10. *Advocacy.* The best promotion of all is a recommendation from a user of the service. Conversely, a former user's comments are harmful if the experience was negative.

Marketing can affect everything to the point of usage. From that point on, however, operations take on an increasingly important role.

Advertising agencies use this type of model to explain the importance of awareness and image campaigns. People first must know about an organization, understand its brand, and have some general information about it before they can be expected to purchase its service. A strong awareness will help drive a stronger perception, which, in turn, will drive preference and ultimate usage. Again, the process does not stop at this point. Customer satisfaction is obviously the key. Low awareness will ultimately produce lower usage; high awareness will ultimately lead to higher usage. Therefore, an organization must examine all options to pinpoint the tactics that, used in combination, will work the best.

Positioning Value of Promotion

Another model, called *marketing ladders*, is also useful in the study of promotion.[32] Customers have a tendency to set similar products in a ladder-like sequence in their minds (**Figure 7.13**). In the rental car business, for example, Avis has worked hard for years to be positioned on this ladder in the number 2 position, while Hertz is number 1. National Car Rental seems to fall in the number 3 spot on the ladder, followed by Budget. All others fall somewhere below the leaders. Each company has either worked hard for its position on the ladder, or it has been positioned by its actions. A consultant traveling on the client's nickel might buy at the top of the ladder, believing that he or she will receive better service and faster check-in and check-out. When traveling on his or her own nickel,

FIGURE 7.13

Ladders in the Minds of Consumers

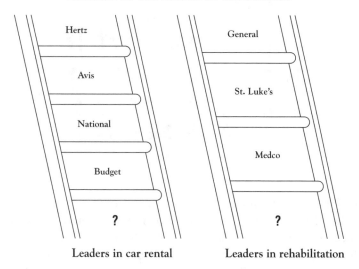

Leaders in car rental   Leaders in rehabilitation

the consultant is more likely to buy somewhere down the ladder, because, although that company offers less value, it also has lower prices.

Ladders are constructed in the minds of consumers, whether they are patients, physicians, or managers. Thirty people selected randomly could probably reach a consensus on a ladder for luxury cars, men's suits, hotel chains, and hospitals. Sometimes, but not always, an organization wants to be at the top of the ladder. For example, no hospital wants to be on the fifth rung of the ladder for a critical procedure such as cardiac bypass surgery. However, Sears is currently trying, through discount pricing, to reposition itself down the retail ladder in order to compete with Kmart, Walmart, and Target.

The ladder concept is an important tool in determining the appropriate strategic position for an organization relative to the needs of its market; some should be positioned as premium, others as middle-of-the-road, and still others as low-end.

The Changing Nature of Promotional Strategy in a Web 2.0 World

In recent years, the environment of marketing communication strategy has shifted dramatically. The "Web 2.0 world" is a new environment of strategy and challenge for healthcare marketers. **Figure 7.14** shows the historical way in which communication strategy occurred in healthcare organizations. This figure depicts a rather simple, unidirectional flow of

FIGURE 7.14

Traditional Marketing Communication Flow

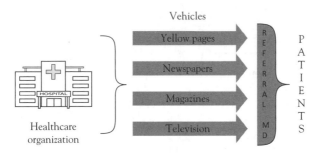

information. Most importantly, it represents a high degree of control by the sender of the information, whether it was a hospital, medical group, pharmaceutical company, health insurance firm, or managed-care entity. The channel for this communication could be a billboard, radio advertisement, or newspaper ad. The key aspect was to develop a message that would be decoded in the intended way by the target market.

The promotional and communication environment in which organizations now operate is different. Control is no longer held by the organization. From a strategy perspective, this is a major issue. Strategy can still be formulated, but it is at a far different level. Examine **Figure 7.15**. This is referred to as the constellation of the Web 2.0 world. The challenge for healthcare organizations (or organizations of any type, whether Toyota, IBM, the American Heart Association, or St. Jude Children's Hospital) is participating in the constellation of conversations that occur on the Internet. For healthcare organizations, this shift is significant. Fitting into a constellation of communication now requires more than thinking of sending or encoding a message, but rather being part of the communication. The use of blogs, podcasts, RSS feeds, YouTube, and other Internet-based social networking tools to build engaged and loyal patients and/or referral sources is part of the strategy that effective healthcare marketing organizations must develop in today's new communication reality.

ADVERTISING

Advertising has increased as a promotional strategy for healthcare organizations. In 2008, hospital advertising expenditures were $1.23 billion.[33] Decisions about advertising revolve around two central issues: copy strategy and media selection. In both instances, the organization must have a

FIGURE 7.15

Communication Strategy in a Web 2.0 Environment

The constellation of the Web

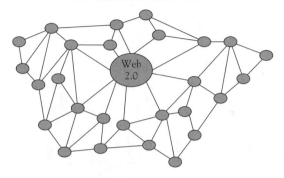

defined target audience on which to focus its advertisements and a differential advantage attractive to that audience.

Advertising Issues: Copy Testing and Media Selection

Unlike public relations pieces, most advertising copy is tested among a sample of consumers representative of the target audience. Copy testing occurs at two stages of the advertising process: pretesting, which is conducted before the advertisement is placed in the media, and posttesting, which is conducted afterward.

In order to determine the advertising copy strategies that should be used, the interest/attention-getting power of an advertisement, or the meaning of an advertisement, many organizations carry out *pretests*. It is often desirable to develop more than one advertisement for consideration. For example, in a very comprehensive pretest and piloting approach, the social marketing firm SUMA/Orchard developed a campaign to test whether interest in breastfeeding could be increased among African American women in a particular region within Texas. As a part of this pretest campaign, two alternative posters were developed that were displayed in Women, Infants, and Children (WIC) offices. In in-depth interviews with 43 women, participants had high recall of the posters, with 74% of the participants remembering one poster that featured a mother with her infant, while 37% recalled the poster of a female African American physician.[34] Pretesting has also been used by the U.S. Agency for International Development (USAID) in the development of materials to help reduce the spread of dengue fever in Vietnam. Public health workers developed a series of six picture cards on ways to reduce the disease (see **Figure 7.16**), which were then pretested

FIGURE 7.16

Sample Pretest Card of USAID Dengue Fever Counseling Cards

Card 2. There is no drug to treat dengue, but you can protect yourself and
your family from getting sick by preventing the *Aedes* mosquito from
breeding and gathering.

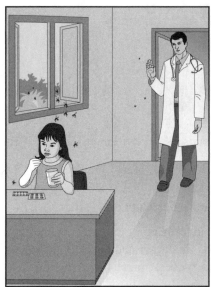 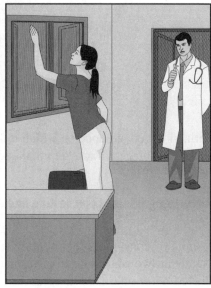

Source: USAID. (2010, November 15–17). *Results of pre-test dengue counseling cards: Mid-BCC–Communications for change in infectious diseases in
Greater Mekong subregion.* Slide 13. Retrieved June 20, 2011, from: http://
mekong.aed.org/docs/Dengue%20Pre-test%20Lao%2011_10.pdf

with mothers aged 24 to 36 who were walk-in clients at a mother and children hospital, with secondary school teachers, and with 12 villagers in the
Mekong region in order to get feedback on the cards. The communications
materials were then improved based on the feedback.

Before any advertisement is placed in the media, an organization should
conduct pretesting to ensure that the market understands the advertisement
in the way that the organization intended. This step is especially important in dealing with the two major market segments for most healthcare
organizations: patients and physicians. Because of the technical vocabu-
lary in health care, patients' ability to interpret advertisements is a central

pretesting concern. When a multispecialty clinic added an endocrinologist to the group, for example, an announcement in the local community paper provided good exposure, but most potential patients did not understand who or what had been added. The point of such an announcement is lost on people who do not understand what an endocrinologist does.

In pretesting an advertisement for physicians, the purpose is less to gauge comprehension and more to determine whether physicians interpret the message as intended. For example, a photo of three male doctors may send the message that a group is all male when, in fact, it may be 20% female. In another case, members of a medical staff may perceive a radio advertisement lead-in that is designed solely to attract attention as unprofessional.

Common *posttesting* procedures focus on recognition or recall. Recognition tests attempt to determine whether the target audience remembers seeing the advertisement. For example, a sample of people may be shown the advertisement for the multispecialty clinic and asked whether they remember seeing the announcement about the endocrinologist. An alternative posttesting procedure is to assess the audience's recall of an advertisement. For example, the Merrimack Hospital decided to run the picture version of the advertisement for its pain clinic in the local newspaper. To test audience recall, random samples of people were called 2 days after the advertisement ran. They were first asked whether they read the local paper. They were then asked whether they recalled any healthcare advertisements during the past week and, if so, what the advertisement was.

Related to the decision about copy is the selection of media. Most clinics and hospitals make media decisions on a local basis. Because of technological advances, however, media that were once out of reach of most local advertisers are now part of any good advertising plan. Cable television, local spot time, and zip code (and metropolitan) editions of national magazines, for example, allow a broader media plan. The selection of appropriate media for advertising requires knowledge of the viewership, readership, and even the travel patterns of the target audience (**Table 7.2**).

The advantage of *newspaper* advertising is coverage. As many clinics and hospitals have found, most adults report reading a newspaper at least once a week, either in print or online.[35] Moreover, newspapers allow for quick, competitive responses. If the competing clinic runs a newspaper advertisement on Monday, the other clinic can retaliate through the newspaper quickly, as advertising space is available on relatively short notice. The major disadvantage of newspaper advertising is the lack of selectivity. Many large newspapers have added zip code editions, but they are primarily in major metropolitan areas. Consequently, when the Rockville Hospital runs an advertisement for its executive fitness program, many

TABLE 7.2 DECISION CRITERIA FOR MEDIA SELECTION

Media Vehicle	Cost of Placement	Selectivity	Message Quality	Lead Time
Newspapers	Relatively expensive	Little selectivity except in major metro areas By zip code or region	Poor photo reproduction Person can spend time with message	Easy to obtain space with short notice
Magazines	Relatively expensive	Great selectivity by lifestyle, interest Reasonably good selectivity by area (particularly metro)	Excellent photo reproduction Person can spend time with message	Often requires contracting for space a month or more in advance
Direct Mail	Relatively inexpensive	Excellent selectivity on criteria required by organization	A function of amount of money spent on printing	Little required except to produce mail piece
Radio	Inexpensive	Reasonable selectivity	Must be short, simple Difficult to hold attention	Little advance notice required
Television	Expensive	Reasonable—a function of time of day and show selected	Excellent for sight and sound Relatively short messages required Hard to hold attention	Often requires substantial lead time
Outdoor	Relatively inexpensive	Little selectivity except by location of billboard	Requires short, simple message	Space availability often necessitates long lead time

nonexecutives also see it. If the program is not intended for this audience, the hospital has paid for wasted coverage.

The proliferation of special-interest *magazines* in the United States allows the potential advertiser to reach specific target audiences. An HMO may run an advertisement in its area's regional edition of *Prevention* magazine. Because the people who read this publication are concerned with health and wellness, an advertisement focusing on the health-maintenance program of the organization may have special appeal. *Runner's World* may be a suitable outlet for a large clinic or hospital that wants to establish a nationally known sports-medicine program. The major disadvantage of placing advertisements in magazines is cost, which can be high. As numerous magazines develop regional/metropolitan editions of their publications, however, costs become more affordable for a hospital or group practice.

Of all the advertising media available to healthcare organizations, *direct mail* provides maximum selectivity. For many organizations, direct mail has become a foundation of one-to-one marketing efforts to remind current customers of services or products. The 347-bed St. Jude Medical Center in Fullerton, California, spends several hundred thousand dollars annually for staff and software to maintain its customized direct-mail program. Direct-mail houses can provide assistance in communicating with defined target audiences, particularly for programs that are tailored to service lines, like bone and joint centers, weight loss programs, or cardiovascular programs. If the Merrimack Hospital decides to focus its pain clinic on individuals who are 60 years of age or older and who have arthritis, for example, a direct-mail house can assist the hospital in sending a brochure on the pain program to that specific group in the desired market area. The major obstacle to advertising by direct mail is its classification as junk mail. The volume of unsolicited mail that households receive is often overwhelming. Well-designed, professional pieces about an issue of importance to the target audience can generate a response, however.

Many clinics and hospitals have turned to *radio* advertisements to generate public awareness of their services. The vast number of radio stations means that some selectivity with regard to the target audience is possible. Spinner Hospital advertises its drug-counseling program for teenagers on the local rock music station, for example. Radio is a relatively low-cost vehicle, and many stations provide assistance in writing and producing advertisements. The major weakness of radio is the ease with which listeners can tune out the message. Long advertisements are not possible, and, even with a short spot, the individual can tune out by hitting a preset button to switch stations.

Although in the past few healthcare managers would have considered *television* for anything but public service announcements, many organizations have now turned to this medium for their advertising. The advantage is the combination of sight and sound. Additionally, television not only can reach a large number of people, but it also provides some selectivity. For most organizations, cost is the major disadvantage of television advertising. Television commercials are expensive to produce, and the cost of placement is often high. Even though low-cost time slots are available at most local stations, the audience that they reach may not be the desired target group. For example, inexpensive time can be purchased from most television stations during the late, late show, which may be perfect for a clinic's sleep program, but is of little value for its fitness program.

Billboards have become popular with many healthcare organizations, because they are effective in increasing public awareness and in supplementing other advertising. A relatively recent study has shown that healthcare content billboards also influence choice and play an important role in reminder and reinforcement. It was also found, however, that it was important to change the content of the billboards after 3 weeks or so to reduce wear-out effects.[36] In the late 1980s, hospitals were the largest growth category in the billboard industry. Costs of billboards vary by market size. A billboard in the Atlanta metro area on the interstate can cost from $3,500 to $10,000 per month. Tenet Healthcare Corporation is a heavy user of billboards for individual hospitals within the system. Billboards should not be the only medium in an advertising campaign, however. A major disadvantage of outdoor advertising is that the message must be short and simple. Also, little selectivity of the people who view the advertisement is possible. In some cities, moreover, it is difficult to obtain billboard space in the desired location.

Increasingly, the Internet is giving advertisers new and exciting ways to advertise. Online advertising is providing many advantages to potential advertisers. It allows sites to track users, how many times a website was clicked on, and how deeply visitors looked at a site. Did the person look at the first page of the medical group's site? Or, did the visitor also look at the page of the orthopedic department and the spine center services? There are many variations to Internet advertising, including:

- *Banners*. Rectangular graphics at the top or bottom of a webpage. They receive less than a 1% click-through rate.
- *Buttons*. These are small banner-type advertisements placed anywhere on a page.
- *Pop-up ads*. These advertisements appear onscreen while a page is being loaded or after the webpage has appeared. Recent technology enables blocking many of these pop-ups, which limits their effectiveness.
- *Email*. Unsolicited email has been referred to as spamming. Many states are passing laws against spamming. While it is an easy way to communicate with prospective customers, it can be considered intrusive.

Direct marketing is an aspect of promotion that can be considered a tactic within this marketing mix variable. It has historically encompassed telemarketing, direct-mail marketing, or direct sales, including those used by companies such as Amway or Mary Kay. The email method of advertising, as is being conducted now on the Internet, is a form of direct marketing. In health care, direct marketing has been commonly used in the form of direct mail campaigns. For example, in 2009 the Cleveland Clinic conducted a direct mail campaign to reach past patients with chronic conditions such as hypertension, diabetes, arthritis, and pain. The push encouraged these consumers to schedule return appointments. The focus of the campaign was on access and a toll-free number for scheduling. The campaign elicited 5,542 patient responses. It was credited with creating a revenue stream of 36 times the amount the Cleveland Clinic spent on it. The Cleveland Clinic saw a 65% response rate when it first used the program from April to November 2009. The success of the campaign led the organization to extend it to other clinical areas, such as pediatrics, heart, and urology.[37]

Once the media type has been selected, the next issue is deciding between one vehicle and another. How can marketers choose one radio or television show rather than another, or one magazine or newspaper rather than another? The best vehicle to buy time or space in is the one that most appeals to the desired target market. The more defined an organization's profile of its target audience, the greater the likelihood that both the media and the vehicle decisions will be effective. A good media profile must include the basic demographics of the buyer. Then, depending on the service, lifestyle, or attitudinal factors, these dimensions help round out the profile to aid in the final selection. On occasion, even with a well-defined profile, a choice must be made between alternatives. In this instance, some simple formulas can be used to guide the final decision.

For choosing between *broadcast* alternatives, a useful formula is the cost per thousand measure (CPM). This is calculated as:

CPM = cost of 1 unit of time × 1,000/number of households reached

The number of households reached is determined by applying the rating against the coverage. For example, a healthcare organization in a community of 100,000 people is considering buying time on a local television show with a rating of 15.2. A unit of time on that show costs $5,200. Because the show covers nearly all the households in the community with television sets—approximately 41,000—the commercial would be seen in 15.2% of these homes, or a total of 6,232 households. The CPM formula is:

CPM = $834

A similar CPM calculation can be the basis for a choice between *print* vehicles. Three variations are often used for print media. The first is the cost per thousand using base-circulation figures:

$$\text{CPM} = \text{cost of 1 unit of space} \times 1{,}000/\text{circulation base}$$

Circulation base is the number of people that will obtain a copy of the material through subscription or general distribution. Potential readers are those people who might view a copy of the material. It is possible to have a circulation base of 1,000 while having 1,500 potential readers due to factors such as family size.

The second calculation is the cost per thousand potential readers:

$$\text{CPM} = \text{cost of 1 unit of space} \times 1{,}000/\text{circulation}$$
$$\text{base} \times \text{number of readers}$$

The third calculation is cost per thousand readers in the target population:

$$\text{CPM} = \text{cost of 1 unit of space} \times 1{,}000/\text{circulation base} \times \text{number of}$$
$$\text{readers} \times \text{percentage of readers in target market}$$

In this calculation, one is looking more at the potential readership in the targeted population. For example, a print vehicle might have a large circulation base. However, only a small subset of those readers is really of interest for the hospital.

Setting Advertising Objectives and Measuring Results

Among the more difficult tasks associated with advertising are setting the objectives and measuring effectiveness of the advertising program. Although it may be hoped that advertising will increase outpatient visits to the ambulatory-care center by 10% during the month of the campaign, the cause-and-effect relationship is not always obvious. Competitive actions and the lag effect can influence the outcome of an advertising campaign. It is necessary to have a set of measurable objectives. Some pre-campaign assessment of the goals is also needed. Logical objectives for an advertising campaign may include:

- To increase name recognition of the Wallace Clinic among people who have moved into the community within the past 6 months from 10% to 25% within 9 months.
- To have 35% of the consumers in zip codes contingent to the hospital express a preference for the hospital's emergency room in the next 2 months.
- To generate 15 inquiries a month from eligible corporations about the hospital's occupational health program.

Advertising objectives should be set with recognition of the fact that the consumer goes through several steps before purchase or usage of a service:

1. *Awareness.* The potential buyer is aware that the product/service exists in the market.
2. *Interest.* The potential buyer is aware of the offering and wants more information about it.
3. *Evaluation.* The customer attempts to evaluate the benefits of one offering versus those of another.
4. *Trial.* The customer is interested in trying the service on a limited basis.
5. *Adoption.* The customer decides to utilize the service on a regular basis.

It is difficult to measure adoption. Several factors may affect utilization, such as the plan offered by the potential patient's employer, the existing medical needs of the patient, or the referral problem faced by the physician. With the episodic nature of medical problems, an organization can never be sure when exposure to an advertisement may lead to eventual utilization.

Although a person's medical need may lag behind his or her awareness of an advertisement for a healthcare service, advertising effects are not unmeasurable. Measures of advertising effectiveness need to be determined before adoption. Possible objectives at earlier stages are listed in **Figure 7.17**.

Without measurable objectives, an organization can never be sure that its advertising is effective. It becomes hard to justify advertising budgets (**Table 7.3**). Before any expenditures are made, objectives must be established.

FIGURE 7.17

Possible Advertising Objectives

Awareness	To increase from 10% to 15% the number of people in Baltimore who know of the outpatient mental health service of Metro Hospital.
↓	
Interest	To generate 15 inquiries a month from eligible corporations regarding our mental health program.
↓	
Evaluation	To have 10% of the possible referring physicians in the five-county area indicate the Martin Clinic as having the most complete diagnostic capabilities in the area.
↓	
Trial	To generate 15 new patients a week in the mall urgent-care setting during January.

TABLE 7.3 PERCENTAGE OF REVENUE SPENT ON ADVERTISING, BY INDUSTRY

Industry	% of Revenue
Accident and Health Insurance	1.2%
Educational Services	9.8%
Pharmaceutical Preparations	4.3%
Surgical, Medical, Instrument Apparatus	0.6%
Wine, Brandy, and Spirits	11.8%

Source: Data from Schonfeld & Associates, Inc. *2011 Advertising ratios & budgets.* Retrieved February 4, 2012, from: http://www.saibooks.com/default.asp

Setting the Budget

Early concerns about advertising often pertained to issues of reimbursement. Advertising may not be a reimbursable expense. Each year, however, more healthcare organizations are realizing that it is an important way to compete. Some studies indicate an ever-increasing budget for advertising.[38] Some organizations spend a significant amount when they compete on a global, or certainly a national scale. In 2009, the Cleveland Clinic doubled its advertising expenditures to $8.5 million from the 2008 level of $3.9 million. Advertisement spending has also increased for healthcare organizations that compete regionally, or even locally. In 2009, Henry Ford increased its advertising expenditures by 15%, while Sarasota (Florida) Memorial Health Care System's advertising budget rose by 10%.[39] Yet, the proliferation of social media has begun to level the field among competitors, allowing smaller hospitals to now compete with larger competitors by strategically using media vehicles that require significantly less outlay of dollars to get their message to the target market. Consumer-friendly websites, Facebook, and Twitter all allow communication with less financial commitment than more traditional media costs.[40] In any case, setting an exact budget amount is difficult, but there are several common approaches.

Many professional organizations determine their advertising budget by calculating what they can *afford.* In developing the operating budget for the coming fiscal year, they allocate dollars to personnel, operations, capital improvements, new equipment purchases, and the like. After all critical categories receive their allocated dollars, these organizations consider spending any additional monies on advertising.

Certainly, the financial viability of the organization might be a constraint in setting allocations for advertising. No banker will lend money for a group practice's advertising campaign. Healthcare organizations that spend just "left-over" dollars on advertising tend to do so only because they think they should advertise, but they do not create specific objectives to direct the campaign. This approach lacks logic.

The budgeting strategy of some organizations is to allocate to advertising a *percentage of their revenue*. Again, this approach has some value in that advertising is tied to the financial performance of the organization. Of all budgeting methods, however, this approach may be the weakest. With this method, revenue results in advertising rather than advertising resulting in revenue. Therefore, an organization may reduce its advertising expenditures at a time when it needs the greatest investment—when demand is down. Likewise, increasing revenue leads to a greater advertising budget, even though this new level of expenditure may not be warranted.

As more healthcare organizations begin to advertise, *competitive parity* is becoming the budgeting model. One clinic observes another clinic's weekly newspaper advertising and, as a countermeasure, begins newspaper advertising. A major competitor's advertising forces an organization to consider a retaliatory strategy. Spending advertising dollars at the same level as the competitor assumes similar organizational objectives. Moreover, it assumes that the competitor's strategy is correct. These assumptions are often incorrect.

Affordability, revenue, and competition must all be assessed, but the overriding weakness of setting an advertising budget by these methods is the lack of objectives. As noted earlier, the effectiveness of advertising can be determined only through prespecified *objectives*. These same objectives should guide the budget determination. For example, if an organization sets an awareness objective, such as that in Figure 7.17—"To increase from 10% to 15% the number of people in Baltimore who know of the outpatient mental health service of Metro Hospital"—the organization must determine how much media exposure is needed to meet this objective. The *tasks* to meet the exposure might be as follows:

- Thirty-three quarter-page insertions in the *Baltimore Sun*.
- Forty 15-second slots on the television during late news on Channel 5.

The costs of these tasks are then calculated. This amount determines the budget.

At this point, the previous factors of affordability, revenue, and competition enter. The organization may find that it cannot financially support the advertising objectives. This discovery may lead to a readjustment of the objectives or a search for more efficient media. If the budgeted amount is well below competitive levels, a critical evaluation of the tasks and the likelihood of success may be necessary.

Of all methods, this approach requires the most planning. The advantage of having an objective-driven budget for advertising, based on accountable performance standards, compensates for the additional investment in management time. Advertising is an expensive and essential part of promotional strategy. Healthcare organizations need to plan this activity as carefully as they plan the establishment of a new medical service.

Conditions for Effective Advertising

Advertising tends to be most effective when buyer awareness is minimal. In this regard, the value of advertising to establish name recognition for a new PPO or walk-in center is unquestioned. Advertising tends to work best when industry sales are rising. Advertising alone, regardless of the level, cannot restore obstetrical business in the face of declining birthrates. Advertising is also effective when the features of the service are not easily observed, and explanation may be required. To some extent, this condition necessitates a good copy strategy; copy can highlight the positive outcomes of joining a plan or going to a particular group practice for medical care. When opportunities for differentiation are strong, advertising is particularly effective. To some extent, this last condition for effective advertising may underscore many questions about the impact of advertising in health care. With so many providers similar in expertise, service level, and the like, advertising is often relegated to a role of underscoring the "me too" nature of the competitors.

Checklist for an Advertising Campaign

In developing an advertising campaign, it is useful to focus on the following questions:[41]

1. What specifically is the organization advertising?
2. Who does the organization want to motivate? Where and why?
3. Which medium should be used? Why?
4. What principal benefit is the audience seeking?
5. What are the intrinsic technical advantages of the product/service?
6. How will the advertisement capture attention initially?
7. How will the advertisement create awareness initially?
8. How will the advertisement create preference initially?
9. How will the advertisement motivate action initially?

SALES

Although we were among the first authors to suggest the use of sales strategies, personal selling is a promotional technique that most hospitals and clinics still do not use to its full potential. As recently as 2001, only 7% of hospitals were reported to have had a formal sales department.[42] In fact, most healthcare organizations have underestimated the effectiveness of a sales force, yet it is growing in terms of its recognized value. In Temple, Texas, Scott & White created its physician relations department in 2007 to call on referral physicians. It tracked a 22.4% increase by improving relationship building and continuing to build goodwill.[43] In recent years, the deployment of physician relations efforts has increased as hospitals have recognized the importance of relationship building and the referral channel as a key strategic resource. **Figure 7.18** shows the budget to support such an effort in surveys that were conducted by Strategic Health Care Marketing and the Corporate Health Group in 2005, 2008, and 2010. The financial value of physician relations is significant. MD Anderson's economic model has demonstrated total payments that include both hospital and professional fees. During fiscal year 2010, the center's physician relations department called on 1,095 referral doctors during a 6-month period; 440 of these doctors had either never referred a patient to MD Anderson or had not referred a patient to the center in the prior 2-year period. Of the 440 who had referred at least one patient after the physician-relations visit, associated revenues totaled more than $12.5 million.[44]

FIGURE 7.18

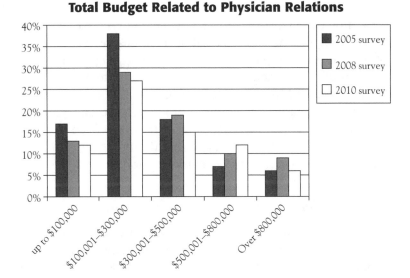

Total Budget Related to Physician Relations

Note: Totals include salaries and benefits of a sales manager, field sales representatives, and any allocated administrative staff; travel, entertainment, meetings, marketing materials/expenses; and any expensed equipment.

Source: Corporate Health Group. *Physician sales and service as a strategic component, competitive maneuver 2010.* Retrieved January 25, 2012, from: http://www.corporatehealthgroup.com/

The Value of Sales

Many people see personal selling as having only one value: to close the sale. In fact, effective personal selling can make many contributions in dealing with the market.

The more technical or complicated the service, the more valuable a sales staff. A salesperson can probably explain many of the programs offered by hospitals and clinics better than an advertisement can. For example, a clinic that establishes an occupational health program commonly runs an advertisement in the local business publication read by company executives. But because the decision to use a particular occupational health program is complicated and may involve several managers, a personal sales strategy may be more effective. The clinic could establish a small sales force to call on local companies. The early sales calls would be to gain knowledge about the organization, such as who is involved in decisions about the healthcare plan, what the occupational health needs of the company are, and which healthcare sources the organization is currently using. With this information, an effective presentation of the clinic's own occupational health services could be made.

A sales staff is as valuable in *maintaining relationships* as it is in selling. This is particularly true for hospitals dependent on physician loyalty and clinics dependent on referrals from physicians and other individuals (e.g., probation officers, social workers, and employee-assistance personnel). In fulfilling this function, the salesperson ensures that the hospital and its staff are meeting physicians' needs. If salespeople uncover problems or areas of dissatisfaction, they can be the links to the administrator or program director. Moreover, the salesperson can act as a conduit of new information regarding the clinic's programs or changes. **Table 7.4** lists several markets on which a sales force may call. Each would be an appropriate place to sell one or more specific programs, although the information, maintenance, and sales purposes may vary.

Role of the Sales Force

The basic purpose of any salesperson is to increase service use, or *close sales*. A hospital sales force for industrial medicine may negotiate contracts with companies. A PPO sales force may recruit physicians for its plan.

Another important role of the sales force is *clarification*. Salespeople can provide an explanation and evaluation of a clinic's new outpatient chemical-dependency program, for example.

An important function of the sales force is *missionary activity*. When a salesperson deals with the referral physician or company contact person,

TABLE 7.4   PROGRAMS OF INTEREST TO SPECIFIC MARKETS

Market	Program/Goals
Companies	Occupational health
High school coaches	Sports medicine
Factory unions	Back rehabilitation
Insurance agents	Industrial health
Physicians	Increased share of patient days

the goal is to help that individual's practice or business through the services provided by the healthcare organization. The salesperson builds goodwill for the organization, as well as a sense of obligation in the primary care physician or contact person.

The final role for salespeople is to monitor the satisfaction of users. A salesperson may regularly call on the physicians who refer patients to the healthcare organization to see that the organization is meeting their needs, for example. The salesperson can be the conduit for any complaints to the administration so that problems can be resolved before the physicians begin to shift patients to another facility. A salesperson may also call on a company benefit officer periodically to ensure that the employee records provided by the HMO meet the company's requirements for its cost review.

The essential requirement for any organization that employs a sales force or liaison group is to track the results of the efforts of these resources that are deployed. A survey conducted in 2006 and updated in March 2009 by healthcare organizations employed physician relations individuals and found a range of tools—with some organizations using multiple tools—used to monitor the results of this resource, as shown in **Figure 7.19**. These tools were found to quantify two basic items: the retention and/or growth of referral volume, and the performance of physician relations staff.[45]

Size of the Sales Force

When establishing a sales force, an organization can use one of several available methods to determine the appropriate size. Conceptually, the most appealing and easiest to implement is the workload method, sometimes called a buildup approach. This method is based on the workload that each salesperson can handle. By measuring that load and dividing it into the total effort necessary to cover the entire market, the number of salespeople required can be determined.

FIGURE 7.19

Tracking Tools Used by Hospitals for Monitoring Physician Relations Efforts

Excel or other spreadsheet	26%
ACT!	21%
Homegrown system	21%
Paper system	14%
Access	13%
Goldmine	12%
Marketware	8%
Other (SalesForce, E–Centaurus, SalesLogix, ContactWise, EchoAccess, Meditech File Maker)	11%

Note: Multiple systems used by some organizations.

Source: McCarthy, A. (2009, March). Tracking the tracking systems for physician relations efforts. *Learning Tools*. Retrieved November 10, 2011, from: http://www.barlowmccarthy.com/resources/physician-relations-sales

First, establish the total time available per salesperson. A sales job in which the salesperson calls on potential industrial accounts for an occupational health program may require working an 8-hour day 5 days per week. Eliminating 4 weeks for vacation, holidays, illness, and other emergencies leaves 48 working weeks in a year. Thus, the total number of hours per year that a salesperson will work on average is 1,920 (40 hours per week for 48 weeks).

Second, apportion the salesperson's time to do all the different required tasks. For this example, the tasks can be grouped into selling, traveling, and nonselling categories (**Table 7.5**). If territories are being established for the first time, the manager's estimates are often used to apportion time to these tasks. When already established territories are being reviewed, the apportionment may be based on the salesperson's reports or time studies.

Third, classify the firm's present and potential customers according to selling effort required. Customers are usually grouped by sales volume, although any basis can be used as long as it distinguishes accounts

TABLE 7.5   APPORTIONMENT OF SALESPERSON'S TIME

Activity	Percentage of Time	Number of Hours
Selling	40%	768
Traveling	30%	576
Nonselling	30%	576
Total	*100%*	*1,920*

according to the differences needed in selling effort. For the occupational health program in the example, customers (both present and potential) are grouped by number of employees (**Table 7.6**). Classifying customers can be a tedious task for a firm with many customers and prospects.

Fourth, specify the length and frequency of calls for each category. The manager may use experimental evidence, personal judgment, or the opinions of the sales force to decide how much time should be spent with an account in each group and how often each account should be visited. Unless potential customers as well as present customers are included in this step, the number of salespersons will not be large enough to allow cultivation of potential accounts. To facilitate the calculation, present and potential customers are treated equally. The manager may then determine that the following call frequencies and call lengths are ideal:

Group 1: 24 calls per year × 45 minutes per call = 18 hours per year

Group 2: 12 calls per year × 30 minutes per call = 6 hours per year

Group 3: 4 calls per year × 30 minutes per call = 2 hours per year

The total time needed to cover all accounts would then be:

Group 1: 10 accounts at 18 hours = 180 hours

Group 2: 25 accounts at 6 hours = 150 hours

Group 3: 100 accounts at 2 hours = 200 hours

Total: 530 hours

Finally, calculate the number of salespersons needed. Each salesperson has 768 hours available on average for selling. Total selling time needed to cover present and potential accounts is 530 hours. By dividing 530 by 768, the result is approximately a 0.7 full-time employee for sales on industrial accounts.

TABLE 7.6   CLASSIFICATION OF CUSTOMERS

Group	Number of Accounts
1—Large	10
2—Medium	25
3—Small	100

This workload method is easy to understand and carry out, and companies have used it with satisfactory results.

Compensation for the Sales Force

In addition to determining the size of the sales force, management needs to choose a method of compensation. There are several elements to a compensation plan for a sales force:

- Salary
- Commission
- Bonus
- Expenses
- Fringe benefits

Commission is a complicated element with several components (**Exhibit 7.1**). Likewise, expense items can vary. **Table 7.7** shows a comparison of the different compensation plans used by various companies.

Advertising/Sales Tradeoff

Many managers find it difficult to achieve a balance between personal selling and advertising. There is no correct formula to solve this problem. Rather, each element has a contribution to make to a proper promotional program.

The consumer's purchase or utilization decision has three stages. First is the prepurchase stage. When a physician decides to send a patient to a referral center, for example, the physician goes through a period of deliberation before deciding on the referral center. The second stage is the purchase or, in this case, the actual decision stage. The third stage is the postpurchase period. At this point, the physician may review his or her decision to examine whether the selection was the appropriate one. Advertising and personal selling have different levels of effectiveness at each stage.

EXHIBIT 7.1

Components of Compensation

Bases for Commission Payments
1. Dollar or unit sales volume (gross or net)
2. Gross margin, contribution to profit
3. Activities or efforts
4. Quotas (which may include above bases)

Rates of Commission
1. Fixed, progressive, regressive
2. Gross versus net
3. Constant versus variable with regard to:
   a. Products
   b. Customers
   c. Territories
   d. Order sizes
   e. Profit margins
   f. New versus repeat business

Starting Points for Commission Payments
1. Zero sales, profits, or activities
2. Some percentage of quota
3. Break-even level of sales volume

As shown in **Figure 7.20**, advertising assumes greater importance in the prepurchase stage than does personal selling. Whatever the strategy, whether it be the distribution of brochures by a referral center to primary care providers or the placement of regional advertisements by a managed-care organization in the *Wall Street Journal*, the purpose of a mass information approach (advertising) is to make as many prospective buyers or users as possible aware of the service.

In the second stage, personal selling assumes greater importance. Rarely has an advertisement closed a big sale. Closing a sale requires personal interaction between buyer and seller. There may be a physician in the region who has never sent a patient to the Holt Orthopedic Group, for example, although Holt has conducted an extensive awareness campaign regarding its services over the past year. After making a few preliminary

TABLE 7.7 Compensation Plans for a Sales Force

Compensation Method (Frequency of Use)	Especially Useful	Advantages	Disadvantages
Straight Salary (10%)	When compensating new salespersons When firm moves into new sales territories that require developmental work When salespersons need to perform many nonselling activities	Provides salesperson with maximum amount of security Gives sales manager large amount of control over salespersons Easy to administer Yields more predictable selling expenses	Provides no incentive Necessitates closer supervision of salespersons' activities During sales declines, selling expenses remain at same level Impedes attracting top salespeople
Straight Commission (5%)	When highly aggressive selling is required When nonselling tasks are minimized When company cannot closely control activities of sales force	Provides maximum amount of incentive By increasing commission rate, sales managers can encourage salespersons to sell certain items Selling expenses related directly to sales resources Quickly eliminate incompetent salespeople	Salespersons have little financial security Sales manager has minimum control over sales force May cause salespeople to provide inadequate service to smaller accounts Selling costs less predictable
Combination (85%)	When sales territories have relatively similar sales potentials When firm wishes to provide incentives and still control activities of sales force	Provides certain part of financial security Provides some incentive Selling expenses fluctuate with sales revenue Sales manager has some control over salespersons' nonselling activities	Selling expenses less predictable Hard to determine points for incentives to begin

Sources: Adapted from Churchill, G. A., et al. (2000). *Sales force management* (6th ed.). Boston, MA: Irwin-McGraw Hill; p. 432; Caruth, D. L., & Hanogloten-Caruth, G. (2002, February). Compensating sales personnel. *The American Salesman, 437*(4), 6–15.

FIGURE 7.20

Impact of Advertising and Sales

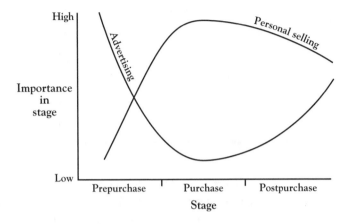

calls on this primary care physician, the Holt representative (i.e., salesperson) may ask the physician to try the group for her next orthopedic referral (i.e., purchase). The salesperson is needed to bring closure by asking for a trial referral.

After the decision stage, advertising and personal selling are still important. Once making a choice from competing alternatives, people often question the correctness of their actions. Advertising may reduce the post-decision anxiety. The referring physician may see another advertisement or brochure for the group and feel at ease about the decision. Even better than advertising is postpurchase personal contact. The more personal the contact with the buyer after the sales transaction, the more satisfied the buyer tends to be with the interaction. In this example, the Holt representative should return to the referring physician to ensure that documentation on the case was received, that the patient's experience was positive, and that there were no problems with this referral. This is also a good time to ask for additional referrals. In deciding on the proper balance of advertising and sales, the organization must consider the feelings of the buyer as carefully as it does its own goals and objectives.

In some situations, however, advertising should receive more attention than sales, and vice versa (**Table 7.8**). For example, the more technically complex the service being sold, the greater the need for personal sales. A salesperson can play a valuable role in explaining the service's benefits to the buyer, especially when these benefits may not be readily observable. In contrast, the more customers or potential buyers in the market,

TABLE 7.8   SALES VERSUS ADVERTISING

Sales	Criteria	Advertising
High	Technological complexity	Low
Few	Potential customers	Many
Push	Marketing strategy	Pull
Complex	Decision-making unit size	Simple
Many	Ancillary services	Few
Great	Degree of risk	Little

the greater the role of advertising. The cost per contact of advertising drops dramatically with more buyers, while the cost of personal selling increases with more buyers. No hospital could have a personal sales force explain the value of its obstetrical service to potential patients, but it may be feasible to have a sales force call on social workers in the community to talk about the hospital's mental health program.

The organization's marketing strategy also influences the relative emphasis on advertising or personal selling. As explained earlier, a pull strategy requires advertising. Salespeople are a prerequisite to a push strategy, however, for they must work with the intermediates (physicians) in the channel.

The more people involved in the decision to use a service, the greater the need for personal selling. Different decision makers may have different criteria for their evaluation of the service. A salesperson can explain the program to each decision maker. Multiple explanations would be difficult to provide in an advertisement.

Ancillary services are post-sales activities that may be required. For example, a company may expect updates on employee utilization of an industrial health program. The referral physician expects documentation on patients sent to a tertiary facility. In these instances, a salesperson can provide the follow-ups; the salesperson is part of the "program" purchased by the buyer.

The greater the risk that the buyer sees in using a program, the more important personal selling is. This risk can be physical or financial. For example, a hospital-based, 1-day surgery program may hold orientation sessions for prospective patients so that a hospital salesperson can explain the procedure and safeguards. Although a physician has recommended

1-day surgery, the patient may view the surgery as serious enough to require more than 1 day of care. A hospital salesperson may need to provide additional information in order to obtain patient compliance and prevent the patient from seeking another physician at another hospital.

Advertising and personal selling are both important components of effective promotion. Healthcare organizations must realize that both elements have a strong impact on the market at varying stages of the buying process.

SUMMARY

Developing a competitive marketing plan involves translating objectives into specific actions or tactics. It is marketing research into the wants and needs of the public that formulates the plan and ultimate tactics. The four Ps of marketing (product, price, place, and promotion) are the foundation of the tactics of the plan. Each element of the marketing plan involves multiple aspects to consider.

It is around the product or service component of the marketing mix from which the core elements of the marketing plan flow. There are multiple considerations around branding that every organization must consider: quality, innovation, and positioning. In health care, branding is an essential element, and service quality is a key issue. In an era of transparency, service quality delivery is a major element to consider in the marketing plan and in the positioning of the organization. All products and services have a defined lifecycle that often cannot be affected by strategic decisions. Rather, they are driven by technological impact, reimbursement, or demographic changes. Organizations must look for new service opportunities or modify existing ones to continue to compete in the marketplace.

This chapter also highlighted an aspect of the product/service mix that is often underappreciated in health care—the importance of branding. There are multiple alternatives that can be implemented, each with its respective strengths.

The distribution component of the marketing mix involves the channel of distribution, the path a service or product takes from producer (or provider) to end user. And, the channel performs or provides multiple functions of value. Some of these functions are now undergoing some dramatic changes. Grading and information are two of the more significant functions where dramatic change is occurring. Further, the decisions of how to deliver healthcare services are also seeing significant change. These shifts are occurring in terms of determining the way in which healthcare services will be delivered. Technology may be having its greatest impact in this element of the marketing mix of health care. A final aspect of the channel that must also be recognized is that there are multiple members of a channel, and each one vies for power. There are multiple sources of power that any one member of the channel can use or try to achieve to control the channel.

The third element of the marketing mix, price, was one that for many years was not believed to be relevant in health care as a reimbursement-driven industry. However, high-deductible plans and transparency of pricing information makes the price component of the marketing plan more essential to consider as a tactic. There are several alternative pricing approaches that any organization can use and that are being used. There is also a psychological and positioning aspect to price that should not go unrecognized.

Promotion is the fourth P of the marketing mix. It comprises advertising, direct marketing, personal selling, and public relations. The most significant change on promotional strategy in the past 10 years has been the Web 2.0 world. While pre-Web allowed marketing strategies to control their message, the challenge today for healthcare organizations is to participate in what is being said about the organization. No longer can one control the conversation. While the media vehicles remain to assist in the implementation of strategy, it is no longer a one-way conversation that can be neatly scheduled and presented to a target market.

All four Ps are utilized in the development of an effective marketing plan. The plan is developed in light of the market's needs and wants, and in consideration of the environment and competitive considerations.

QUESTIONS FOR DISCUSSION

1. Quality has been said to have two dimensions. Describe the two dimensions and how a multispecialty group practice might consider making these operational or visible to its patients or potential patients in its marketing strategy.
2. Describe the alternative branding approaches available to a healthcare organization. What are the advantages and disadvantages to each approach?
3. Explain the difference between the push strategy and the pull strategy in the channel of distribution. How are they used with regard to the pharmaceutical industry today? Which approach seems to be used with greater frequency: push or pull? Why is this the case?

4. You are part of the senior leadership team of a major healthcare system. In the strategic planning meetings, the team realizes it is essential to control the physician referrals as much as possible. During a meeting, one group member says, "The physicians are our channel; we have to control them. We are the largest health system in town, we have all the power, and we must exert it!" The chief executive officer has asked you to meet with the team the next morning and give an overview of how the health system might exert power. Provide an overview of the sources of power, give an example of each for the health system over the physicians, and then provide your recommendation as to which one might be the most appropriate to use, along with your rationale.

5. There are several alternative pricing strategies, such as bundled pricing or price skimming. Identify three such strategies, define each one, and provide an example showing how they can be implemented in the healthcare context.

6. You have been called into a medical group as a marketing consultant. The president of the group has asked you about the group's advertising budget for the coming year, as it is in a highly competitive market where there has been a significant amount of advertising on billboards, and now online. The president asks, "How much should I spend? Five percent of the group's revenue? 10%? Give me a plan! The partners have a meeting tomorrow afternoon. I would like you to meet with us and give us your preliminary thinking. I have sent you a listing of our competitors and a copy of the ads that everyone is running, but we are in our budget cycle now." How would you respond?

NOTES

1. Berry, L. L., Parasuraman, A., Zeithaml, V. A., Adsit, D., Hater, J., Vanetti, E. J., & Veale, D. J. (1994, May). Improving service quality in America: Lessons learned (1993–2005). *The Academy of Management Executive, 8*(2), 32–52.

2. Emani, S., Yood, R., & Dugan, E. (2005). Patient loyalty, trust, and satisfaction: Data and observations from a medical group practice. *Abstract of the Academy of Health Meetings, 22*(3393).

3. Berry, L. L., & Bendapudi, N. (2003). Clueing in customers. *Harvard Business Review, 81*(2), 100–106.

4. Chandran, R. (2010, July 4). In India, for India: Medical device makers plug in. Reuters. Retrieved February 29, 2012, from: http://www.reuters .com/article/idUSTRE6640F120100705?feedType=RSS&feedName=every thing&virtualBrandChannel=11563.

5. Herrick, D. M. (2006, September 21). Update 2006: Why are health costs rising? National Center for Policy Analysis. Retrieved February 29, 2012, from: http://www.ncpa.org/pub/ba572.

6. Goodman, J. (2010, July 26). Where are the innovators in health delivery? Kaiser Health News. Retrieved February 29, 2012, from: http://www .kaiserhealthnews.org/Columns/2010/July/072610Goodman.aspx.

7. Jensen, J. (1989, March 10). Consumers consider quality in deciding on a hospital, but measurements differ. *Modern Healthcare, 19*(10), 88, 90.

8. Hart, C. W. L. (1988, July–August). The power of unconditional service guarantees. *Harvard Business Review, 13,* 54–62.

9. Berry, L. L., & Seltman, K. (2007, May–June). Building a strong service brand: Lessons from the Mayo Clinic. *Business Horizons, 50*(3), 199–209.

10. Knox, R. (2007, November 7). India's middle class gets brand-name health care. National Public Radio. Retrieved February 29, 2012, from: http://www.npr.org/templates/story/story.php?storyId=16077448.

11. MassDevice Staff. (2010, September 28). Biospace Med rebrands as Eos Imaging. Retrieved February 29, 2012, from: http://www.massdevice.com/ news/biospace-med-rebrands-eos-imaging.

12. Wallack, S. S., Thomas, C. P., Flieger, S. P., & Altman, S. (2010, February). Part I: The Massachusetts health care system in context: Costs, structure, and method used by private insurers to pay providers. Retrieved February 2012, from: http://www.mass.gov/eohhs/researcher/physical-health/health -care-delivery/health-care-cost-trends/2010/prelinimary-reports/part-i-the -massachusetts-health-care-system.html.

13. Robins, R. (2006). Brand matters: The lingua franca of pharmaceutical brand names. Interbrand Wood Healthcare. Retrieved February 29, 2012, from: http://www.marketing.cmru.ac.th/doc/A48B251Cd01.pdf.

14. Fianrelli, M., & Pillai, N. (2007, May 15). Retail health clinics. Hospitals and Health Networks. Retrieved February 29, 2012, from: http://www .hhnmag.com/hhnmag_app/jsp/articledisplay.jsp?dcrpath=HHNMAG/ Article/data/05MAY2007/070515HHN_Online_Finarelli&domain =HHNMAG.

15. Weinick, R. M., Pollack, C. E., Fisher, M. P., Gillen, E. M., & Mehrotra, A. (2010). Policy implications of the use of retail clinics, Technical report. Retrieved February 29, 2012, from: http://www.rand.org/pubs/technical_ reports/2010/RAND_TR810.pdf.

16. Gagnon M.-A., & Lexchin, J. (2008, January). The cost of pushing pills: A new estimate of pharmaceutical promotion expenditures in the United States. *PLoS Medicine, 5*(1), e1.

17. Kravitz, R. L., Epstein, R. M., Feldman, M. D., Franz, C. E., Azari, R., Wilkes, M. S., et al. (2005). Influence of patients' requests for direct-to-consumer advertised antidepressants. *JAMA, 293*(16), 1995–2002.
18. CBO. (2011, May). Potential effects of a ban on direct-to-consumer advertising of new prescription drugs. CBO Economic and Budget Issue Brief. Retrieved February 29, 2012, from: http://www.cbo.gov/sites/default/files/cbofiles/ftpdocs/121xx/doc12164/5-25-prescriptiondrugadvertising.pdf.
19. American Medical Association. (2007). Competition in health insurance: A Comprehensive study of U.S. markets, 2007 update. Retrieved February 29, 2012, from: http://www.ama-assn.org/ama1/pub/upload/mm/368/compstudy_52006.pdf.
20. Dafney, L., Duggan, M., & Ramanarayanan, S. (2010, May). Paying a premium on your premium? Consolidation in the U.S health insurance industry. NBER Working Paper No. 15434. Retrieved February 29, 2012, from: http://www.nber.org/papers/w15434.
21. Rice, B. (2007, January 22). Economic credentialing: When hospitals play hardball. Medical Economics. Retrieved February 29, 2012, from: http://www.mbbwi.com/PDF/sneddon_med_econ.pdf.
22. Higman, S. A., McKay, F. J., Engstrom, P. F., O'Grady, M. A., & Young, R. C. (2000). Fox Chase Network: Fox Chase Cancer Center's community hospital affiliation program. *The Oncologist, 5*(4), 329–335.
23. Ginsburg, P. G. (2007). Shopping for price in medical care. *Health Affairs, 26*(2), w208–w216.
24. McNamara, M. (2009, February 11). Want to pay less at the doctor? Negotiate. Retrieved February 29, 2012, from: http://www.cbsnews.com/stories/2007/01/24/eveningnews/main2395899.shtml.
25. Workforce Management. (2006, September 26). WellPoint launches hospital cost comparison tool. Retrieved February 29, 2012, from: http://www.workforce.com/section/news/article/wellpoint-launches-hospital-cost-comparison-tool.php.
26. St. Luke's Iowa Health System. (2011). Hospital cost savings plan for expectant parents. Retrieved February 29, 2012, from: http://www.stlukes.org/Documents/PatientInfo/Billing/costsaving-1210.pdf.
27. Francis, T. (2007). Hospital charge card: Don't leave the ward without it. *Wall Street Journal Health Blog.* Retrieved February 29, 2012, from: http://blogs.wsj.com/health/2007/08/23/hospital-charge-card-dont-leave-the-ward-without-it/.
28. Langabeer, J. (1998, November–December). Competitive strategy in turbulent healthcare markets: An analysis of financially effective teaching hospitals. *Journal of Healthcare Management, 6,* 512–526.
29. Lasik MD. (n.d.). Lowest price guarantee. Retrieved February 29, 2012, from: http://www.lasikmd.com/vancouver/price-financing/lowest-price-guarantee.

30. Robinson, R. (2011, March 28). How CaroMont is like the cable company. *Gaston Gazette.* Retrieved February 29, 2012, from: http://www .gastongazette.com/articles/healthcare-56307-state-knee.html.

31. Tellis, G. J. (1987, Fall). Creative pricing strategies. *Journal of Medical Practice Management, 3*(2), 120–124.

32. Ries, A., & Trout, J. (1981). Positioning: The battle for your mind. New York: McGraw-Hill; p. 33.

33. Newman, A. A. (2009, May 3). No actors, just patients in unvarnished spots for hospitals. *The New York Times.* Retrieved February 29, 2012, from: http://www.nytimes.com/2009/05/04/business/media/04adco.html.

34. SUMA/Orchard Social Marketing, Inc. (n.d.). Final report on pilot project WIC breastfeeding promotion outreach campaign targeted to African Americans. Retrieved February 29, 2012, from: http://www.dshs.state .tx.us/wichd/bf/pdf/Executive-20Summary.pdf.

35. 74% of U.S. adults read newspapers at least once a week in print or online. (2009, November 17). *Nielsen Wire.* Retrieved February 2012, from: http:// blog.nielsen.com/nielsenwire/consumer/74-of-u-s-adults-read-print-news -at-least-once-a-week/.

36. Fortenberry, J. L., McGoldrick, P. J., & French, G. E. (2010, March/April). Is billboard advertising beneficial for healthcare organizations? An investigation of efficacy and acceptability to patients? *Journal of Healthcare Management, 55*(2), 81–96.

37. Washkuch, F. (2010, May 17). Marketers provide simple healthcare solutions. *Direct Marketing News.* Retrieved February 2012, from: http://www.dmnews.com/marketers-provide-simple-healthcare-solutions/ article/170217/.

38. American Medical Association. (2006). Hospital ad spending rising. Retrieved February 29, 2012, from: http://www.ama-assn.org/amednews/ 2006/02/27/bicb0227.htm.

39. Thomaselli, R. (2010, June 28). Health-care reform stokes spending by top hospitals, clinics. *Advertising Age.* Retrieved February 29, 2012, from: http://adage.com/article/news/health-care-reform-stokes -spending-top-hospitals-clinics/144696/.

40. Warren, J. (2009, November 29). Hospital marketing: Competing with smaller ad budgets. Retrieved February 29, 2012, from: http:// marketingyourhospital.com/2009/11/29/hospital-marketing-how-to -compete-with-smaller-ad-budgets/.

41. Thalhuber, J., & Clasen, N. (1987). If Sears can do it, so can we. A retail approach to health care advertising. In John K. Wong (Ed.), *Leadership, Proceedings, Academy of Health Services Marketing.* Chicago: American Marketing Association; p. 63.

42. West, W. (2004). Healthcare sales: Relationship marketing at its best. *Healthcare Marketing Report.* Retrieved February 29, 2012, from: http:// www.corporatehealthgroup.com/ftpuser/CHG%20Library/Physicians%20

Relations/Healthcare%20Sales-Relationship%20Marketing%20at%20
Its%20Best-Healthcare%20Marketing%20Report%209-04.pdf.

43. Health Management Technology Management e-newsletter. (2010, April 27). Physician referrals increased by 22.4 percent. Retrieved February 29, 2012, from: http://www.healthmgttech.com/newsletter/index.php/ newsletters/general/physician-referrals-increased-by-224-percent.html.

44. Green, L., & Choe, C. (2011, June). Return on relationship. *The Liaison.* Retrieved February 29, 2012, from: http://www.physicianliaison.com/ sharedfiles/AAPL/Brochures/aaplNewsletter2011June.pdf.

45. McCarthy, A. (2009, March). Tracking the tracking systems for physician relations efforts. *Learning Tools.* Retrieved February 2012, from: http://www.barlowmccarthy.com/resources/physician-relations-sales.

CHAPTER 8

STEP 5: INTEGRATION OF THE MARKETING PLAN WITH THE BUSINESS PLAN AND THE STRATEGIC PLAN

WHAT YOU WILL LEARN

- Marketing plans, business plans, and strategic plans are not built in an organizational vacuum.
- Working with the management team is critical to implementation of the marketing plan.
- The marketing plan must be in concert with the strategic plan and vision, but the marketing plan is a part of a specific product- or service-based business plan.

THE NECESSITY OF INTEGRATION

Step 5 is the process of integrating the marketing plan into the business plan or the entity (**Figure 8.1**). First, the plan must be integrated with the other major functions of operation, human resources, and finance. Second, the plan has to be integrated within the context of other business plans and programs to make sure that internal competition is minimized, resources are maximized, and the business is most efficiently managed. Such integration is commonly referred to as portfolio management. As a result of discussions in these two areas, marketing plans may be accepted, modified, or completely rejected; and the business, therefore, could be eliminated.

If an organization consists of a group of cardiologists, it is likely that the group will have a strategic plan and one marketing plan for the group—a rather straightforward situation. However, if the organization is a hospital with obstetrics, general surgery, cosmetic surgery, outpatient services, and many other programs, each program should have a marketing

FIGURE 8.1

Step 5: Integration of the Marketing Plan

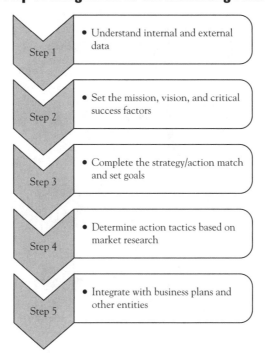

Step 1　• Understand internal and external data

Step 2　• Set the mission, vision, and critical success factors

Step 3　• Complete the strategy/action match and set goals

Step 4　• Determine action tactics based on market research

Step 5　• Integrate with business plans and other entities

plan because each program's markets or customer base is different. In this situation, the coordination of marketing tactics is critical, and that is why integration of marketing plans and business plans is even more important.

The process of integration is dynamic based on personalities, politics, available resources, and the tone of the organization. This step can require the development of a revised marketing strategy, which may be different from the original strategy. A marketing strategy may be revised as a result of resource allocations, coordination with other market plans, or the integration of the plan with the organizational mission.

INTEGRATION OF PLANS WITH OTHER MANAGEMENT FUNCTIONS

Marketing serves as a key first step in the development of a comprehensive business plan. As indicated in **Figure 8.2**, the marketing plan serves as a basis for the operational plan (how services will be provided), the human resources plan, and the finance plan (e.g., budget, cash management). Also, marketing plays a role in helping to formulate the overall

FIGURE 8.2

Business Planning Process and the Key Role of Marketing

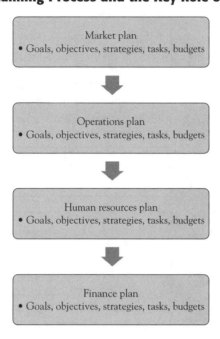

corporate mission and goals. Marketing planning includes understanding the environment and devising ways to connect the market with the services provided by the corporation.

Although most hospitals and many clinics have people with marketing responsibility, few of these people have been able to act as the key agents in developing business plans. Often, instead, market data are analyzed, advertising budgets are developed, and sales forecasts are made after the business plan has been approved. Many organizations choose to use marketing as a support in the implementation of decisions initiated in other areas. Marketing provides key input, but does not play a role in the early decisions on service viability. Therefore, an important question that faces marketing in health care is: To what extent can marketing integrate itself into the organization at a high level in order to maximize its value?

Successful healthcare businesses of the future will have market, finance, and operations planning well integrated in the early stages of service development. Early integration of these functional plans will result in a total business plan with an increased likelihood of success. All the concerns of each functional area described as follows are legitimate. Each one needs to be discussed. The key for marketing is to be sensitive to these disciplines, to resolve concerns, and to understand that marketing is part of a larger business unit on which success depends.

Integration with Operations

Operations is concerned with providing clinic or hospital services on a day-to-day basis. Marketing often means change—change in service, in location, or in policy. As is to be expected, these changes often affect routine operations. In the hospital, nurses may be asked to call on physicians' offices, change work schedules, and modify the way they interact with patients. The dietary department may be asked to offer 24-hour room service, while the admissions department may be asked to have physicians' offices linked directly by computer. Within physicians' offices, operations are the physicians' services. A marketing plan may require the physician staff to change office hours, modify the length of appointments, or provide health education.

In order to carry out these changes, a variety of operational areas, such as staffing, equipment, schedules, union agreements, historical relationships, coordination with other departments, productivity analyses, coverage, and call systems, must be examined. However, many managers resist change. If developed without early operations input, the marketing plan will probably be blocked or not implemented in critical operations areas. More important, valuable ideas on how to change or establish a competitive advantage in service delivery will probably be lost. Therefore, instead of going to the family-practice department and simply telling its staff that office hours must be extended, marketers should meet with family-practice human resources and show them the consumer research data that indicate a demand for service after normal hours. With the family-practice staff as team members, the potential impact of this marketing opportunity can be mutually assessed. These individuals can be informally surveyed for ideas they may have for designing an after-hours coverage system to capture this business. In this role, marketing serves as a catalyst to integrate organizational direction with the day-to-day provision of service. Furthermore, marketing can take into account the fact that market segments exist both externally and internally.

Integration with Human Resources

Human resources is concerned with providing the proper talent, maintaining fair systems for managing and compensating employees, and developing the appropriate culture for the organization. As marketing concepts become more widespread, the human resources function will be forced to find solutions to difficult problems. First, human resources will have to find a way to create an entrepreneurial environment within the existing bureaucratic structure of most hospitals. Second, human resources will have to develop new compensation systems, such as bonus plans, commission programs, and incentives. Although common in traditional industries, these alternatives are rarely used in health care. Third, major changes in strategy and operations will make it necessary for human resources to reevaluate long-standing middle-management needs. For example, do hospitals need separate departments for electrocardiography, electroencephalography, cardiology, physical therapy, occupational therapy, and respiratory therapy? Could one manager handle all these services with well-trained supervisors in each area? Does the hospital need separate department heads for food, housekeeping, and admissions, or would an executive innkeeper be more capable? Fourth, human resources will need to consider the needs of top management.

Drastic human resources changes are likely under a market-responsive system. For example, if a hospital manages the "hotel functions" through an executive innkeeper and the clinical business areas through a product (brand) manager who has a master's degree in business administration, what will become of the assistant administrators?

Most of these changes will take time to be integrated into the organization. Marketing should not develop a marketing plan in November that calls for program managers to provide plans for commission sales by January. Alternative compensation systems to reward sales efforts in accordance with organizational goals and other marketing plans that affect human resources must be tested.

Human resources can provide valuable input for the successful implementation of marketing plans. As with the operations group, marketing should consider human resources a partner in problem solving.

Integration with Finance

Finance is concerned largely with the preservation and growth of capital. To a financial manager, the marketing plan often represents a degree of risk for which the reward should be appropriate. The higher the perceived risk, the larger the return on investment should be. Finance looks at risk in relation to the probability that targets can be reached within a reasonable time and with a large enough return on investment (**Figure 8.3**).

Finance often evaluates the marketing-plan risks in relation to the potential return to be obtained by investing capital in "safe" areas, such as bonds. For example, $1 million invested in a health-food store with no net income for 4 years is weighed against $1 million in high-grade bonds at 6%. If a safe investment can immediately generate a 6% return, it stands to reason—from the perspective of finance—that anything with a higher risk should generate more than a 6% return. The long-term position of the

FIGURE 8.3

Risk-Return Philosophy

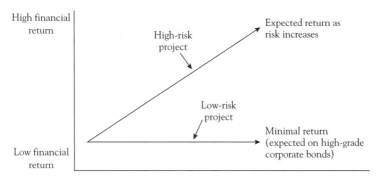

organization, however, may be to extend itself from medicine to health. The short-term losses of the health-food store may result in a more profitable position for the organization as a whole in the long run.

Finance is concerned with meeting projected sales, controlling costs, dealing with competitors, and predicting the state of the economy in 3 years. From the finance manager's perspective, the risks inherent in most marketing plans are large in relation to those of a "safe" investment. Integrating the finance view is therefore essential to developing realistic business (and specifically marketing) plans. Although finance is primarily responsible for budgets, revenue forecasts, and cash flow, the finance perspective is valuable beyond these areas. Finance often gives a critical second opinion, and these experts excel at developing creative strategies for syndicating new ventures. In general, therefore, finance is helpful in weighing risk and evaluating alternative marketing plans.

By nature, finance is often conservative. Its goal is to protect capital from bad risks, and as most finance people know, many ventures are bad risks. Marketing should not try to avoid this critical examination by finance, however, particularly when capital resources are scarce.

INTEGRATION WITHIN THE ORGANIZATION'S PORTFOLIO

Each proposed marketing plan and its related business plan must be integrated with other proposed marketing plans and business plans, and all of this work should be within the context of the strategic plan.

Figure 8.4 shows how each business within an organization has a marketing plan and how these plans, taken together, form the portfolio of the hospital or clinic.

FIGURE 8.4

Portfolio of the Organization

Enterprise-wide strategic plan followed by:		
Cardiac business plan	Obstetrics business plan	Rehabilitation business plan
Marketing	Marketing	Marketing
Operations	Operations	Operations
Finance	Finance	Finance

Note: Integrated strategic and business plan model. All business plans created in context of overall enterprise strategic plan.

Integrating the portfolio involves determining:

1. Whether the proposed plans overlap.
2. Whether the proposed plans compete with each other.
3. Whether the proposed plans duplicate resources.
4. Whether the proposed plans represent the correct balance of activity for the clinic or hospital.

In 1981, for example, American Express Company purchased the brokerage house of Shearson. With this purchase, American Express was able to offer a full line of financial services: a financial card through American Express, insurance through Fireman's Fund (which it also owns), and investment advice through Shearson. Many of these services, such as the American Express Gold Card, were directed to upper-income individuals. Although each business unit had independent responsibility for the development of its own marketing and business plans, integration did occur. The company coordinated sales of the three product categories to the same upper-income market segment. The company also explored cross-selling activities: A Shearson broker could recommend a Gold Card, for example, and a Fireman's Fund independent agent might have passed on information about the Shearson brokerage firm. Similar legitimate opportunities exist in the healthcare industry. For example, an obese patient in the emergency room for a sprained ankle may be given a brochure for a hospital-sponsored weight-loss program.

Checking for program integration involves making sure that the organization takes full advantage of marketplace opportunities. Home health care should support respiratory care. Obstetricians should support internists. A clinic should seek to serve entire families rather than individual family members.

In the integration process, the marketing focus shifts somewhat from a particular business plan to the organization's overall plan. With this more complete organizational focus, the marketing professional and other organizational executives should shift from concern for competitive advantages in a given business plan to concern for balance of the product line, total growth of the organization, and the best use of resources.

When hospitals develop plans, management should be impartial; the plans should not reflect the strong artificial influence of two or three specialty areas by representatives on the planning committee. Hospitals need to balance their portfolios between sources of business today and sources of business in the future. Often, cash generated from high-profit clinical services should not be invested back into those areas, but into new areas in the hope that they will become the high-profit areas of the future.

Completion of this step and development of the other elements of the business plan will change the original marketing plan. These changes occur as more people participate in refinement of the plan. The final step is to develop a set of rules for deciding which plans can be approved.

SUMMARY

As the process of developing a marketing plan draws to a close, senior management of the organization is advised to take a step back and assess to what extent the proposed marketing plan fits within the context of the entire organization. Sometimes organizations create powerful marketing plans, but they are outside of the bounds or mission of the clinic. The following questions are helpful in making sure that the marketing plan under consideration makes sense for the organization:

1. Does this marketing plan complement the organization's other services?
2. Do the other management functions complement the marketing plan?
3. Is the plan a major contribution to the organization?
4. Is the organization spending too much time/effort on this plan for the expected return?
5. As a result of the integration process, do the combined plans offer balance, and are they responsive to the market?

QUESTIONS FOR DISCUSSION

1. What element of the strategy process is most important?
2. What should a business plan for a charitable organization focus on?
3. Who should participate in the strategic planning process? Who should participate in the business-planning process?

CHAPTER 9

STEP 6: THE APPROVAL AND MONITORING PROCESS

WHAT YOU WILL LEARN

- Financial and analytical skills are required to approve and monitor the plan.
- The job of marketing continues during the implementation of the overall plan.
- Clear evaluation guidelines should be established in advance.
- A robust strategic process is continuous.

AN END AND A BEGINNING

Approval and monitoring is the last step in the development of the planning process and the first step in implementation (**Figure 9.1**). The marketing job is not over; it is just beginning.

APPROVAL PROCESS: ESTABLISHING GUIDELINES FOR SELECTING AMONG ALTERNATIVE PLANS

Many organizations find that they have more proposed business plans than they can support, and they therefore need guidelines for selecting the business plans they will implement. These guidelines are the "game rules." They should be developed before a formal marketing planning document is drawn up, and these rules should be available to senior staff as parameters for business planning. Just as physicians develop criteria for evaluating medical case management before the cases are managed, business plans should be developed after the evaluation criteria have been specified. Prespecification

FIGURE 9.1

The Overall Strategic, Marketing, and Remaining Business Plan Model

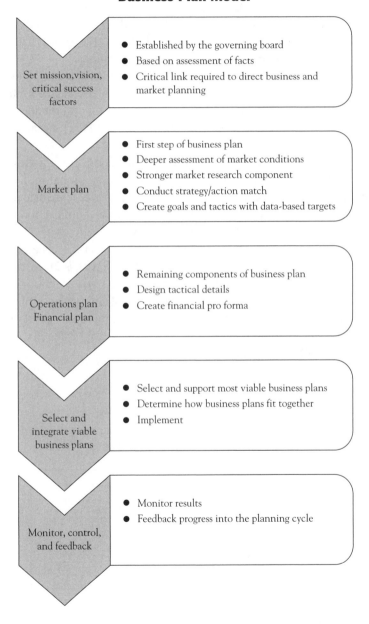

Set mission, vision, critical success factors
- Established by the governing board
- Based on assessment of facts
- Critical link required to direct business and market planning

Market plan
- First step of business plan
- Deeper assessment of market conditions
- Stronger market research component
- Conduct strategy/action match
- Create goals and tactics with data-based targets

Operations plan Financial plan
- Remaining components of business plan
- Design tactical details
- Create financial pro forma

Select and integrate viable business plans
- Select and support most viable business plans
- Determine how business plans fit together
- Implement

Monitor, control, and feedback
- Monitor results
- Feedback progress into the planning cycle

of guidelines has several advantages: It saves time by eliminating projects that do not meet predetermined standards, it avoids the implementation of unwise "pet" projects, and it informs the staff of the tasks required to meet the organization's mission. Step 4 helped guide us through the selection of new product offerings through use of a checklist of criteria, such as facility equipment and process familiarity, market stability, market trend, number of potential customers, effect on present products, and so on. This same general approach can be used to choose marketing plans.

A quantitative method can be used to evaluate business plans. This approach uses a numerical scoring system. Those plans that score highest are approved. Each organization must develop its own criteria and scoring system according to its specific guidelines and needs. The management and board can then determine which plans to approve.

For many healthcare services, however, decision criteria cannot be provided with quantitative scales. The mix of organizational motivations, which often include the desire to survive, as well as more intrinsic motives that relate to community service, goodwill, and the public good, makes using a strict numerical system difficult.

A less structured evaluative method concentrates on the general advantages or disadvantages of one plan over another (**Figure 9.2**). In this approach, guidelines are less specific and quantifiable. Instead, the idea is to evaluate general positive and negative attributes of the business plan. This approach to evaluation, in which the process is used more as a point of reference for decision making than as a strictly quantitative evaluation, is more common in healthcare organizations.

FIGURE 9.2

A Qualitative Approval Process

Criteria (examples)	Check one item per criterion	
	+ Positive evaluation	– Negative evaluation
• Return on investment	_____	_____
• Volume of revenue generated	_____	_____
• Competitive advantage	_____	_____
• Location	_____	_____
• Match with lifecycle	_____	_____
• Available technical know-how	_____	_____
• Financial risk	_____	_____
• Competition ability	_____	_____
Overall evaluation:		

FIGURE 9.3

Selecting Among Alternative Business Plans

Criteria (examples)	A Proposed plan for home health + –	B Proposed plan for heart surgery + –	C Proposed plan for vision center + –
• Return on equity			
• Volume of revenue			
• Competitive advantage			
• Certificate of need			
• Capital required			
• Ease of entry			
• Research time required			
• Knowledge of business			

Whatever method is selected, it is important that it be developed in advance and that all plans be evaluated against it. **Figure 9.3** gives an idea of how several alternative plans could be evaluated using a qualitative method. Doing so allows for a rational determination of the mix of plans that makes the most sense.

Return on Equity

One of the most common criteria for evaluating alternative projects is return on equity—that is, the percentage of return realized from the owners' investment. A $1 million investment with a net income of $100,000 translates into a return of 10%. Several more precise methods of calculating return are available. Generally, projects that have an average return in excess of 20% over the life of the investment score favorably. Projects that have an average return of 10% or less score low. Any return on equity must be tied to the organization's cost of capital, however. As the perceived risk of a project increases, or as the length of time increases before profits are realized, the expected return usually increases. Although return on equity is a good indicator of how well the investment is doing overall, other criteria must also be considered.

Margin

Margin is another measure of company performance. Estimated margins can be used as a basis for evaluating alternative projects. **Table 9.1** lists margins for selected healthcare organizations.

TABLE 9.1 Margins for Selected Healthcare Sectors*

	2011 Margin
Medical products (devices)	17%
Pharmaceutical	15%
Healthcare facilities	4%
Health insurance	4%

*Margin equals net income/sales.
Source: Data from Fortune 500: Who's on top by sector. (2011, May 23). *Fortune, 163*(7), 33–38.

Volume of Sales

Small projects or new service offerings can generate large returns on investment. Often, however, organizations must look beyond return on equity to make sure that the project is of sufficient magnitude in terms of absolute gross revenue dollars to add to the organization's product line. An important issue is whether the service generates cash flows that are large enough for management to spend time on them in the first place. Each organization must determine the exact parameters of this criterion. In some hospitals, projects that do not expect to have annual revenues of $1 million within 3 years would be rejected, whereas in other organizations, projects that generate gross revenues of $300,000 are considered acceptable.

Return on Sales

Another criterion that is often incorporated into the selection process is return on sales. When used in conjunction with the previously mentioned criteria, return on sales helps to provide a balanced analysis of the financial value of the marketing plan. If an eyeglass store has sales of $2 million and a profit of $400,000, the return on sales would be 20% ($400,000/$2,000,000 = 20%). The reason for considering both return on equity and return on sales can best be illustrated by the following example. A hospital is considering a business plan for a health-food chain and a plan for a large retail drugstore. The alternative results are shown in **Table 9.2**.

The health-food chain has a low gross margin and, as a result, generates a relatively small profit on each dollar of sales compared with the drugstore. Nevertheless, because the investment required is lower for the health-food store, the percentage of return on equity for each project

TABLE 9.2   Comparison of Return on Sales and Equity

	Health-Food Chain	Drugstore
Sales	$5,000,000	$5,000,000
Net income	$100,000	$500,000
Total equity investment	$500,000	$2,500,000
Return on sales	2%	10%
Return on equity	20%	20%

is the same. Thus, it is useful to look at several financial criteria when evaluating alternative marketing and business plans.

Existing Competition

An objective evaluation of the number of competitors and the threat that they pose is also a useful criterion for plan approval. Clearly, if there are few competitors in a market that is known to be capable of sustaining a clinic office, a business plan suggesting such an action would get a positive score. However, a business plan with few innovations that proposes entry into an intensely competitive area would get a low rating. At times, however, it is a good strategy not to enter the market first. If the service is completely new and untried, it may be useful for someone else to enter first and bear the necessary expense of educating the market. The second entrant would be able to learn from the first, avoid some high media costs, and catch the market as it moves from the introduction phase to the growth stage of the marketplace lifecycle.

Technical Protection

Business plans that entail new services or products that have patent protection, regulatory protection, or technical advantages should generally be evaluated positively. Patent protection is the exclusive use of a product or service through research and development, and ultimately the acquisition of proprietary rights. This protection is rare in a clinic setting. Regulatory protection refers to the necessity of obtaining a certificate of need before establishing a service. This form of protection has been valuable in the past for healthcare providers, but its value has diminished with the elimination of these regulations in many states. Technical know-how is the special capabilities, equipment, personnel, and similar advantages that an organization has. Others could develop this capability, but it is expensive, risky, and difficult to do. As new technological advances rapidly appear in the market, the length of time in which a marketing plan can be based on this advantage is limited.

Additional Factors in the Analysis

The examples that have been discussed in this section illustrate the type of analysis that an organization should carry out as it considers each individual business plan. Screening criteria can be summarized by asking:

1. Is the return on the investment adequate?
2. Does the plan enhance the organization's political power?
3. Are estimated revenues sufficient and profitable?
4. Does the plan require capital? How much?
5. Does it require research time?
6. Is a certificate of need required?
7. Does the plan have a competitive advantage in the marketplace?
8. Will the proposed new product or service appeal to a solid market segment?
9. Is it easy for a competitor to duplicate?
10. Is the proposed process one with which the organization is familiar?
11. Does the product enhance stability of the other products offered by the organization?
12. Does it promote product competition?
13. Does the plan provide for long-range growth?
14. Does it provide for adequate market share?

In order for the marketing plan and subsequent business plan to develop to the greatest level of precision and potential, criteria such as those suggested here should be agreed upon before the marketing and business plans are begun.

During this evaluation, it is also important to analyze marketing and business plans for logic and consistency. For example, it is difficult to have high profits and high growth in the same product in the same year. The growth stage of the product lifecycle often requires high expenses for capital needs, new staffing, promotion, and start up. These costs diminish net income in the short term. Also, it is generally not likely that an organization can seek high-growth opportunities and at the same time require stability. Aggressive investment in a product in a mature market is rarely logical. Instead, investment in this stage of the market lifecycle should be minimized. Generally speaking, a review of the logic of a plan should cover the following six areas identified by Jain:[1]

1. Internal consistency (Is the plan consistent with company ideas and direction?)
2. Consistency with the environment
3. Appropriateness in light of available resources
4. Reasonable degree of risk
5. Appropriate time horizon
6. Workability

These guidelines will help in developing appropriate criteria for selecting those plans that can best meet the goals of the organization.

MONITORING SYSTEMS

Monitoring the Strategic Plan

The strategic planning process is often an event that culminates with a board retreat in the fall of the year around budget time. And from that moment on, the strategic plan is not mentioned again until the next year. This is not the way to operate a strategic planning process.

Once the strategic plan has been approved, the management team and the board should monitor progress on a regularly scheduled basis. Recognizing that the completion of the strategic plan may take many months to approve, it is likely that, on a monthly basis, it may seem that progress is slow and plodding. Nevertheless, keeping the strategy and progress in front of the management team is important. Many organizations use a simple technique to keep the strategic vision in front of the organization.

At the monthly board meeting, or once a month at the management team meeting, place the strategic plan on the agenda as a standing item, just like an organization would have approval of minutes or review of financial statements as standing items. In other words, the board knows that every month it should expect to see a report on progress that is being made toward the successful implementation of the plan. Many boards include the mission, vision, and critical success factors in the board package of information, located just behind the cover or agenda page. Using this methodology, the strategic plan and vision of the company will not get lost in the whirlwind of day-to-day concerns regarding running the business. Further, this methodology will foster continuous understanding of the board and leadership in terms of what the organization is trying to accomplish.

Monitoring the Business Plan

If the prior steps have been properly followed, a precise, measurable, and targeted marketing plan will have been developed and approved. As the organization begins to implement the marketing plan and business plan, the use of monitoring systems is necessary. Over the long run, the organization will be monitoring results that are broad in scope. These evaluation systems include return on equity, which is discussed earlier in this chapter. Most of the monitoring systems that are specific to a marketing plan are short term and are designed to test plans and, if necessary, suggest how they can be adjusted. These types of day-to-day monitoring systems help determine the strategies that should be employed in future marketing plans.

One basic monitoring tool that is fundamental to the enterprise is the calculation of performance in relation to budgeted plan. Such a tool is required in any organization.

As **Table 9.3** indicates, each month the organization should prepare an income statement that shows what was planned (column A), what happened (column B), the difference between the first column and the second column (column C), and actual performance last year (column D). This sample statement is a quick and timely snapshot of the performance of a home health business. It shows that the business had a profit for the month and that business has grown since the previous year. It also shows that net income was less than expected because of lower than anticipated sales and higher than anticipated expenses. The conclusion to be drawn is that greater emphasis needs to be placed on increasing sales volume,

TABLE 9.3   HOME HEALTH INC. BUDGETED/ACTUAL INCOME/EXPENSE STATEMENT, MAY 201_, IN THOUSANDS OF DOLLARS

	(A) Budget	(B) Actual	(C) Variance	(D) Last Year Actual
Sales	$100	$90	$ 10	$50
Expenses:				
Salaries	$ 50	$51	$ (1)	$40
Travel	$ 4	$ 5	$ (1)	$ 3
Office supplies	$ 3	$ 2	$ 1	$ 2
Medical supplies	$ 14	$20	$ (6)	$10
Rent	$ 3	$ 3	—	$ 2
Utilities	$ 1	$ 1	—	$ 1
Total expenses	**$ 75**	**$82**	**$ (7)**	**$58**
Net income (loss)	**$ 25**	**$ 8**	**$(17)**	**$ (8)**

perhaps through the development of a more aggressive sales strategy, or on reducing operational expenses, or both.

Although this type of income/expense statement is valuable, other monitoring systems are more specific to the marketing area. It is worthwhile, for example, to track sales by a specific business or service area. **Table 9.4** shows total sales volume for a month, net income by laboratory test, and the percentage return on sales. This format helps to pinpoint those areas that generate strong profits and those that are in difficulty. Lab test 3 has strong sales, but has a negative income. This information can be helpful in adjusting prices, eliminating services, or modifying the commission plan to encourage sales in higher margin areas.

Another monitoring tool is required when a sales force is in place. It is helpful to look at the activity of each salesperson and the outcomes of those activities. **Table 9.5** charts the activity of and important productivity measures for each salesperson and the total sales force. Column A lists

TABLE 9.4 SALES ANALYSIS FOR A LABORATORY, IN THOUSANDS OF DOLLARS

	Gross Sales	Net Income	Return on Sales*
Lab Test 1	$30	$ 6	20%
Lab Test 2	$35	$ 6	17%
Lab Test 3	$60	$(5)	–8%
Lab Test 4	$50	$ 3	6%

*Return on sales = net income sales

TABLE 9.5 DOCTORS HMO INC. BIWEEKLY ANALYSIS OF SALES FORCE, IN THOUSANDS OF DOLLARS

(A) Salesperson	(B) No. of Calls	(C) Sales	(D) Call-to-Sales Ratio	(E) Revenue Generated	(F) Revenue Budgeted	(G) Variance
M. E.	12	1	8%	$25	$40	$(15)
K. E.	15	0	0%	—	$40	$(40)
B. M.	10	3	30%	$90	$40	$ 50
B. H.	17	2	12%	$42	$40	$ 2
Total	*54*	*6*	*11%*	*$157*	*$160*	*$(3)*

the names of each salesperson. Column B summarizes total sales calls. Column C provides data on actual sales, with column D providing a useful ratio of calls to sales (sales/number of calls = call-to-sales ratio). Column E presents the revenue each salesperson generated; columns F and G show budgeted revenue and variance from the budget. This analysis shows that, although salesperson K. E. makes many calls, she sells no HMO contracts. However, salesperson B. M. makes relatively few calls, but has a high call-to-sales ratio, which, in turn, generates revenues well beyond those budgeted. Such an analysis indicates that it is necessary to look not only at sales calls, but also at actual sales and dollars generated in order to get an accurate picture of the performance of the sales force.

This type of analysis should be done on a monthly basis at a minimum. The data are easy to collect and track, so problem areas can be quickly pinpointed. Tracking individual performance in this way can result in support for the sales force. Possibly the low producer in Table 9.5 is new and needs to attend training sessions. Maybe this person's sales territory is not appropriate, or the low producer could learn by spending time with the high producer to observe how higher levels of sales are achieved. In any case, this system allows for fast analysis and concurrent actions designed to meet the objectives of the marketing plan.

In advertising, the usefulness of monitoring systems depends on the advertising objectives. Some advertising is directed toward educating potential buyers about a new service or the use of an existing service. In these cases, it may be difficult to tie an advertising campaign to immediate sales. When the advertisements are specifically about a product or service, monitoring becomes more precise and valuable. If, for example, a health-food store located on the first floor of a medical-arts building runs advertisements in the newspaper that include a coupon, a monitoring system could be developed to test which of several different advertisements (each with a different coupon) is the biggest draw.

In the analysis in **Table 9.6**, three different advertisements were developed at different costs. Because they each contained a different coupon, it was possible to track the volume of sales that each generated. Column B is the cost of each advertisement. Column C is the amount of sales attributed to the coupon in each of the three different advertisements. Column D shows which advertisement was the most efficient by calculating the cost of the advertisement in relation to sales revenue generated. The small advertisement cost 20 cents for each dollar generated. The medium advertisement was more efficient in that it cost 18 cents to generate a dollar in sales. The large advertisement was not as efficient in generating sales: Each dollar of sales cost 31 cents in advertising.

TABLE 9.6 ADVERTISING ANALYSIS FOR HEALTH-FOOD STORE

(A) Ad Description	(B) Cost per Ad	(C) Coupon Sales per Ad	(D) Ad Costs per $1 of Sales
Small Ad, 2 × 10	$1,000	$5,000	$.20
Medium Ad, 3 × 10	$2,000	$11,000	$.18
Large Ad, 4 × 10	$4,000	$13,000	$.31

$$\frac{\text{Cost per Ad (column B)}}{\text{Sales per Ad (column C)}} = \text{Ad cost per \$1 of sales (column D)}$$

Numerous monitoring systems can be used for evaluating advertising. It is wise to use several approaches, because many variables can affect advertising. For example, the same size advertisement can generate different responses because of the graphics. An advertisement's impact may also fluctuate according to which day it appears in the paper, where in the paper it appears, or when it appears on television and what television station is used. Advertising agencies are helpful in evaluating which media methods to use, how to monitor performance, and when to make changes.

These monitoring examples illustrate some of the different ways in which a marketing plan can be evaluated on a continuous basis. The development of specific monitoring systems for a specific service depends on the strategies used in the business and marketing plan.

THE BALANCED SCORECARD

As the entire strategy and business plan come together, sometimes the strategy is out of balance with reality. In the excitement of charting the direction for the organization, leadership oftentimes loses track of reality, including financial commitments, internal system capability, understanding true customer requirements, and the need to bring people along in terms of skills and training. Kaplan and Norton noticed a gap between the exuberance of pie-in-the-sky strategy versus on-the-ground, day-in and day-out execution of the strategy. Recognizing this issue, they developed a model that is now widely used called the *balanced scorecard*.[2] The Kaplan model requires that organizations measure themselves around four specific areas: finance, customers, process, and learning. Kaplan argues that sometimes organizations become too dominated by finance or by customers; therefore, healthcare organizations must balance themselves to

FIGURE 9.4

Strategic Plan with Balanced Scorecard

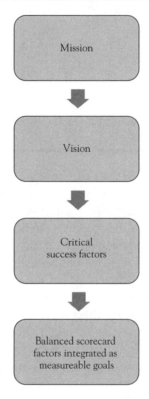

consider the four functions of finance, customers, process, and learning. **Figure 9.4** shows how the balanced scorecard fits with the strategic plan, and **Figure 9.5** shows the elements of a balanced scorecard integrated into the strategic plan.

In Figure 9.5 the Kaplan categories are listed across the top of the chart and the critical measurement areas are listed underneath. In this example, in the customer category there are two measureable marketing-related targets, in the process area there is an important marketing target related to customer wait times, and in the finance area the targets related to margin and return on investment (ROI) are also important to marketing.

What this tool accomplishes is that it prods the organization to consider its vision in light of these four elements. The model requires the organization to keep these elements in front of the organization at all times and to measure results using these four categories. Some organizations

FIGURE 9.5

How the Balanced Scorecard is Presented with Measurement

Mission: Provide hospital care to the community.

Vision: By 2015, be known as the safest hospital in the region, with 80% of the community staying in town for their care, and be recognized as a regional center for eye/ophthalmology care.

Critical Success Factors:

#1 Recruit recognized eye group.

#2 Become more efficient in resource use.

#3 Invest in safe medical practice and technology.

----Balanced Scorecard Thinking, Modified to Reflect Important Healthcare Attributes-----

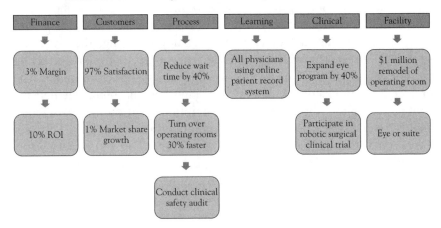

use a rigorous and formal balanced scorecard measurement system. Other organizations simply keep the balanced scorecard categories in mind as they form their strategic goals.

Hospitals and clinics often overcomplicate things, including the balanced scorecard model. When implemented in a hospital, the balanced scorecard measurement tool frequently becomes more intricate than necessary, with dozens if not hundreds of measurements being taken; organizations seem to get caught up in measuring for the sake of measuring, consequently losing sight of using the balanced scorecard as a tool to accomplish the vision. In fact, authors Steven Hillestad and Eric Berkowitz have observed on many occasions that managers filling out balanced scorecard measurements, when asked why they are doing the measurement, do not know why. When this happens, the process is cumbersome, and it has lost its value of closely knitting daily operations with the vision of the company. Extensive published materials, seminars, and training modules are available to better understand the balanced scorecard model and to determine what level of involvement is best for a particular organization.

An organization's mission, vision, and critical success factors can be converted to goals with the *influence of* the balanced scorecard as a guideline.

THE NEED FOR CONTINGENCY PLANS

Contingency planning covers problems that arise when events do not occur as expected. A contingency plan is based on uncertainty, on the possibility that the outcome will not be the one anticipated. In the past, contingency planning was not at all common. However, because of growing uncertainties in an increasingly complex business environment, increasing numbers of organizations are setting contingency plans.

In organizations that practice contingency planning, the "what if" strategies are usually well thought out, but the detailed plans of action are not usually as well developed as the primary operating plans. The greater the perceived risk of the plan, however, the more detailed the contingency plans should be. The assumptions portion of the situation analysis is the basis for the development of contingency plans. This section should include the major assumptions regarding significant events in which the degree of uncertainty is great and the risk of being wrong is high. In the financial area, it may be assumed, for example, that inflation for the next 3 years will average 12% per year. If the degree of uncertainty about this assumption is perceived to be high, contingency plans would include financial forecasts that show the impact of the expected rate of inflation and for the effect of a higher rate of inflation (e.g., 15%).

PLANNING FOR NEXT YEAR

Analysis of the implementation and use of this year's marketing plan (and entire business plan) for each of the organization's service areas will be a valuable resource for next year's planning cycle. The monitoring systems and financial statements provide insight into opportunities in the market, the likelihood of reaching profit expectations, the degree of competitive turbulence, and the ability to execute marketing plans correctly. This type of information will help the organization to fine-tune its business direction and strategies. Therefore, marketing planning must be integrated and interactive. It is integrated in the sense that it works with all elements of the organization. It depends on finance, operations, and personnel. It feeds data to the planning department in order to help set strategic direction.

The plan is interactive in that its development depends on feedback, give and take, and constant modification. It is not a process in which finance is involved only temporarily or to which operations contributes in a prescribed way. Instead, constant input from all areas is required. The cycle of marketing planning and modification is also constant. In this way, marketing remains responsive and competitive.

SUMMARY

Approving the marketing plan is not complete until the entity has a firm understanding regarding how the plan will be monitored. In this chapter, only a sampling of the possible methods to evaluate progress has been presented. Checklists of the essential elements should be part of the ongoing monitoring and review process of a marketing plan. The figures and tables provide some ideas on how to actually go about setting up ways to monitor progress. As in the for-profit business world, accountability has become more important and rigorous. In health care, as competition for resources becomes more intense, monitoring results will become even more important.

QUESTIONS FOR DISCUSSION

1. Should the organization have specific criteria for determining whether the strategic plan should be approved? If yes, what should they be?
2. What specific and measurable criteria should be part of the marketing plan?
3. Who should monitor performance of the business plan?
4. What is the value add of a balanced scorecard?
5. What should happen if in 5 months there are major changes in the data assumptions that were used to build the strategic plan?

NOTES

1. Jain, S. C. (1981). *Marketing planning and strategy*. Cincinnati, OH: South-Western; p. 224.
2. Kaplan, R. S., & Norton, D. P. (1996). *Translating strategy into action*. Boston, MA: Harvard Business School Press; Kaplan, R. S., & Norton, D. P. (1993, September–October). Putting the balanced scorecard to work. *Harvard Business Review*, 2–16.

FURTHER READING

1. Beik, L. L., & Buzby, S. L. (1973, July). Profitability analysis by market segments. *Journal of Marketing, 37,* 48–53.
2. Dunne, P., & Wolk, H. I. (1977, July). Marketing cost analysis: A modularized contribution approach. *Journal of Marketing, 41,* 83–94.
3. FitzRoy, P. T. (1976). *Analytical methods for marketing management.* New York: McGraw-Hill.
4. Hillier, F. S., & Heebink, D. V. (1965, Winter). Evaluating risky capital investment. *California Management Review, 8,* 71–80.
5. Hulbert, J. M., & Tay, N. E. (1977, April). A strategic framework for marketing control. *Journal of Marketing, 41,* 12–20.
6. Kirplani, V. H., & Shapiro, S. S. (1973, July). Financial dimensions of marketing management. *Journal of Marketing, 37,* 40–47.
7. Mossman, F. H., Fischer, P. M., & Crissy, W. J. E. (1974, April). New approaches to analyzing marketing profitability. *Journal of Marketing, 38,* 43–48.
8. Sevin, C. H. (1965). *Marketing productivity analysis.* New York: McGraw-Hill.

Chapter 10

Conclusion

WHAT YOU WILL LEARN

- Organizations must balance strategy with precise tactics.
- Organizations need to recognize the issues that frequently plague good strategy.
- Strategy and plans often fail, but many of the common failures can be avoided.

STRATEGY VERSUS TACTICS

It should be recognized that there is a debate between strategy and operational execution. Some experts suggest that if the strategy is not correct, then operations will quickly lead to failure. Others argue that an organization can have a mediocre strategy, but if the tactical or operational team is excellent, then operations can essentially make up for a poor strategic analysis.

This text is about connecting strategy at the corporate level, along with connecting marketing at the product or service-line level. It is important to conduct an impartial analysis that helps the organization discover opportunities to exploit any weaknesses that need to be fixed. Strategy must be understood in light of the data and facts that have been uncovered during this analysis. Once the marketing analysis is completed and strategy is well defined, an organization can concentrate on tactics and ongoing operational evaluation. In essence, this text looks at all of the elements necessary to help create success in the market, with an emphasis on market analysis and strategic options. Does this mean that we view strategy as more important than tactical operations? The answer to that question is an emphatic *no*. We believe that a successful organization is a combination of good strategy and good tactical operational execution. That said, we also understand that some organizations are strong in analysis and weak in execution, while others have a more intuitive analytical bent and a much stronger execution of sales, advertising, and pricing. Yet, in a majority of cases, although hospitals and clinics spend a lot of time talking about market strategy, they often seem to have less interest or inclination to concentrate on the tactical application of marketing concepts. The reality is that strategy discussion is often more exciting and feels more professional, while tactical application is more mundane and therefore garners less interest.

Hours and hours of meetings do not equal a sound strategy. In fact, many hours in a strategy session with limited or misinterpreted data can be dangerous and can lead to bad assumptions, which result in bad strategy, which drives inappropriate tactics. Consider the following example: A company that produces an antidepressant developed a dosage that requires the patient to take the drug only once per week rather than once per day. The drug company, along with a pharmacy in Florida, teamed up with a local doctor to send out a direct mailing with a sample of the antidepressant contained in the envelope. The mailing went to the doctors' patients who had been diagnosed as depressed. Obviously, the partners assumed this was a good strategy, and they followed up with tactics that were designed to accomplish their goal. Unfortunately, they failed to consider data indicating that patients view medical records, especially mental health records, as sacred and private. This tactical strategy was based on bad assumptions and bad (or limited) data. Patients reacted swiftly and vehemently against the partners; they were upset that depression medicine was sent without their prior approval or knowledge; this tactic placed the patients at risk of having employers, family members, and friends discover their mental health histories. This example shows that solid tactical execution without a sound strategy can be dangerous. Therefore, we have concentrated on strategy and a solid vision as the first step in achieving market success. Meanwhile, we clearly understand that a sound strategy without solid tactical application is, in fact, a wasted strategy.

PLANNING ISSUES

Given that the strategy and its tactical application are important, we now turn to a series of issues that frequently arise as organizations create and begin to execute their plans. This is not a complete list of issues organizations face as they go about the business of trying to increase market share or as they try to create new services and products. These issues also do not necessarily arise during any specific step in the planning process.

Assumed Assumptions

Assumed assumptions sounds like a tautology, yet such assumptions can create serious problems when putting a strategic or marketing strategy into place. Assumed assumptions are based on a belief that they are true, not on facts that would prove that they are true. Market plans are often replete with assumptions that the team believes must be true when, in fact, they are supported by little, if any, data. Customer relations management (CRM), by which a company has a highly organized and detailed information system to access and track customer information, is an example where there is a tendency to make assumptions because a strong CRM program sounds good and feels good; therefore, we assume it must be something for which the customer hungers. The underlying belief is that customers are searching for better service and more personal, customized service. Many times that is the case, but it is not necessarily always the case. Take cancer services, for example. Broadly speaking, cancer services are offered in three areas: cancer prevention and screening, cancer treatment, and post-cancer care, including end-of-life issues. Some healthcare marketing people have assumed that in cancer care, customer service is critical. In fact some have suggested that customer service deserves the most attention as the hospital tries to build market share in the cancer program. Obviously, making these types of assumptions creates a direction for the organization: The hope is that it will develop into a robust and exciting, customer- and family-friendly environment. But are these assumptions correct? Does CRM affect customer decision making? Will improving CRM result in satisfied customers? Maybe yes and maybe no.

The key in making assumptions about cancer services and other services is, in fact, not making assumptions at all. Instead, attempt to figure out exactly what patients, family, and referral doctors are saying and thinking in order to determine how they are behaving. **Figure 10.1** provides an example of how cancer patients in several markets really think. It arrays the broad categories of cancer care along the horizontal axis and the importance of customer service along the vertical axis. In broad terms, when people are accessing the health system for a routine colonoscopy or a routine mammogram, customer service requirements rate high.

FIGURE 10.1

**Customer Relationship Management and Categories
of Cancer Care**

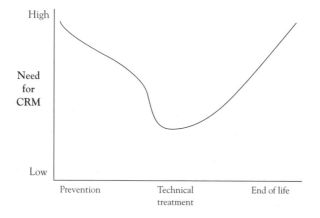

Timeliness, pleasant staff, parking access, and a feeling of warmth and privacy are all important. The second category, cancer treatment, however, can be much different. Although there are many different treatment protocols and possible outcomes, as the treatment becomes more complex and the results have a greater life-and-death impact, people have a much greater tendency to look for skill and technical expertise, and they place a much lower emphasis on customer service issues. The cancer program that offers warmth and caring at the expense of technical skill might find itself losing patients to a university hospital that is not known for the bedside manner of its physicians, but, in fact, has access to the latest protocols and technical equipment.

As cancer patients demand a higher and higher level of treatment, they may forego service amenities if, indeed, a tradeoff is required. Making assumptions about what cancer patients are looking for without any market research is an example of an assumed assumption. Cancer patients expect a seamless system of care and they expect the care to be integrated so that treatment providers are working together. But that is a minimal and, in the mind of the patient, elementary and basic requirement. More sophisticated customer services have different levels of importance to the patient depending on what stage of care the patient is in at any given time. Good marketers will seek, without being overly intrusive, to understand patients' decision-making process in order to determine how they select doctors, hospitals, and other healthcare providers.

Expect the Unexpected

Market plans are developed with 20/20 hindsight knowledge and with no knowledge of what will happen in the future. From the moment the team begins to implement the plan, assumptions are questioned, and the data change; the team then needs to adjust to the new situation. On September 11, 2001, the World Trade Center and the Pentagon were attacked by terrorists. This event immediately changed entire businesses throughout the United States. The travel and leisure business came to a halt, while security agencies and security-monitoring companies grew exponentially. Building a market plan on a narrow set of assumptions is the equivalent of walking a tightrope: One small mistake can result in a fatal fall. Instead, those developing the market plan should err on the side of making conservative assumptions so that there is enough cushion to survive slower than expected growth.

Instead, we often see the opposite. Hospitals, clinics, and health plans usually have targets that must be achieved before a business plan is approved. A team is assembled to work on the plan, and soon the team leader becomes "invested" in the product or service. Team members want this product to be offered because they feel it is a good one; as a consequence, the product is pushed forward. In the process, the team glosses over data, assumes some assumptions, creates aggressive sales forecasts without creating the tactics necessary to hit the forecast; and next, the pricing assumption is cranked up just a bit so that even more revenue can be pumped into the pro forma financial statement. All the while, the team knows what the organizational target is and, consciously or not, is scheming to hit that target rather than figuring out whether creating the new product makes sense within the organization and in the marketplace. Usually these kinds of plans are based on a thin set of assumptions; if any of them do not properly fall into place, the program will not work. And more often than not, at least a few of the assumptions will not hold. If the plan has 10 critical assumptions, maybe only 8 of those assumptions will prove to be true.

Figure 10.2 demonstrates how strategy assumptions can change over time because of changes in data. Within weeks after a new strategy is unveiled, the community's major employer might shut down, or the legislature might change healthcare regulations, or Medicare funding might improve, or a lead doctor might leave. The arena within which we compete and operate is not unchangeable, and we have to allow for modifications in our strategy and plans. Expect, and plan for, the unexpected. Have a business plan that allows for adjustments and that is flexible enough to accommodate unforeseen circumstances. A marketing plan must allow the organization to bend but not break when the unexpected happens.

FIGURE 10.2

Possible Changes in Assumptions Based on Changes in Data Over the Lifetime of a Marketing Plan

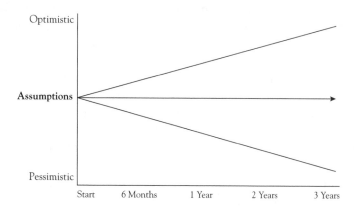

Limit Initiatives

Healthcare people love lists! Strategy in health care usually translates into a long list of initiatives, coupled with dozens of tasks to be carried out with precious little staff and capital. Part of the reason for this outcome is that a typical large clinic or hospital has many clinical lines supported by many high-powered professionals, and it is simply too difficult to suggest that in the current planning cycle resources be channeled to one or two clinical lines instead of a dozen. Nevertheless, having too many initiatives often results in a lack of focus and eventually in performance that is often marginal.

How many marketing initiatives can a typical hospital manage? For the purpose of this discussion, assume a hospital has 300 beds and that even though it is operating in a suburban environment where there are competitors, it is busy. Given that the hospital needs to maintain ongoing marketing efforts for well-established programs, it can probably launch one or two major marketing efforts per year unless it decides to devote an unusual set of resources to initiating more. A successful launch depends on having staff talent available to support the effort, financial resources that the hospital is willing to commit to the launch, and an overall commitment from the organization to support the new service by providing a call center, nursing support, physician champions, and other resources.

Some organizations choose to take another route. They understaff and underfund long-range and short-term efforts, and yet they expect the marketing team to support an ever-widening array of products. This approach does not work. For example, if the marketing department had an advertising budget last year of $1 million and those funds were supporting four different areas, it is difficult to see how this year's budget of $1.1 million can now be expected to support nine different areas. Other organizations use the approach of trying multiple initiatives with the expectation that the strongest will survive. In the process, it increases expectations for staff and also spreads resources more thinly as each new initiative is launched.

Other organizations take a serious look at their vision and their product portfolio and attempt to focus resources on those offerings that have the greatest return on investment and that move the organization closer to its vision. In this model, when a new marketing effort is launched, new resources are provided. Successful and sustainable marketing efforts are built with the commitment of appropriate resources, including staff and direct funding.

Marketing as a Team Player

Sometimes marketing is expected to create miracles for the organization, and sometimes marketing is kept in the back hallways and is used only to create colorful brochures. Both models are wrong. Marketing is a member of the team, and it is neither the superstar nor the water boy.

Sometimes marketing is asked to go head-to-head against a cross-town rival through a deluge of ads touting the message of the day, such as "we have good doctors," "our place is friendly," or "we deliver quality." But these messages are hollow if the doctors fail to show up on time, if the building looks shabby, or if the organization has been in the headlines because of patient safety issues. Great advertising for marginal organizations with clinical and services issues is unlikely to create a miracle.

At the other end of the spectrum, marketing staffs are often placed in the backwater of the healthcare system and are brought out only to implement tactics devised by another group without being able to analyze the situation or to contribute their point of view. A university physician received a grant to study asthma in young children. He decided to use the student newspaper to recruit subjects for his research. Why? Because, he said, it was fast and cheap. Consequently, instead of engaging marketing to help create a strategy and to ask some probing questions, he used marketing as a messenger to go to the student newspaper to get them to write about his research program. He was angry when he failed to reach his quota of research subjects within the time allotted. He should instead have engaged marketing in suggesting other channels that could have been used to recruit people. Through this discussion, the physician might have come to understand that posting information at daycare centers, working with grade-school nurses, and talking with pediatricians would have reached 5-year-old asthmatic children better than advertising in a university's student newspaper.

Too many times, it seems, marketing people get trapped. They are willing to run ads touting a hospital's service when, in fact, the service is out of control. In such instances, the marketing staff should suggest that advertising money be diverted from marketing to help improve the service level. Instead, however, most marketing groups move headlong into a promotion campaign that does not match community experience or that is viewed with disdain internally. Other marketing people are too willing to sit in the backwater of the organization, taking orders for brochures, without asking questions and without offering advice.

Marketing is a contributing member of a management team when it moves away from taking orders and moves toward offering professional judgments and opinions. Marketing can contribute to an organization when it is involved with clinical lines that have a good track record and involves medical professionals who are highly regarded within the community. In other words, marketing works when it is able to provide valuable support to the organization and when the organization is able to offer a set of products and services that are respected and valued by the community. Good marketing is about good value for patients; it is not about pushing dubious services with unproven outcomes.

Marketing is part of the team within healthcare management. It is not a backroom function destined to carry out the orders of others, and it is not a hero creating market share through advertising while, in fact, the hospital's product line is in serious trouble. To become part of the team, marketing must be respectful of the contribution of the other members of the organization. At the same time, marketing cannot be bashful about expressing a professional judgment and offering an opinion when all management wants is someone to carry out orders.

THE FUTURE OF STRATEGY AND MARKETING

Healthcare delivery today is sometimes standing flat-footed when it comes to offering fresh ideas about systemic healthcare issues. Health science is making great leaps forward with technology, gene therapy, DNA research, and new pharmacology-based answers. But healthcare delivery is doing little to resolve access issues, stabilize financing, and control utilization. As noted author Ian Morrison bluntly stated, "Strategy innovation has stalled in health care. No one has really envisioned a radical new future for U.S. health care that combines compassion, caring, cure, and coherence."[1]

In the early 1970s, marketing was introduced to health care with much fanfare, only to fall on hard times as it became apparent that it is difficult to move market share and build strong new programs, even with the best marketing strategy and tactics. Today, healthcare delivery seems to be imploding. The healthcare environment is shifting from the managed-care environment of the 1990s and the first decade of the 21st century to one of accountable care organizations and healthcare systems in which a large number of physicians at the primary care and at the specialty level are employed. At the same time, the benefits promised by mergers and integration have not materialized in a way that has become readily visible either to the organizations or to the buyers and patients that interact with these new entities providing the care. New health insurance products such as high-deductible plans have also entered the market, while companies have increasingly placed more of the purchasing decisions on consumers by shifting cost of the insurance (and ultimately the care) to them. For healthcare organizations, the pace of this change has resulted in organizations having little time to think about strategy in general, and about market strategy in particular. At the same time, medical inflation is again surging forward, hospitals are filling with patients but losing money, staff shortages are everywhere, and doctors are not happy.

In many communities, the issues faced today seem to be the same as those faced 30 years ago. Our agendas often seem tired and old. This is the context that marketing will function in for the next several decades. What is the future of marketing in this situation?

Healthcare delivery revolves around customers, product/service delivery, access to care, and how care is paid for. Marketing is about customers, product design, delivery of service, access to services, and pricing of services. The marketing agenda and the national and local healthcare agenda overlap in every aspect. Because of this overlap, marketing could participate in shaping health care at both the institutional and the societal level. Whether marketing is able to participate is another question. In order to assist at any level, marketing must deal with its own set of issues. Marketing, if it exists at all in a healthcare organization, is often thought of as playing a secondary role. Such thinking is relatively rare in every industry except health care. Yet, in order for marketing to work effectively, it must be part of the senior leadership group. The question is whether this is an earned role or an assigned role. In other words, should we prove that we deserve to be at the senior management table, or do we just ask to be assigned to the table because in other industries that is the norm?

Marketing in health care has a checkered past. Sometimes it was useful, and often it was just seen as more overhead. Many marketing professionals had a narrow understanding health care, and these professionals were often not considered team players. With that background, marketing is going to need to prove that it deserves a place at the table. How? The following elements are essential for marketing professionals if they are to participate in the leadership of health services delivery.

Be the Voice of the Market

Marketing has, as its principal task, the responsibility to constantly strive to understand the views of the marketplace and to bring those views into the decision-making process of the organization. This is a powerful responsibility that provides a tremendous opportunity for marketing professionals to deliver fresh information designed to help organizations make good decisions. At least that is the theory. In reality, many marketing professionals are not trained or particularly interested in consumer decision-making theory, market research, or customer preference data. As Levitt said, "How curious that so seldom is heard an encouraging word about customers and marketing."[2] Yet, marketing must take a front-and-center role in understanding and, if possible, being the voice of the customer. Marketing's principal value to an organization is its ability to search out and explain customer data. Providing knowledge about customers is the first and most important contribution we can make to our organizations.

Earned Role versus Assigned Role

Participation at the senior management table is a reward for value-added performance. Individuals become a part of this team because they have skills and knowledge that they bring to the table. Marketing has a deep understanding of the marketplace, coupled with skill in devising appropriate tactics. Understanding and applying the strategy/action match is an example of a skill. Marketing and the strategy team should participate at the highest levels of senior management, just as they routinely do in virtually every for-profit sector of the economy. But in health care, that position needs to be earned. It can be earned by constantly providing a stream of knowledge about the behavior of the marketplace, and by devising tactics to match customer behaviors and requirements.

Accountability

Effective marketing executives have a set of methods that they can demonstrate to the organization and that the organization can see as logical and reliable and as complementing the tools other team members use to run the organization. For example, these methods can be used to quantify demand for a new clinic or to project a salesperson's compensation based on performance. Using these tools helps integrate marketing within the management team. Marketing is part science and part art, but too often marketing professionals have applied the art and have forgotten about the science. They have developed advertising strategies that are "soft," that are not connected to goals of the organization, and that lack a performance-tracking mechanism.

Marketing must be held accountable for its actions and tactics, just as other members of the management team are held accountable for their bottom-line performance, financial-control systems, or quality- and safety-tracking methods. Marketing can optimize its performance by utilizing methods and models to study customers and the marketplace, and by embracing the analytical side of the marketing profession. By using actual data, marketing can make critical judgments about appropriate tactics while keeping in mind pricing, advertising, distribution, and product development. At this critical decision point, the marketing staff connects the marketplace data with the tactics instead of creating a marketing scheme that seemingly appears out of nowhere. The final critical element is to establish reliable systems to connect the marketing strategy to the rest of the organization and to monitor results. The ideas of integration and ongoing evaluation help marketing create a connection to the organization, and they also create expectations for results from the marketing efforts.

Marketing can seem mysterious and fuzzy to many people. Healthcare workers are trained in the sciences, and the management team is trained to be accountable and to expect accountability. Given these different perspectives, it is no wonder that marketing is often viewed as being outside the mainstream of senior management. If marketing is to enter that mainstream, it should eliminate as much mystery and fuzziness as possible and focus on data.

Be Bold and Have Ideas

Organizations, particularly established bureaucracies, tend to think in a conservative fashion. Obviously, they want to protect themselves and continue to operate in the way that has become comfortable to them. They tend to change when threatened, usually by outside factors. And when threatened, organizations often hope that the threat will go away and that business as usual can remain. Such organizations are inclined to embrace information that is not troubling and to ignore data that pose a challenge. For years, hospitals believed that instituting a freestanding surgical center was a bad idea, in large part because they were afraid they would lose volume and revenue if these centers started to take hold. Instead of embracing the concept and retaining market share, they avoided it. Now, thousands of nonhospital-based surgical suites have opened in profitable clinical areas such as orthopedics, plastic surgery, and eye services. Walk-in, urgent-care centers are increasingly located in retail supermarkets. In this case, hospitals are not unlike record companies that said, "We make our money being in the CD business; why would we want to abandon CDs for cloud-based music?"

One of the principal tasks of the marketing professional is to constantly scan the environment and customer data for early signs of new ideas and structural shifts in the marketplace. If marketing is doing this job effectively, by definition it will be bringing to the organization information and ideas that might not fit into the organization's comfort zone. The new ideas will often challenge conventional wisdom. Marketing people must be unafraid to challenge what organizations are doing today, and they must be vigilant about what is on the horizon. They must be bold because they may be a lone voice in an organization that does not want to hear about the new idea that could upset its equilibrium. The doctors in a clinic are there to work with the patients who present themselves for care on a daily basis. The doctors are often rooted in the here-and-now, and they do not have the time or skill set to discern the changes that are over the horizon. Marketing's position can be a lonely one. Arguing in 1997 that the Internet was going to create a sea of change was a lonely position to take—there was no smartphone, no iPad, no blogs, no online patient appointment systems; the post office was how we sent messages; and there were no robot surgical suites. By 2000, the Internet was changing both business and family life in profound ways, and today it is where we learn, shop, navigate, communicate, and evaluate where to go for doctors and hospitals. Suggesting in the 1980s that managed care would be important was considered outrageous; in the 1970s, many physicians thought that for-profit urgent-care centers were unethical and unnecessary; and in the early 2000s, many primary care doctors thought that retail medicine was a fad. Yet, all of these ideas have become a routine part of our environment. Marketing people, using data and tools for scanning the marketplace, are often lonely early observers of trends and opportunities for an organization. Many times their observations suggest that the organization must rethink its core products and shift its operations to a new model. Upsetting the organizational equilibrium is an essential and respected aspect of marketing accountability.

Up until now, hospitals and doctors have focused their attention on growth via more doctors and more facilities in more locations. Capital has flowed into profitable health care like a gusher of water. But now, public policy conversation and demographic changes suggest that we cannot afford to continue on a revenue model that is based on providing more and more units of care. Health care is in the middle of the policy debate, and the focus is on slowing healthcare resource consumption. Policy leaders are working on ways to focus providers on pay for performance or ways to become more prudent with limited healthcare dollars. The accountable care organization (ACO) is one model that would have physicians take care of a population of patients and get paid based on health outcomes of those patients. Providing more and more services, visits, and tests to each patient would no longer be as profitable. Providing better outcomes would drive incentive payments. Under this model, does that mean that marketing and business plans would no longer have a purpose? No, not at all; marketing has a purpose. Moving toward new models like ACOs requires new strategies and more rigor in terms of looking at options. Assuming we move toward a health outcomes–based model, what might marketing look like in the future?

Instead of focusing on building new clinics, the marketing team might concentrate more on strategies to communicate how patients can stay healthy or how patients should access care when they need it. Maybe the marketing team does research to figure out how to provide financial incentives to patients when they are prudent about their healthcare decisions or if they are willing to see a less expensive health professional for a routine pediatric check. In this new world, marketing would be involved in market research to find out what incentives will work to help people take their medicine, or quit smoking. We will spend more of our time on issues of public health and public service, like the researchers at the Wharton Business School are doing to try to figure out how to help improve organ donor rates in New England and the United States.[3] Instead of trying to get more use out of magnetic resonance imaging (MRI) equipment, the new environment could be about consolidating two machines from two different locations into one location and figuring out how to make the experience a value add to patients and the providers. Or, when a patient goes online to view medical test results, marketing will have worked with software engineers to provide targeted information to patients when it appears they have started to search for a physician upon seeing the test results. In this case, the marketing staff and software engineers are working together to help the patient navigate the clinic's website, using intuitive software to anticipate what the patient will do next online, and can even anticipate the patient's potential frustration because of the way he/she is navigating the system.

In short, all of the marketing tools that were required in a brick-and-mortar world, where success equaled more tests, will be required in a world where the incentives have changed and models are different. Strategic planning, business planning, and marketing will need to shift their strategies, learn new models, and establish different criteria for success. The baseline tools presented in this text can provide the framework to make good decisions today, during the transition, and tomorrow.

The opportunities in health care have never been greater. The industry is faced with scientific breakthroughs along with challenges around access and cost. This sector is one of the largest, and people see opportunity in it. The marketplace will continue to change and present challenges. At the same time, marketing will be expected to function with accountability and prudence. This text has been designed to provide tools, models, tactical ideas, and suggestions for control systems that improve the profession's contribution to healthcare management. Now it is time to contribute to our respective organizations.

QUESTIONS FOR DISCUSSION

1. Why do healthcare organizations tend to take on more initiatives than they have capital to support?
2. What are the core reasons for strategic planning failure?
3. Is a profit target a legitimate aspect of a not-for-profit organization's vision?
4. In what ways is strategy development in a hospital or multi-group physician setting more complex than other business entities?

NOTES

1. Morrison, I. (2000). *Health care in the new millennium.* San Francisco: Jossey-Bass; p. 199.
2. Levitt, T. (1991). *Thinking about management.* New York: Free Press; p. 113.
3. Wharton School, University of Pennsylvania. (2011). How to encourage people to become organ donors: An incentive system with heart. Retrieved February 28, 2012, from: http://knowledge.wharton.upenn.edu/article .cfm?articleid=2854.

APPENDIX A

CONSOLIDATED LIST OF KEY QUESTIONS TO ASK IN ANALYSIS

CONSOLIDATION OF KEY QUESTIONS USED IN CONDUCTING AN INTERNAL/EXTERNAL ANALYSIS

The internal/external analysis is a key component in developing the strategic and marketing plan, and it is the foundation from which the strategy/action match is determined. It is also important in determining which specific action-oriented marketing tactics are appropriate.

THE ENVIRONMENT AND THE MARKET

1. What kinds of external controls affect the organization? Local? State? Federal? Self-regulation?
2. What are the trends in recent regulatory rulings?
3. What are the main developments with respect to demography, the economy, technology, government, and culture that will affect the organization's situation?
4. Who are the organization's major markets and publics?
5. How large is the service area covered by the market?
6. What are the major segments in each market?
7. What are the present and expected future profits and characteristics of each market or market segment?
8. What is the expected rate of growth of each segment?
9. How fast and far have markets expanded?
10. What is the role of the Internet in terms of impacting consumer decision making?

11. Where do the patients come from geographically?
12. What are the benefits that customers in different segments derive from the product (e.g., economy, better performance, displaceable cost)?
13. What are the reasons different market segments are buying the product (e.g., product features, awareness, price, advertising, promotion, packaging, display, sales assistance)?
14. What is the organization's market standing with established customers in each segment (e.g., market share, pattern of repeat business, expansion of customers' product use)?
15. What are the requirements for success in each market?
16. What are the customer attitudes in different segments (e.g., brand awareness, brand image)?
17. What is the overall reputation of the product in each segment?
18. What reinforces the customer's faith in the company and product?
19. What circumstances force customers to turn elsewhere for help in using the product?
20. What is the lifecycle of the product?
21. How would our company be impacted by gene therapy or advanced DNA–related innovation?
22. What product research and improvements are planned?
23. Are there deficiencies in servicing or assisting customers in using the product?

THE COMPETITIVE ENVIRONMENT

1. How many competitors are in the industry? How are competitors defined? Has the number increased or decreased in the previous 4 years?
2. What is the organization's position (size and strength) in the market relative to competitors?
3. Who are the organization's major competitors?
4. What trends can be foreseen in competition?
5. Are other companies likely to be enticed to serve the organization's customers or markets? What conglomerates or diversified companies may be attracted by the growth, size, or profitability of these markets?
6. Who are those companies on the periphery—those that serve the same customers with different but related products, including related pieces of equipment? (It is impossible to list all related items, but those closest should be included.) Can they become competitors, or possibly partners?

7. What other products or services provide the same or similar functions? What percentage of total market sales does each substitute product have?
8. What product innovations could replace or reduce sales of the organization's products? When will these products be commercially feasible? (Information about potentially competitive products can be found by searching the records of the U.S. Patent Office and foreign patent offices.)
9. What are the choices afforded patients? In services? In payment?
10. Is competition on a price or nonprice basis?
11. How do competitors (segment/price) advertise?
12. Might competitors in other geographical regions or other segments who do not currently compete in the organization's markets or segments decide to come into the market?
13. Who are the customers served by the industry?
14. Who are the suppliers to the industry? Are they changing strategies? Why?
15. How does your web presence compare to the competition's?
16. What is your web ranking relative to the competitors in terms of hits and page views?

INTERNAL CAPABILITY

1. What has the historical purpose of the organization been?
2. How has the organization changed over the past decade?
3. When and how was it organized?
4. What has the nature of its growth been?
5. What is the basic policy of the organization? Is it health care or profit?
6. What has the financial history of the organization been?
7. How has it been capitalized?
8. Have there been any problems with accounts receivable?
9. What is the return on investment?
10. How successful has the organization been with the various services it has promoted?
11. Is the total volume (gross revenue, utilization) increasing or decreasing?
12. Have there been any fluctuations in revenue? If so, what caused them?
13. What are the organization's present strengths and weaknesses in management capabilities? Medical staff? Technical facilities? Reputation? Financial capabilities? Image? Medical facilities?

MARKETING ACTIVITIES

1. Are there specialized training programs for key personnel that emphasize the marketing concept?
2. Do the CEO and other key personnel have marketing experience?
3. Does the marketing department have a key role in the planning activities of the organization?
4. Does the person with marketing responsibility report directly to the CEO or top administrator?
5. Is market research appreciated as an ongoing task necessary for the development of effective marketing plans?
6. Are policies and procedures in place to coordinate the marketing activities with the other ongoing activities of the organization?
7. Does the organization have a high-level marketing officer to analyze, plan, and implement its marketing work?
8. Are the other persons who are directly involved in marketing activities competent? Do they need more training, incentives, or supervision?
9. Are the marketing responsibilities optimally structured to serve the needs of different activities, products, markets, and territories?
10. What is the organization's core strategy for achieving its objectives, and is it likely to succeed?
11. Is the organization allocating enough resources (or too many) to accomplish its marketing tasks?
12. Are the marketing resources allocated optimally to the various markets, territories, and products of the organization?
13. Are the marketing resources allocated optimally to the major elements of the marketing mix (i.e., product quality, pricing, promotion, and distribution)?
14. Does the organization develop an annual marketing plan? Is the planning procedure effective?
15. Does the organization implement control procedures (e.g., monthly, quarterly) to ensure that its annual objectives are being achieved?
16. Does the organization carry out periodic studies to determine the contribution and effectiveness of various marketing activities?
17. Does the organization have an adequate marketing information system to meet the needs of managers in planning and controlling various markets?

PRODUCTS AND SERVICES

1. What are the organization's products and services, both present and proposed?
2. What are the general outstanding characteristics of each product or service?
3. How are the organization's products or services superior to or distinct from those of competing organizations? What are the weaknesses? Should any product be phased out? Should any product be added?
4. What is the total cost per service (in use)? Is the service over- or underutilized?
5. Which services are most heavily used? Why? Are there distinct groups of users? What is the profile of patients/physicians who use the services?
6. What are the organization's policies regarding number and types of services to offer? Regarding needs assessment for service addition/ deletion?
7. What is the history of the organization's major products and services?
   a. How many did the organization originally have?
   b. How many have been added or dropped?
   c. What important changes have taken place in services during the previous 10 years?
   d. Has demand for the services increased or decreased?
   e. What are the most common complaints about the services?
   f. What services could be added to make the organization more attractive to patients, medical staff, and nonmedical personnel?
   g. What are the strongest points of the services to patients, medical staff, and nonmedical personnel?
8. Does the organization have any other features that individualize its services or give it an advantage over competitors?

PRICING STRATEGY

1. What is the pricing strategy of the organization? Cost plus? Return on investment? Stabilization? Demand?
2. How are prices for services determined? How often are prices reviewed? What factors contribute to a price increase/decrease?
3. What have the price trends been for the past 5 years?

4. How are the organization's policies viewed by patients? Physicians? Third-party payers? Competitors? Regulators? Managed-care organizations?
5. How are price promotions used?
6. How would a higher or lower price affect demand?

SALES FORCE

1. Is the sales force large enough to accomplish the organization's objectives?
2. Is the sales force organized along the proper principles of specialization (e.g., territory, market, product)?
3. Does the sales force show high morale, ability, and effort? Is it sufficiently trained and motivated?
4. Are the procedures adequate for setting quotas and evaluating performance?

PROMOTION STRATEGY

1. What is the purpose of the organization's present promotional activities (including advertising)? Protection? Education? Search for new markets? Development of all markets? Establishment of a new service?
2. Has this purpose undergone any change in recent years?
3. Is the Internet strategy customer friendly?
4. Does the Internet strategy allow consumers to interact with the organization and schedule appointments, update records, and maintain other important consumer information?
5. To whom has advertising been largely directed?

   a. Donors?
   b. Patients? Former? Current? Prospective?
   c. Physicians? On staff? Potential?

6. Is the cost per thousand viewers, listeners, or readers still favorable?
7. Are the media delivering the desired audience?
8. What media have been used?

   a. Web media?
   b. Social media?

9. Are the objectives (reviewed in question 1) being met?
10. What advertising copy has had the most favorable response?

11. What methods have been used for measuring advertising effectiveness?
12. What is the role of public relations? Is it a separate function/department? What is the scope of its responsibilities?
13. Has the public relations effort led to regular coverage?
14. Are the public relations objectives integrated with the overall promotional plan?
15. Are procedures established and used to measure the results from the public relations program?

DISTRIBUTION STRATEGY

1. What are the distribution trends in the industry? What services are being performed on an outpatient basis? What services are being performed on an at-home basis? Are satellite facilities being used?
2. What factors are considered in location decisions?
3. How important is distribution in establishing a competitive advantage for a particular service?
4. How is the organization using the Internet to distribute its product?

CONCLUSION

1. What are the three to five most important factors from this assessment that will impact the organization's strategy and market plan?

APPENDIX B

SAMPLE STRATEGIC AND MARKETING PLAN

CASE STUDY: THE METZ CLINIC IN THE COMMUNITY OF GREENTREE

The following is a sample strategic plan and marketing plan for a clinical organization located in Greentree, a suburban community located south of the river that divides Greentree from the larger community of Brighton. Before providing the actual plan, an overview of the community and the clinic organization are provided. Not all work papers, data, or complete market information are provided; however, enough material is detailed to allow for an understanding of the rationale for the strategy and market plan.

BACKGROUND SITUATION

The Community

The Metz Clinic has been in the community of Greentree for many years, and the eight physicians who practice at the Metz Clinic are oriented toward primary care. The Metz Clinic refers patients almost exclusively to a 400-bed general hospital called Arcola Health System, located across the river in the larger city of Brighton (**Figure B.1**).

The service area of Brighton has 900,000 people, with five hospitals and extensive primary and specialty physician services. Fifty percent of the physicians are in two major health systems, one of which, Arcola Health System, already has a clinic in Greentree. Physician income is stable, but not increasing for physicians at the Metz Clinic.

FIGURE B.1

Map of Greentree and Brighton

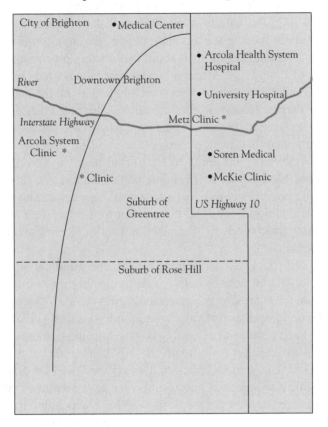

The Metz Clinic

The Metz Clinic has not changed much over the years. It has grown ever so slightly, recently adding one more full-time physician and some part-time, subspecialty consultant services. Three of the physicians are in their early 60s, and there have been rumors that they want to be bought out. In general, the group members complain about having to be on call too often, but overall the practice seems to run itself on a day-to-day basis. However, the doctors have watched the growth of other clinics in the community, and they are very much aware that their incomes are not increasing. Dr. Loftlen, a 39-year-old internist, has raised concerns about what the future holds for the group, such as: What would happen if three doctors retired, and why are the incomes of the doctors behind national averages? Dr. Loftlen convinced the group to have group meetings and to discuss how the clinic could be more proactive regarding its future. At the first meeting, Dr. Quigly made it clear that he wanted to retire in 4 years and did not want to see anything happen that might upset his plans. Dr. Loftlen said that she had read about two doctors practicing in the tiny community of Long Lake, Minnesota, and how they started the concept of the Retail Quick Clinic, which was soon adopted by all the national chain drugstores, Target, grocery stores, and others. She noted that a clinic does not need to be large to have an impact on medical care across the country. She also indicated that as more people age and care becomes even more expensive, innovators are going to try to find new ways to deliver care, and either the Metz Clinic will become one of the leaders, or it will be a follower. She pointed out that just a few years ago newspapers were very profitable, and almost overnight, the Internet took away their profitability and, for many, their survival. "Let's get in front of change, and not be left behind," she said.

"Honeywell, Intel, General Electric [GE], and all kinds of other companies are looking at how to deliver quality health care—at lower costs. These people are working on home-monitoring devices, videophone systems, and mobile devices that can monitor body systems—all of which are designed to keep people out of nursing homes, hospitals, emergency rooms, and doctors' offices. Let's get involved; let's help guide the research; we can be part of the new model of care. It's exciting," said Dr. Loftlen. Fred Mac, the clinic manager, was not so sure. "We have no money in the bank, patient visits are flat, and people want to retire," he countered.

Dr. Loftlen responded by painting a picture that involved about the same number of physicians in the clinic, but adding 25 revenue-producing nurse practitioners who would get paid to monitor hundreds of patients per day, and make house calls to help patients avoid unnecessary and expensive emergency room visits. "Imagine," said Dr. Loftlen, "our clinic working with GE, Intel's Health Guide monitoring device, Medtronic for remote cardiac monitoring, and Epic Systems Corporation (Epic)— a Madison, Wisconsin based medical record technology company—for medical record systems. Imagine that we are the monitoring center for thousands of patients, 95% of which can be taken care of by lower cost, revenue-generating nurses, and every day we help our patients monitor lipids, blood sugar, hemoglobin, body temperature, CRP, and TSH for thyroid issues, with only the most interesting and complex patients or those with changes in status actually needing to come into the office. Imagine each of us getting paid to oversee the monitoring of 75 patients per day per nurse using Internet, telephone, and home-visit tools, and only 15 of those patients will need to be seen in person by a clinic doctor."

Dr. Quigly looked skeptical. Dr. Ross could not imagine a model where he did not actually see all of his patients in an exam room. Nevertheless, Dr. Ross said, "I am not sure about all of this, but it is exciting enough to talk about. Does anyone have any factual data?"

Consequently, the group decided to begin to gather data about the community and the practice.

EXTERNAL AND INTERNAL DATA

The Environment

1. The population of Greentree was 27,000 in 2005, and is 33,000 today.
2. The number of physicians in Greentree was 9 in 2005, and has risen to 18 today. Eight of the 18 are from the Metz Clinic.
3. Twenty percent of all clinic patients are government paid (Medicare/Medicaid).
4. Eighty percent of all new health-insurance policies written in the greater metropolitan area in the past year involved coverage for second opinions.
5. The population is growing, but the real estate crash of 2008 still has people concerned.
6. Family income appears to be flat, while medical costs continue to rise at twice the rate of inflation. The Metz clinic has seen many patients drift away to a new nurse-driven model at the local pharmacy, and it wonders how it can change its model to compete.
7. Some companies are paying for house-call visits if it avoids the need for an emergency room visit.
8. Many articles are being published in the popular press about "push button" care or "remote control" clinical testing from home.

Market Segments

Tables B.1 to B.4 illustrate the market dynamics in Greentree. Some of the key market considerations include the following:

1. Twenty-six percent of the community consists of households with people living alone (single, separated, widowed, or divorced).
2. Forty percent of all households have both adults working.

TABLE B.1   GENERAL TRENDS: GREENTREE

	2005	2012	2017 Projected
Population	27,000	33,000	45,000*
Physicians	8	18	
Metz physicians	7	8	
% Commuting to Brighton for work	42%	58%	
Population of Brighton	557,000	589,000	588,000*

*Estimated before real estate crash of 2008.

TABLE B.2   SAMPLE CHARACTERISTICS OF GREENTREE

Age		Number of People in Household	
35 and under	40.5%	1	26.5%
36–55	23.5%	2	30.0%
Over 55	35.5%	3 or more	43.5%
Religious Affiliation		Length of Time in Neighborhood	
Catholic	37.0%	Less than 5 years	35.0%
Protestant	32.5%	5–10 years	18.0%
Jewish	2.5%	More than 10 years	47.0%
Other	3.0%		
No affiliation	23.0%		
Refused	2.0%		
Age by Area	North	West	South	East
35 and under	44.3%	27.2%	35.5%	34.7%
36–55	21.5%	24.3%	12.9%	30.4%
Over 55	33.9%	48.5%	51.6%	34.9%

3. Twenty-two percent of all households indicated in market research studies that they would switch hospitals if their physician selected a hospital that they did not like; and the hospital used by the Metz Clinic is viewed as good quality.

4. The typical resident in Greentree averages 2.5 visits to a primary care physician per year.

TABLE B.3 MARKET SEGMENTS

	% of Greentree Population	% Metz Clinic Patients
1. Women	54	64
2. Two-income households	40	12
3. Over 50	35	76
4. People who perceive need for more specialty care	41	45
5. People who seek convenience	65	30
6. HMO patients	12	0

TABLE B.4 HEALTH INSURANCE STATUS

Q: What is your health insurance coverage?

Plan	Percentage
Company plan	23.8%
Blue Cross	21.8%
Health, Inc.	17.1%
Medicare	15.5%
Don't know	3.6%
Refused to answer	4.1%

5. Forty-five percent of all people are under age 55.
6. Thirty-eight percent of the community drives 7 miles to the metropolitan area to visit physicians.

Market Share and Market Research

Tables B.5 to B.8 are the result of a pro-bono class project market research study conducted by graduate students at the local university:

TABLE B.5   MARKET SHARE AND SATISFACTION OF GREENTREE HEALTHCARE CONSUMERS

Q: Where do you obtain your medical care and how satisfied are you with your care?

Clinic Used	Market Share	Percentage Very Satisfied
Metz Clinic	7%	87%
Soren Medical	12%	95%
Arcola Health System	6%	96%
McKie Clinic	7%	89%
Other metro clinics*	38%	92%
No established doctor**	30%	–
	100%	

*Includes patients who travel to Brighton to obtain care
** Includes people who do not indicate that they have a regular doctor

TABLE B.6   CONSUMER USE OF AFTER-HOURS SERVICES

Q: If a doctor's office in Greentree offered clinic services after business hours, how likely is it that you would visit that office instead of a pharmacy-based urgent clinic, assuming the clinic fee is within 20% of the pharmacy's urgent clinic fee?

	Total	Single Parent	Dual Working	Households Over 65
Very likely	35%	35%	42%	40%
Somewhat likely	25%	30%	34%	15%
Somewhat unlikely	30%	20%	11%	20%
Not likely at all	10%	15%	13%	25%
	100%	*100%*	*100%*	*100%*

TABLE B.7   COMMUNITY VIEW OF METZ CLINIC

Q: I am going to tell you the name of a medical clinic. Tell me the first word that comes to mind when you hear the name Metz Clinic.

Never heard of them	25%
Don't know much about them	30%
General practitioners	27%
My doctor's office	7%
I hear they are OK	8%
You will get surgery if you go there	3%

TABLE B.8A INTEREST IN A NEW METHOD TO GET CARE

Q. I am going to tell you about a different form of visit to a doctor and I would like you to tell me how interested you would be in this service. Assume you are not feeling well and you need medical attention. You access your doctor's office by bringing up their website on your smart phone or home computer. The web-based clinic site asks you what your temperature is. With each answer you give, another question is asked. There are a total of five questions, and everything takes less than 2 minutes to answer. Based on your answers, the screen gives you the option to see a nurse practitioner at the clinic with an expected charge of $30, the nurse and doctor with an expected charge of $70, just the doctor at $90, or a home visit by a nurse for $80. How interested would you be in using this form of medical care?

	Under Age 30	Over Age 30
Very interested	45%	39%
Somewhat interested	27%	21%
Not sure	10%	20%
Not interested	13%	10%
Not at all interested	5%	10%

TABLE B.8B CLINIC VISIT WITH A NURSE

Q. Assume you decide you need to visit the clinic after accessing the clinic's website on your smart phone. When you get to the medical office, you are escorted to an exam room where you log in again and your information shows up on a large wall-mounted, flat-panel screen. Based on the answers you gave at home, as you wait for the nurse to arrive, you are able to see some preliminary information about your particular concern, including possible tests the nurse might want to order and some possible prescriptions that might be ordered along with the cost of filling the prescriptions. It is 85% likely that the nurse is able to make a determination of your condition without the need for you to see a physician. How interested would you be in this method of providing care?

	Under Age 30	Over Age 30
Very interested	47%	36%
Somewhat interested	28%	21%
Not sure	10%	17%
Not interested	10%	14%
Not at all interested	5%	12%

Internal Assessment

1. The net income of the partners dipped 4% last year, and overall income per physician remains at about 20% below the Medical Group Management Association (MGMA) mean.

2. Relative value units (RVUs) produced per doctor continue to run at 8% below MGMA mean.
3. Receivables have increased 15% within the past 2 years.
4. The partners are satisfied with the composition and responsiveness of the professional staff, patient satisfaction, and the service area within which they are practicing.
5. The staff believes that the location and convenient traffic pattern of the clinic are better than those of competitors.
6. In the areas of visibility within the community, financial condition, and coverage, the clinic is probably not performing as well as the competition.
7. With regard to quality of service, the clinic is performing equally as well as the competition.
8. The clinic has good financial information, including RVUs per physician, accounts receivable by month, gross charges by payer, collection rates, profit by physician, and profit per full-time equivalent (FTE), in addition to the standard income statement and balance sheet (**Table B.9**).
9. Net patient revenue at the Metz Clinic in the past year was $2.95 million, with the physicians averaging W-2 income of 39–42% of net patient revenue or an average take-home income for a family practice doctor of about $136,000 per year (**Table B.10**).
10. The building is 15 years old and is in need of major repair and expansion estimated at $2 million.

TABLE B.9   CLINIC STAFFING

	Current Year
Physician staff	8 FTE
Family practice	3
Internal medicine	2
OB-GYN	1
General surgeon	1
Urology	0.5
Cardiology	0.5
Office staff	5 FTE
Technical and nursing staff	10 FTE
Total	*23 FTE*

TABLE B.10 CLINIC FINANCIAL INFORMATION

	2009	2010	2011
Total relative value units (RVUs)	62,100	61,800	62,700
Net revenue collected (in millions)	$2.8	$2.85	$2.95
Overhead expense as a percentage of net revenue collected	55%	54%	55%

SUMMARY OF DATA IMPORTANT TO THE METZ CLINIC STRATEGY PROCESS AS VOTED ON BY THE PHYSICIAN OWNERS

■ **Comment:** The data outlined here are fairly typical; there are a lot of data, but some of them are not all that useful. Some of the data may have come from the local Chamber of Commerce, other data from the hospital marketing department, and still more from the local newspaper or other community sources. A portion of the data might be opinion or wishful thinking. In any case, it is relatively easy to capture information, but what is more important is to determine what data are most helpful to the conversation and what data can be discarded. For example, in this data set, religious preference is probably not critical to the conversation. After gathering data, the group met to discuss and agree on those data points that were most important to them. The following is their list of critical data elements. ■

- Metz Clinic physician income is 20% below national mean, and Metz Clinic income is declining.
- Metz Clinic market share seems to be steady at 7%, but not growing.
- The clinic is not well known in the community, with 55% knowing little or nothing about the group.
- The market has positive views about an after-hours clinic business, with more than 35% of people saying they are very likely to use a clinic-based system.
- The consumers are open to a new model of care involving technology and nurse practitioners, with around 35–40% saying they are very interested.
- Dozens of companies are working on systems, software, and hardware designed to avoid clinic visits, emergency room visits, and hospital stays.
- Patient satisfaction level is 87%, and it is below that which other clinics in the community have achieved.
- The community of Greentree is positioned to grow in a dramatic fashion, with population increasing from 33,000 today to 45,000 in just 6 years.
- Health systems are active in the community.

METZ CLINIC FIVE FORCES EXERCISE

■ **Comment:** The clinic has agreed on what they think the important facts of the situation are. Sometimes, this is a difficult discussion, because human nature might prevent some people from believing the meaning of the data. But after several conversations, the clinic has come to understand that they are an average group, with less-than-average awareness and community support, but located in a community that could soon grow quickly. The group found Tables B.6, B.7, B.8A, and B.8B to be very interesting, but the group was skeptical about the validity of the data. Dr. Loftlen thought it would be wise to look at the data from yet another angle. She had attended a "mini-MBA for physicians" course at the local hospital, where she learned about a process called the Five Forces model. The model asks five questions, which she posed to the group, and the following section represents the model questions and the group's answers. ■

Question 1. Is there a threat of substitution for our services?

Yes. There is a threat from grocery stores, drugstores, and online services such as WebMD that seem to want to provide more and more basic clinical evaluation. It is estimated that 40–50% of our clinic visit volume could be performed by this type of substitution provider.

Question 2. Is there a threat of new entry into the community by a competitor?

Yes. The health systems in Brighton will be increasingly interested in the community of Greentree because of the possibility of growth. As Greentree grows, more providers will be interested in entering the community.

Question 3. Do our suppliers have too much power?

No. Multiple options exist to find different suppliers, such as radiology, pathology, and nursing coverage, if necessary.

Question 4. Do our buyers (patients/health plans) have excessive power?

Yes, possibly. The Metz Clinic is not a large organization and the health plans do not need to have small clinics in their panel of providers. Patients seem to have plenty of options, and it would appear that more competitors will come to the community, thus making the current volume of clinic business more difficult to maintain.

Question 5. Is there an unusual amount of competitive rivalry?

Mixed. The clinic does not feel competitive rivalry. However, it is possible the clinic has been out of touch with what is going on in the community.

With the Five Forces analysis and the market research data, the clinic had already gathered it was time to converse around a strategy for the future. Dr. Loftlen convened seven meetings over a period of 5 months. At first, the group was reluctant to get too involved, but over time the group was pleased to get the issues out in the open. Some members of the group wanted to sell the practice, others wanted it to stay the same, and still others wanted to grow the practice or move the practice into the city. Dr. Loftlen wanted to be in the forefront of medical innovation. The conversation was intense and difficult, but the data were helpful in keeping the group objective and on task. Finally, after months and months of discussion, the group reached the following preliminary strategic plan.

METZ CLINIC STRATEGIC PLAN

Our Mission

We provide primary care medical services to the community of Greentree.

Our Vision for the Future

By the year 2020, we will be the dominant provider of primary medical services for the residents of the city of Greentree. We will have 12 physicians and 30 revenue-generating nurse practitioners on staff, and we will practice in an expanded facility at our existing location. We will be known for state-of-the-art, algorithm-based electronic and interactive patient- and clinic-based care management designed to provide safe, effective, and cost-efficient care with a focused and monitored nurse practice model as the frontline of care. We will have incomes that exceed the MGMA mean by 20%.

Critical Success Factors

- The ability to create, develop, and install state-of-the-art medical record and transaction technology, including patient previsit applications at home and/or at the clinic
- That patients will be comfortable with patient input via technology and understanding of algorithm methods
- That we can successfully integrate a dominant nurse practice model, with 66% of our total revenue generated from nurse practice and 33% of total revenue generated from physician practice
- That the clinic can reliably depend on Epic to move from beta test to business application within 3 years

■ **Comment:** The *mission* of the Metz Clinic is very clear. They will continue to be a provider of primary care, and they will be located in Greentree. They are not in the freestanding surgical business or the wellness business, and they are not providing care outside of their local community.

The *vision*, on the other hand, may seem a little obscure to an outsider. Even to the members of the clinic the vision is not exact. While everyone understands what the desired future state looks like, they are not sure how the strategy will unfold over the next few years. The strategy is not as far reaching as some of the leaders wanted, yet it is a new direction for the clinic.

What is the Metz Clinic vision all about? The practice model involves each primary care physician supervising three to five nurse practitioners, each of whom are seeing and billing patients under the supervision of the physician. At first, a couple of the physicians called this a "pyramid scheme," and they thought it might be unprofessional. But when the leader of the group reminded the doctors that architects, lawyers, and accountants all use a model where junior professionals generate large fee volumes that are a significant portion of the firms' income, the doctors came around to support the concept. Tables B.8A and B.8B were interesting enough to the doctors that they decided to make the concept a part their vision. The clinic's plan is to work with a firm called Epic Systems Corporation. The clinic would sign an exclusive arrangement to become a beta tester, and ultimately an operating site, for highly interactive patient and clinic coordination using a series of computer-assisted questions to patients through protocols that were originally designed at the Mayo Clinic and at the Johns Hopkins University. Immediately, as each question is answered, the user-friendly decision tree on the screen is adjusted, guiding the patient to the next question on a new screen. The patients would be able to access the algorithm from home or at the clinic.

In the meantime, the physician could simultaneously be looking at three screens, for three patients, who are in three different exam rooms where they are being cared for by three nurse practitioners. The doctor might determine that everything is OK in exam rooms one and two, but he would be able to head to exam room three to provide further examination to a patient where the data have raised some concerns.

The three nurse practitioners and the physician would be able to see 15 patients an hour on average, and the fees generated per hour would exceed $1,000, not including laboratory and other tests. Patient satisfaction scores could be very high.

As the doctors consider this vision, they realize that success will hinge on several *critical success factors*. First, they wonder if the market will accept spending more time with a nurse and less time with the physician. Second, it will be critical that Epic deliver on their promises.

The clinic decides to do some research before committing to this strategy. It is this commitment to the research that distinguishes a market-based strategy from a nonmarket-based model. Instead of just moving ahead, the clinic decides to do extensive research with consumers in Greentree regarding the use of nurses and patient-friendly, high-tech displays to see if consumers will support that method of care delivery.

Second, the physicians decide to do comprehensive due diligence on Epic to see if they have the funding and technical wherewithal to deliver on its promises. Epic, through its Dubai funding sources, agreed to post a $40 million bond to be paid to the Metz Clinic in Greentree and in six other clinics in the United States, Canada, and Spain if the project fails.

Approximately 9 months after gathering the initial data, the clinic physicians approved the strategic plan outline. Soon thereafter, the clinic completed the plan by adding the following strategic goals to the aforementioned outline. ■

Strategic Goals

Implement by 2015 the Epic/nurse practice model.

- Conduct extensive market research to test concept funded by Epic. Complete in 2012.
- Educate patients and provide them with access to patient clinical pathway material. Complete in 2012–2013.
- Budget: $52,000.

Create staffing model and begin to educate staff assuming an Epic partnership.

- Determine nurse practice model. Complete in 2013.
- Educate staff on new model and Epic. Complete in 2013.
- Demonstrate Epic capability. Complete in 2013.
- Establish model clinical exam room and clarify operating method(s). Complete in 2014.
- Budget: $12,000.

Obtain margin of 5% and improve physician income to national average in 3 years.

- Review and modify pricing structure. Complete in 2012.
- Hire coding consultant to recommend changes. Complete by 2013.
- Create capital requirements plan assuming Epic model. Complete by 2012.
- Negotiate Epic deal by 2012.
- Budget $45,000 for legal and consultants.

■ **Comment:** The completion of the strategic plan allows the clinic to move on two parallel and coordinated tracks. Track one is to begin to implement the strategic plan and the goals and tactics. The clinic could use the balanced scorecard as a benchmark model, but at this moment it has decided to place this method on hold until it becomes more comfortable with strategic planning in general. The clinic will begin to more carefully track patient requirements and their receptivity to the Epic model. The clinic will also begin to develop, create, and implement all the internal systems necessary to realize the dream—clinic leaders understand this could take years. Finally, the clinic realizes that it needs to pay more attention to financial performance. All of these activities are long run in nature, and everyone understands that while the dream is important, the daily business must move on.

The second track is the creation of a business plan, the first step of which is to create the marketing plan—recognizing that the marketing plan is guided by the

Continued

strategic plan. Hence, the strategic plan works toward the future, while the marketing plan and overall business plan work in concert, but on a more focused and current basis.

As the Metz Clinic considers its marketing plan, it first looks at the strategic plan for guidance—and indeed, the strategic plan provides strong directional support. For example, as the marketing plan is thought through, executives at the clinic know that the Metz Clinic is committed to its current location, it will remain in primary care, and the clinic does not intend to become a huge medical facility. Finally, clinical pathways and electronic interactions with patients using a large number of nurse practitioners will be the future. With this backdrop in mind, the marketing team can go to work to design a plan that supports the clinic today and the strategic plan for tomorrow.

The following is the marketing plan developed for next year for the clinic. Once the marketing plan is completed, operations and finance will add their components. If the combined business plan makes sense, then it will be approved. ■

THE METZ CLINIC MARKETING PLAN 2012

Overview

The Metz Clinic is experiencing stable, but not growing, patient visits, less-than-average patient satisfaction, declining physician income, 7% market share from Greentree, and low market awareness of the clinic.

At the same time, the clinic would like to stay in its current location, grow, and become regionally known for its innovative use of nationally acclaimed clinical guidelines, supported by state-of-the-art electronic systems and a very strong, revenue-based nurse practice program. The clinic realizes that achievement of this overall strategy will take time.

Overall Market Situation

The data suggest that the strategy/action match condition is *maintenance*. This means that the market conditions are steady, but not growing. Market strategies appropriate to this condition will be utilized, including working on consumer awareness (but not engaging in large-scale advertising), making sure fees are competitive, and keeping all facilities in good condition (but not expanding facilities at this time).

It is also understood that the new strategic plan calls for a significant shift in practice style, including the role of the physician, the use of unproven electronic systems, and the expanded role of nurse practitioners. While these systems will be developed over several years, significant market research will be conducted now to monitor and determine likely market reaction and endorsement of these changes. Using research, we would hope to determine if the plan will work in general, and what, if any, course corrections need to be made to have a successful strategic plan. The primary vendor or systems, Epic, will provide funding for the research outlined here.

Goal #1: Improve patient satisfaction scores from 85% to 95% satisfied.

Tactics:

Conduct exit interview with 500 patients to determine basis for patient issues.

- Responsible: JM
- Completion target: February
- Budget: none

Using patient exit interview data, make selective changes.

- Responsible: LL
- Completion target: April
- Budget: none

Establish front-door greeter program.

- Responsible: JM
- Completion target: year end
- Budget: $15,000 for staffing

Address and solve privacy complaints in the admissions area.

- Responsible: MP
- Completion target: February
- Budget: expected $5,000 for partitions

Goal #2: Improve positive community awareness of the clinic from 20% to 50%.

Tactics:

In conjunction with the local newspaper, write a weekly health-related column.

- Responsible: JM
- Completion target: year end
- Budget: none

Purchase billboard space across the street from the clinic.

* Responsible: JM
* Completion target: March
* Budget: $24,000

Participate in the new resident good-neighbor program packages.

* Responsible: JM
* Completion target: March
* Budget: $15,000

Goal #3: Provide onsite mobile magnetic resonance imaging (MRI) services 3 days per week.

* Responsible: LL
* Completion target: September
* Cost: $84,000 for pad area for equipment. Radiology. LTD provides mobile equipment and marketing effort. Clinic is paid per click.

Goal #4: Introduce the concept of clinical pathways and algorithms to every patient who has visited the clinic more than one time.

Tactics:

Provide free copy of American Medical Association clinical flowcharts for consumers to all eligible patients.

* Responsible: KP
* Completion target: July
* Budget: estimated at $13,000

In the lobby of the clinic, sell the Epic home edition consumer-packaged pathways software at cost as a vehicle to introduce patients to the technology.

* Responsible: JM
* Completion target: August
* Budget: none

Send a letter to every patient indicating that the clinic is teaming up with the Cleveland Clinic, Johns Hopkins, and the American Medical Association to bring state-of-the-art clinical pathways to the practice.

* Responsible: LL
* Completion target: mid-summer
* Budget: $8,000

Goal #5: Create a program called 50:50 to introduce new 50-year-old patients to the clinic.

Tactics:

Build a program called 50:50 where patients 50 years old or older can get their blood pressure checked, receive tests for cholesterol and diabetes, and spend 10 minutes with a nurse practitioner for $50.

- Responsible: LL
- Completion target: year end
- Budget: break even

Establish a media day with the press to promote the 50:50 program.

- Responsible: JM
- Completion target: July
- Budget: $2,000 for special event

Goal #6: Develop a comprehensive market research effort to determine and track community interest in aspects of the Metz Clinic strategic plan.

Tactics:

In conjunction with Epic, survey 350 patients and 350 nonpatients to determine at least the following:

Understanding consumers have of clinical variance among physicians
Understanding consumers have of national clinical guidelines
Comfort level with physician opinion versus published clinical guidelines
Support and understanding of nurse clinicians
Comfort with proposed technology from Epic
(Intend to do a concept pretest with and without the equipment)

- Responsible: JM
- Early findings: by April
- Budget: paid by Epic $123,000

■ **Comment:** This market plan takes its cues from the key elements of the strategic plan, including the introduction of tactics that would help to introduce patients to algorithm-based clinical decision making. This plan also takes the lead to look at market research to see if the strategic plan idea will work in the first place.

Continued

Further, the plan introduces a new MRI mobile service (designed to generate large margin revenue) and the 50:50 program designed to generate new, and likely higher volume demand, through the over-50 market. Meanwhile, the plan also recognizes that the market is flat at the moment, and clinic volumes are flat, so the program is relatively conservative in that no sales force is hired and no extensive media plan is put in place. This is an incremental growth plan designed to help lay the foundation for the new nurse practice–focused service sometime in the future, while trying to add some new patients now and new revenue services like the MRI and 50:50 programs. Once the community begins to grow rapidly again, and the clinic's Epic project is in place, the marketing strategy will likely shift from the current position of maintenance to a new position of growth and more resources, in which heavy advertising and sales would likely be used.

In the meantime, every tactic has a responsible person assigned to it for accountability, a target outcome is assigned, and a budget is allocated.

Overall, the strategic plan is ambitious and is moving into a world with which the community and the Metz Clinic are not familiar. The clinic is, in a sense, rolling the dice. However, the strategic plan is long term and the nurse practice/algorithm/Epic strategy would develop over several years. But more important, the strategy depends on what the market research data are saying as they are gathered and tracked. The clinic has indicated that the rollout of the new strategy for the future is contingent on a robust market research investment today. In other words, it is a classic market-based approach. If the clinic is not able to provide to the market a clear advantage with the new strategy, then presumably the strategy would be modified or a different path would be examined.

With the completion of the market plan, the operations group now can complete its plan, and then finance can create a finance plan, including a budget and cash flow forecast, and capital requirements study. Assuming all of these elements fall into place, the organization will have a long-term strategic road map and a shorter term, day-to-day business plan. ■

CASE QUESTIONS FOR DISCUSSION

1. To what extent does the Metz Clinic have a strategy? Does it have a mission and a clear vision? Are the critical success factors clear?
2. To what extent is the vision too optimistic, or is it too conservative?
3. To what extent does the clinic understand its environment, the market, and competition? (Key market data are presented.)
4. Does the strategy/action match seem logical?
5. Are the marketing objectives specific, and do they make sense given the condition of the market?
6. Are tactics specific, appropriate, and backed with enough power to meet the marketing objectives?
7. Is the plan logical, realistic, and cohesive?
8. What added data would be helpful to determine if the strategy is likely to succeed?

A P P E N D I X   C

MODEL SHORT-FORM CONSOLIDATED STRATEGIC AND MARKETING PLAN FOR SMALLER CLINICAL ORGANIZATIONS

Some organizations do not have the need or capability to manage what can be a complex process of strategic and business planning. Particularly in single clinical–line organizations or small hospitals located where competition is limited, it may be more practical to use the following approach. This model is particularly useful when management support is limited.

The model outlined in this appendix captures all of the elements described in the text, but as the execution of the strategic and business plan proceeds, the management support necessary for implementation is reduced. This "short-form" version still assumes a clear mission and vision. It assumes that data have been collected, including market research data. This model also suggests that tools such as the Five Forces model and strategy/action match are used before goals and tactics are crafted. Finally, this model assumes that there are critical success factors that must be achieved. But beyond that, the model is simplified so that strategic and tactical goals are consolidated into the same document. Also, while not specifically referenced, the short form strongly suggests that the concepts contained in the balanced scorecard model are thought through and integrated into the plan.

Using the Metz Clinic data, mission, vision, and critical success factors from Appendix B, the following simplified version is presented here—noting specifically that the chief executive officer (CEO) is the key individual accountable for this plan versus a team of executives or providers.

METZ CLINIC
COMBINED STRATEGIC AND BUSINESS PLAN

METZ CLINIC STRATEGIC PLAN

Our Mission

We provide primary care medical services to the community of Greentree.

Our Vision for the Future

By the year 2020, we will be the dominant provider of primary medical services for the residents of the city of Greentree. We will have 12 physicians and 30 revenue-generating nurse practitioners on staff, and we will practice in an expanded facility at our existing location. We will be known for state-of-the-art, algorithm-based, electronic and interactive patient- and clinic-based care management designed to provide safe, effective, and cost-efficient care with a focused and monitored nurse practice model as the frontline of care. We will have incomes that exceed the Medical Group Management Association (MGMA) mean by 20%.

Critical Success Factors

- The ability to create, develop, and install state-of-the-art medical record and transaction technology, including patient previsit applications at home and/or at the clinic
- That patients will be comfortable with patient input via technology and understanding of algorithm methods
- That we can successfully integrate a dominant nurse practice model, with 66% of our total revenue generated from nurse practice and 33% of total revenue generated from physician practice
- That the clinic can reliably depend on Epic Systems Corporation (Epic) to move from beta test to business application within 3 years

METZ CLINIC BUSINESS PLAN

Current Patients and Internal Operations

Improve satisfaction to 95%.

- Conduct satisfaction survey and address issues.
- Establish front-door greeter program; budget $15,000.
- Solve privacy complaints in admissions area; budget $5,000.

Clinic Future

Implement nurse practice model by 2015.

- Conduct extensive market research to test viability; budget $130,000+ paid by Epic.
- Educate patients and provide them with free access to patient clinical pathway material.
- Sell Epic consumer laptop software to interested patients.

Growing Today

Improve awareness to 50%.

- Publish weekly health article in newspaper; start in February.
- Purchase billboard space for $2,000/month.
- Participate in new resident neighbor package by March; cost $15,000.
- Add MRI service 3 days per week; capital cost $85,000; complete by September.
- Establish 50:50 program of tests and visits to people age 50 or older for $50.

Investing in Our People

Create staffing model and begin to educate staff, assuming Epic future.

- Determine nurse practice model by October.
- Educate staff on how new model of nurse/doctor would work—ongoing.
- Demonstrate Epic electronic capability by August.
- Establish model exam room with full Epic flat screens and software; November start.

Finance

Obtain margin of 5% and improve physician income to national average in 3 years.

- Review pricing structure and implement changes in 1st quarter.
- Hire coding consultant to recommend changes by June; budget $45,000.
- Create capital requirement plan assuming Epic implementation.
- Negotiate Epic deal by February; legal fee budget of $21,000.

INDEX

Note: Page numbers with *f, e,* and *t* indicate figures, exhibits and tables respectively.

A

O

P